Penile Augmentation with Injectable Hyaluronic Acid

Du Geon Moon

Penile Augmentation with Injectable Hyaluronic Acid

Springer

Du Geon Moon
Department of Urology
Korea University Guro Hospital
Seoul, Korea (Republic of)

ISBN 978-981-95-5384-6 ISBN 978-981-95-5385-3 (eBook)
https://doi.org/10.1007/978-981-95-5385-3

This Springer imprint is published by the registered company Springer Nature Singapore Pte Ltd.
The registered company address is: 152 Beach Road, #21-01/04 Gateway East, Singapore 189721, Singapore

Preface

Penile augmentation (PA) has a long history intertwined with cultural, social, and psychological factors. Across diverse civilizations, the phallus has symbolized masculinity, power, and fertility, leading to numerous attempts at enhancement throughout history. Early methods included mechanical traction, herbal remedies, and even crude techniques such as snake bites, reflecting cultural beliefs about virility rather than scientific understanding.

In the twentieth century, medical advancements introduced surgical approaches such as dermal-fat grafting, PMMA injections, silicone-based fillers, and suspensory ligamentolysis. However, despite initial enthusiasm, these methods were associated with severe complications, including paraffinomas, fibrosis, necrosis, and unnatural deformities, leading to psychological dissatisfaction and functional risks for patients. These limitations created a pressing need for a safer, minimally invasive alternative that could provide reliable and aesthetic outcomes.

The introduction of hyaluronic acid (HA) fillers into aesthetic medicine transformed soft-tissue augmentation, and I recognized their potential in penile enhancement. Over the past two decades, I have pioneered the clinical application of HA-based Glans Penis Augmentation (GPA) and Penile Girth Enhancement (PGE), developing precise injection techniques, refining filler characteristics, and optimizing patient selection criteria. These innovations have provided a predictable, reversible, and biocompatible alternative to previous augmentation techniques.

This book is a culmination of my 25 years of clinical expertise, offering a comprehensive guide to PA with HA. Unlike generalized discussions on penile augmentation, this work is dedicated exclusively to HA-based methods, consolidating scientific insights, technical refinements, and practical "tips and tricks" that I have developed through extensive clinical experience.

Having previously authored *Penile Augmentation* (Springer) and *Illustrated Textbook of Penile Surgery (Gunja Pub, Korea)*, I aim to take this book further by providing a step-by-step, experience-driven reference for practitioners worldwide. As interest in HA-based penile augmentation grows—particularly in Western markets—this book serves as both an educational resource and a clinical manual, ensuring that practitioners can achieve safe, effective, and aesthetically superior outcomes.

While the field continues to evolve, standardization, long-term studies, and international collaboration remain crucial for further legitimizing HA-based PA. By sharing my expertise, I hope this book contributes to shaping best practices and advancing the field of noninvasive penile augmentation for future generations of clinicians.

Seoul, Korea Du Geon Moon

Contributed Books: Penile Augmentation, Springer 2016

Part II

Chapter 7. Penile Girth Enhancement with Dermofat Graft
Nam Cheol Park, pnc@pusan.ac.kr
Chapter 13. Penile Girth Enhancement with Injectable HA gel
Du Geon Moon, dgmoon@korea.ac.kr

Part IV

Chapter 21. General Principle of GA
Du Geon Moon, dgmoon@korea.ac.kr
Chapter 22. Glans Penis Augmentation by Filler
Du Geon Moon, dgmoon@korea.ac.kr

Acknowledgments

During the preparation of this book, I received valuable support from Prof. Sun Tae Ahn, who contributed to the development of Part I. I am also grateful to Prof. Min Gu Park for his insightful input on Chap. 11 of Part III, titled "Premature Ejaculation: Integrating Pathophysiology and Current Treatment Modalities."

Competing Interests The author has no competing interests to declare that are relevant to the content of this manuscript.

Contents

Part I

General Perspectives

1 Introduction

Contents

1.1 Necessity of Hyaluronic Acid Fillers in Penile Augmentation: Toward a Safer and More Effective Approach

Penile augmentation (PA) has long captured both clinical and societal interest, reflecting persistent concerns about penile size, aesthetics, and sexual confidence. Across decades, various surgical and nonsurgical techniques have been explored to fulfill this demand, ranging from autologous fat grafting and dermal-fat flaps to synthetic materials such as polymethylmethacrylate (PMMA) microspheres and liquid silicone [1, 2]. Despite their initial popularity, these methods were associated with significant limitations, including asymmetry, reabsorption, nodular formation, granulomatous reactions, and even severe deformities leading to surgical revision [3]. These complications, coupled with variable patient satisfaction, underscored a critical need for safer, minimally invasive, and reversible alternatives in penile enhancement.

1.2 The Rise of Hyaluronic Acid Fillers in Aesthetic Medicine

The introduction of hyaluronic acid (HA)-based fillers marked a transformative advancement in aesthetic medicine. Originally developed for facial rejuvenation, HA fillers rapidly gained global acceptance owing to their excellent biocompatibility, biodegradability, and reversibility [4]. Their unique properties allow smooth integration into soft tissues without provoking severe inflammatory responses. Additionally, hyaluroni-

D. G. Moon, *Penile Augmentation with Injectable Hyaluronic Acid*,
https://doi.org/10.1007/978-981-95-5385-3_1

dase enables rapid enzymatic degradation in cases of overcorrection or adverse reactions, further enhancing their safety profile [5].

These attributes have positioned HA fillers as a cornerstone in soft tissue augmentation, and their application has naturally expanded beyond facial aesthetics into urology and sexual medicine. In recent years, clinicians have explored their utility in penile girth enhancement (PGE) and glans penis augmentation (GPA), with promising outcomes.

1.3 Necessity of HA Fillers in Penile Augmentation

Conventional materials used for penile augmentation, such as autologous fat, dermal grafts, PMMA, and silicone-based fillers, have consistently demonstrated unpredictable long-term results and high rates of complications [6–8]. Fat grafting, while initially appealing, often results in significant resorption, irregular contours, and asymmetry [9, 10]. Synthetic materials like PMMA and silicone, although durable, carry risks of chronic inflammation, foreign body reactions, and irreversible deformities [11]. These limitations highlight the need for a material that is both effective and forgiving in case of complications.

HA-based fillers fulfill this need. Multicenter trials and longitudinal studies have demonstrated their efficacy in increasing penile girth with a favorable safety profile and high patient satisfaction rates [12, 13]. Moreover, HA fillers have shown additional functional benefits, such as reducing hypersensitivity in patients with premature ejaculation (PE) when applied to the glans, further broadening their clinical utility [14].

In this context, HA fillers emerge not merely as an alternative but as a preferred option for penile augmentation—providing a balance between efficacy, safety, and reversibility that conventional materials could not achieve.

1.4 Purpose of This Book

This book was conceived to address the growing global demand for a focused, evidence-based resource on penile augmentation with HA fillers. Unlike prior publications, which often include historical perspectives and broad overviews of various techniques, this text concentrates exclusively on *HA-based penile augmentation*. It reflects over two decades of pioneering clinical experience and research in this field, with particular emphasis on the author's contributions to the development of GPA and PGE using injectable HA gel.

Designed as a *practical guide for urologists, sexual medicine specialists, and aesthetic practitioners*, this book provides comprehensive coverage of patient selection, anatomical considerations, injection techniques, postoperative management, complication handling, and optimization strategies. The aim is to equip clinicians with the knowledge and skills necessary to incorporate HA fillers safely and effectively into their practice.

1.5 Structure of the Book

The content is organized into two major sections for clarity and practical relevance:

- *Part II: Penile Girth Enhancement (PGE)* explores the evolution of techniques, clinical studies, safety data, and practical tips for achieving optimal aesthetic outcomes.
- *Part III: Glans Penis Augmentation (GPA)* focuses on the unique anatomical and functional considerations of the glans, technical nuances, and clinical results, including applications in managing premature ejaculation.

By presenting both PGE and GPA comprehensively, the book offers a holistic framework for physicians seeking to adopt HA-based penile augmentation.

1.6 Future Perspective

As interest in minimally invasive approaches to penile augmentation continues to rise globally, HA-based fillers are poised to become the standard of care. Their unique combination of biocompatibility, reversibility, and favorable clinical outcomes positions them as the ideal solution for both cosmetic and functional indications. This book aspires not only to provide practical guidance but also to inspire further research and innovation in the field of sexual medicine. By emphasizing patient safety and ethical practice, it aims to contribute to the responsible advancement of penile augmentation techniques in the years ahead.

References

1. Perovic S, Djordjevic M. Penile lengthening. BJU Int. 2000;86(9):1028–33.
2. Chen Y, Jiang Y, Li X, Wang B, Guo X, Mai Z, et al. Penile enhancement: a comprehensive and current perspective. Curr Urol. 2022:10.1097.
3. Abo-Hedibah SA, Badawi AN, Aly SA, Ismail SR, Elmokadem AH. Penile girth augmentation by injectable fillers: a comprehensive review of imaging features and inflammatory complications. Abdom Radiol. 2021;46(4):1703–17.
4. Carruthers JD, Glogau RG, Blitzer A. Advances in facial rejuvenation: botulinum toxin type a, hyaluronic acid dermal fillers, and combination therapies--consensus recommendations. Plast Reconstr Surg. 2008;121(5):5S–30S.
5. Gold M. The science and art of hyaluronic acid dermal filler use in esthetic applications. J Cosmet Dermatol. 2009;8(4):301–7.
6. Zhao Y, Qiao S, Sun X. Long-term follow-up of penile augmentation using silicone injections: clinical outcomes and patient satisfaction. Andrology. 2017;5(5):990–7.
7. Falagario UG, Piramide F, Pang KH, Durukan E, Tzelves L, Ricapito A, et al. Techniques for penile augmentation surgery: a systematic review of surgical outcomes, complications, and quality of life. Medicina (B Aires). 2024;60(5):758.
8. Xu T, Zhang G, Bai W, Li Q, Yang A, Lin Q, et al. Complications and management of penile girth enhancement with acellular dermal matrix. J Sex Med. 2019;16(12):2011–7.
9. Lee SW, Lee WH. Penile girth enhancement with autologous fat transfer. Penile Augmentation 2016:65–69.
10. Del Vecchio D, Rohrich RJ. A classification of clinical fat grafting: different problems, different solutions. Plast Reconstr Surg. 2012;130(3):511–22.
11. Le Penske W, Leslie DC, Latini JM, Lerner LB. Injectable penile enhancement procedures: a review of agents, risks, and complications. Urology. 2024;189:126–34.
12. Ahn ST, Shim JS, Bae WJ, Kim SW, Kim JJ, Moon DG. Efficacy and safety of penile girth enhancement using hyaluronic acid filler and the clinical impact on ejaculation: a multi-center, patient/evaluator-blinded, randomized active-controlled trial. World J Mens Health. 2021;40(2):299.
13. Yang DY, Ko K, Lee SH, Lee WK. A comparison of the efficacy and safety between hyaluronic acid and polylactic acid filler injection in penile augmentation: a multicenter, patient/evaluator-blinded, randomized trial. J Sex Med. 2019;16(4):577–85.
14. Kwak T, Jin M, Kim J, Moon D. Long-term effects of glans penis augmentation using injectable hyaluronic acid gel for premature ejaculation. Int J Impot Res. 2008;20(4):425–8.

Anatomy of the Penis

2

Contents

2.1 Gross Structural Anatomy of the Penis

The penis is a complex organ composed of external and internal structures designed for reproduction and sexual function. Externally, the penis includes the glans, shaft, and root, which together form the visible and anchoring portions of the organ [1, 2]. The glans penis, forming the distal tip, is highly vascularized and densely innervated, making it the primary sensory structure for tactile and sexual stimuli [3]. Surrounding the glans is the prepuce or foreskin, a mobile fold of skin that protects the sensitive surface when retracted [4].

The shaft of the penis contains three cylindrical erectile bodies: two corpora cavernosa positioned dorsally and a single corpus spongiosum located ventrally. These structures are encased by the tunica albuginea, a tough, fibrous sheath that contributes to the rigidity of the penis during erection [5, 6]. Encircling these erectile tissues is Buck's fascia, a dense connective tissue layer providing structural support and housing key neurovascular components, including the dorsal arteries, veins, and nerves [2]. The shaft is covered by highly elastic skin, allowing significant expansion during erection and augmentation procedures [7].

D. G. Moon, *Penile Augmentation with Injectable Hyaluronic Acid*,
https://doi.org/10.1007/978-981-95-5385-3_2

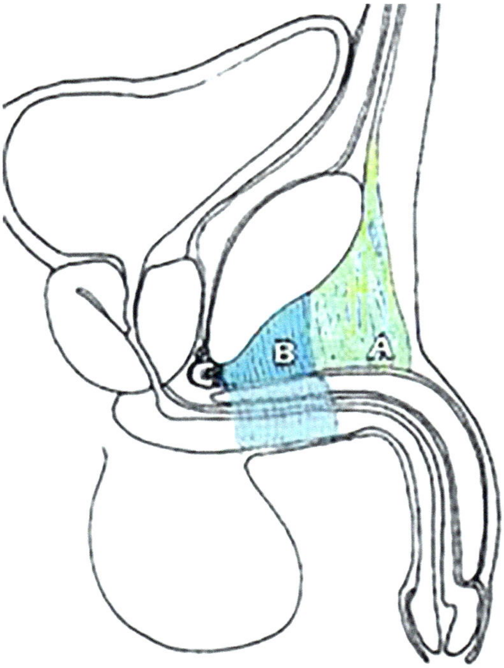

Fig. 2.1 Suspensory apparatus of the penis. Diagrammatic sagittal section representing the different distinct parts of the suspensory ligament of the penis. (**a**) Fundiform ligament and (**b**) suspensory ligament of the penis

The root of the penis, or radix, is embedded within the perineum and attached to the pubic bone by the suspensory ligament and fundiform ligament [8]. The crura of the corpora cavernosa extend posteriorly and anchor the penis to the ischiopubic rami, while the bulb of the corpus spongiosum lies centrally, fixed to the perineal membrane. These anchoring structures ensure the stability of the penis during penetration and provide a base for erection [9] (Fig. 2.1).

Additionally, the superficial layer of Dartos fascia lies immediately beneath the skin, composed of smooth muscle fibers and elastic connective tissue [10]. This fascia plays a pivotal role in thermoregulation by contracting and relaxing to adjust the surface area of the scrotum and penile skin. The elasticity of Dartos fascia also makes it an ideal layer for filler placement, contributing to uniformity and natural aesthetic outcomes.

2.2 Microscopic Anatomy of the Penis

On a microscopic level, the penis comprises a variety of specialized tissues, each contributing to its unique functionality. The corpora cavernosa is formed by a network of trabecular smooth muscle and connective tissue that encloses vascular sinusoids. These sinusoids are lined by endothelial cells and play a critical role in erection by filling with blood under the influence of nitric oxide and other vasodilators [11]. The ability of these sinusoids to distend is central to achieving and maintaining penile rigidity.

The corpus spongiosum differs from the corpora cavernosa in structure and function. It is composed of more elastic connective tissue and a denser network of blood vessels to maintain patency of the urethra during erection [12]. The terminal portion of the corpus spongiosum expands to form the glans penis, which is covered by a thin layer of epithelium. The glans is rich in sensory nerve endings, including free nerve endings, Merkel cells, and Pacinian corpuscles, which detect fine touch and pressure stimuli [13].

The tunica albuginea, encasing the corpora cavernosa, has a bilayered composition: an outer longitudinal layer and an inner circular layer of collagen fibers [5, 6]. This structure allows the penis to resist high intracavernosal pressures during erection. The septum of the tunica partially divides the two corpora, allowing communication through fenestrations for blood flow coordination between the compartments.

Elastic and collagen fibers are also abundant within Buck's and Dartos fascias. The elastic properties of these fibers contribute to the penis's ability to expand and contract while maintaining its structural integrity. These characteristics are particularly important for augmentation, as fillers must integrate with these tissues without disrupting their natural function [2, 14] (Fig. 2.2).

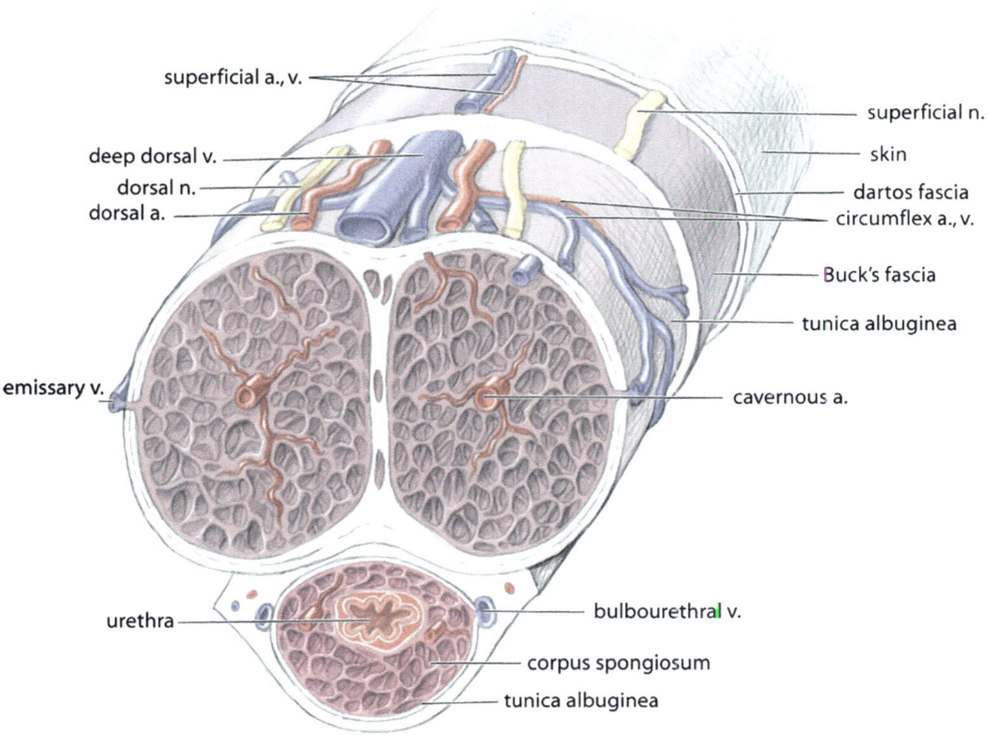

Fig. 2.2 Fascial coverings, vessels, and nerves in cut section of penis: The body of the penis is composed of three cylinders: two corpora cavernosa and one corpus cavernosum. These three cylinders are covered with three dense layers: the skin, Buck's fascia, and the tunica albuginea. Between the skin and Buck's fascia lie the loose superficial fascia (dartos) and superficial vessels. Between Buck's fascia and tunica albuginea lie the deep vessels and dorsal nerves (© Ahmed T. Hadidi 2022 [14]. All Rights Reserved)

2.3 Vascular and Neural Supply of the Penis

The vascular supply of the penis is extensive and includes both arterial and venous components critical for erectile function. The internal pudendal artery, a branch of the internal iliac artery, serves as the primary source of arterial blood [15]. It gives rise to the cavernosal artery, which supplies the corpora cavernosa; the dorsal artery, which supplies the glans and penile skin; and the bulbourethral artery, which supplies the corpus spongiosum and urethra [1]. These arteries branch extensively, ensuring adequate perfusion of all penile tissues during both flaccid and erect states.

Venous drainage is equally intricate. Superficial veins, including the superficial dorsal vein, drain the skin and subcutaneous tissues into the external pudendal vein. Deeper structures, such as the corpora cavernosa and corpus spongiosum, are drained by the deep dorsal vein, which empties into the prostatic venous plexus. The emissary veins connect the sinusoids within the corpora cavernosa to the deep dorsal vein, facilitating efficient blood outflow [16].

Lymphatic drainage of the penis is divided into superficial and deep systems. Superficial lymphatics, responsible for draining the skin and prepuce, converge at the superficial inguinal lymph nodes. Deeper structures, including the glans and erectile tissues, drain into the deep

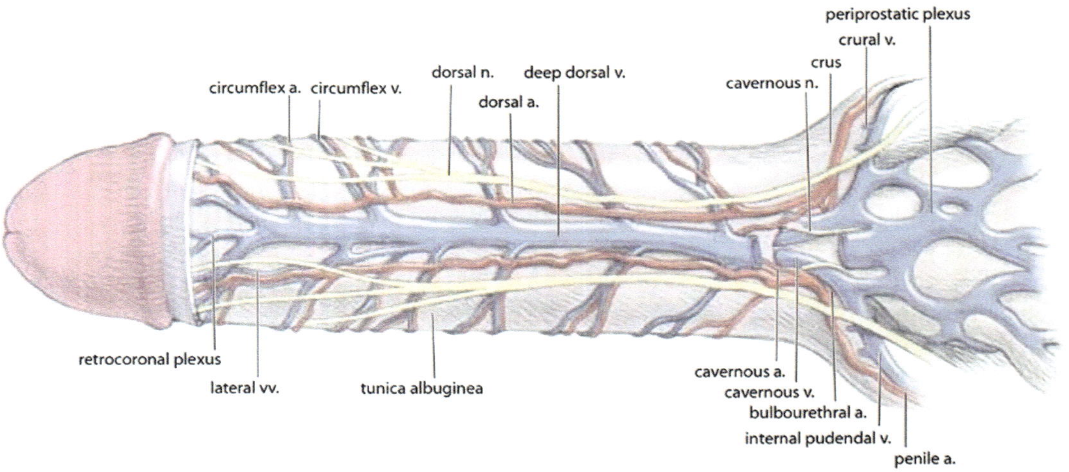

Fig. 2.3 Relations of nerves and vessels on the dorsum of the penis (© Ahmed T. Hadidi 2022 [14]. All Rights Reserved)

inguinal and external iliac lymph nodes [17, 18]. This system is clinically significant in understanding and managing conditions such as penile lymphedema or malignancy.

Neural supply to the penis is provided by both sensory and autonomic nerves. The dorsal nerve of the penis, a branch of the pudendal nerve, is the primary sensory nerve, innervating the glans and shaft [3]. It travels alongside the dorsal arteries within Buck's fascia. Autonomic innervation is supplied by the cavernous nerves, which arise from the pelvic plexus and carry parasympathetic fibers (from S2 to S4) and sympathetic fibers (from T11 to L2) [11]. These nerves regulate vascular tone and erectile function, highlighting the importance of avoiding damage to these structures during augmentation procedures [14] (Fig. 2.3).

2.4 Functional and Structural Roles of Buck's and Dartos Fascia

Buck's fascia is a dense, fibrous connective tissue layer enveloping the corpora cavernosa, corpus spongiosum, and neurovascular bundles. Extending from the penile root to the glans, it provides a critical structural framework and serves as a protective barrier [19]. The fascia's role in encapsulating the dorsal arteries, veins, and nerves makes it a vital anatomical feature for procedural accuracy. Filler placement above Buck's fascia ensures minimal risk to deeper structures while promoting uniform distribution [20].

Dartos fascia, situated superficially beneath the penile skin, is composed of elastic fibers and smooth muscle. Its primary functions include allowing skin mobility and participating in thermoregulation by adjusting the scrotal and penile surface area. The fascia's elastic properties also accommodate the even distribution of fillers, contributing to aesthetically pleasing and natural outcomes [20]. Its continuity with the scrotum and lower abdominal wall underscores its importance in maintaining the functional and structural harmony of the external genitalia.

The interplay between Buck's and Dartos fascias is central to the structural and functional integrity of the penis. Buck's fascia maintains the rigidity and alignment of the erectile tissues, ensuring effective blood flow during erection. In contrast, Dartos fascia provides flexibility and surface mobility, preventing tissue distortion and facilitating filler integration. Understanding the roles of these fascias allows practitioners to achieve optimal outcomes in penile augmentation while minimizing risks such as vascular compromise, asymmetry, or overfilling.

2.4.1 Glans Penis Anatomy

The glans forms the distal end of the penis. Historically considered as the anterior bulge of the corpus spongiosum of the urethra, it covers the tip of the corpora cavernosa. In contrast to the penile shaft, the glans is formed solely through the continuous expansion of the urethral corpus cavernosum without a surrounding white membrane. The glans has a relatively minor role in the process of penile erection, but preservation of the core structures of the glans penis contributes to the maintenance of superior penile function in surgical techniques of various penile surgeries [21–23]. The conical shape of the glans is functional to its role in sexual intercourse, which consists of promoting penetration [24]. The structural dimorphism and the variations in the ratio of dense connective tissue components of the fibrous skeleton are considered to contribute to the varying degrees of flexibility, distensibility, and rigidity of the human glans penis. It is evident in a histological study, central ligamentous structure penetrated the glans penis by the course of the fossa navicularis in 91% of the individuals [25]. A firm trunk with buckling collagen bundles (red striped areas) supports the maintenance of shape and force during coitus (Fig. 2.4).

The arterial vascularization is supported by the internal pudendal artery, via the dorsal artery of the penis [26]. The structure of the arterial tree is manifestly terminal, an aspect not to be underestimated during invasive maneuvers on the glans. The venous system is ensured by the tributary branches of the deep dorsal vein, which after passing the root of the penis disappears into the dorsal vascular plexus of Santorini [26]. The glans mucosa has a great wealth of sensitive nerve branches. The glans mucosa is rich in sensitive nerve branches. Underneath a stratified squamous epithelium, the dermis is made up of a dense layer of connective tissue as in typical skin. The innervation comes mainly from the branches of the genitofemoral nerve and the internal pudendal nerve and continues as the dorsal nerve of the penis. Nerve endings are predominantly corpuscular. Yang and Bradley [27] conducted an anatomical study revealing the presence of two branches of the dorsal penile nerve. One branch consists of nerve fibers that travel distally along

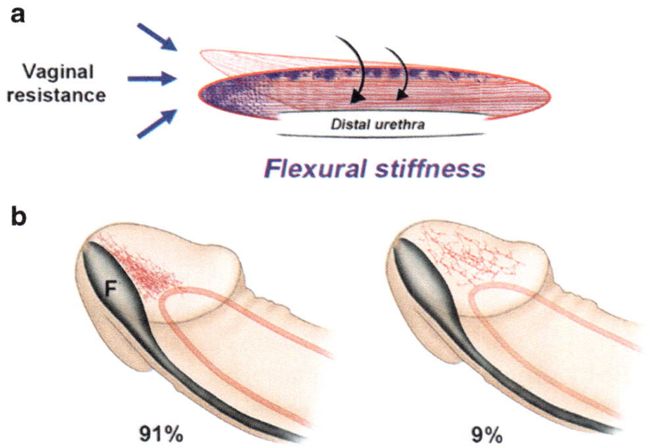

Fig. 2.4 Schematics of ligamentous tissues of the human glans penis. (**a**) A firm trunk with buckling collagen bundles (red striped areas) supports the maintenance of shape and force during coitus. Flexibility during thrusting due to peripheral arrangement of elastic fibers (purple) could provide the required flexural stiffness. (**b**) Dense connective tissues consisting of concentrated collagen bundles formed compact trunks in the central glans (91% of cases) or were dispersed as sparse bundles penetrating the sinusoidal space (9% of cases). Red networks in the glans and the penile shafts indicate the fibrous frame consisting of collagen bundles. F, fossa navicularis

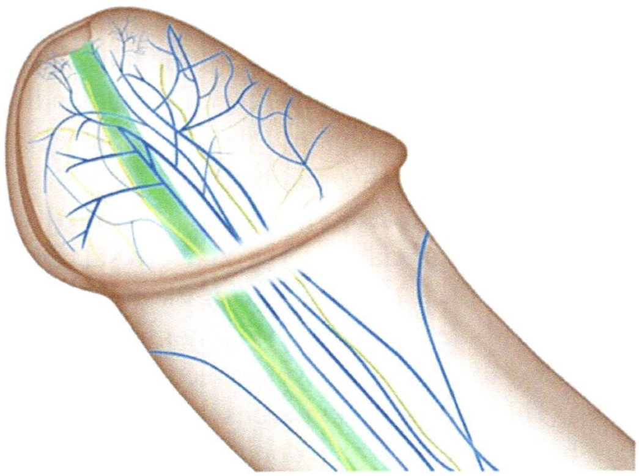

Fig. 2.5 (**a**) Blue and yellow indicate the dorsal nerves of the penis, green indicates the urethra. (**b**) The nerves in the urethral orifice are more densely distributed

the lateral side of the dorsal deep penile vein and the dorsal deep penile artery, forming a vascular nerve bundle with these structures. This branch serves as the main trunk of the DNP in the penile shaft, penetrating and terminating at the glans of the penis. The other branch originates from the main trunk of the DNP and travels laterally and ventrally to the penile shaft, ultimately terminating in the urethral corpus cavernosum and urethral mucosa [27]. This suggests that different axons control the glans compared with the shaft, with the lateral and ventral aspects of the shaft being regulated by nerves originating from the dorsal midline to the ventral region of the penis. Some branches of these nerves penetrate the corpus cavernosum, while the nerves controlling the glans are primarily concentrated along the midline of the penile shaft. Upon entering the glans, this portion of the nerve branches out extensively [13] (Fig. 2.5).

2.4.2 The Special Epithelium of Glans

During the process of embryonic development, there is a gradual separation of the stratified squamous epithelium of the connective tissue of the glans from the prepuce [28]. As a result, the glans acquires a distinct epithelium, consisting of stratified squamous epithelium and a dense connective tissue layer on its surface. In contrast, the penile shaft is covered by regular skin. Dorsal surface of the glans and the coronal sulcus are covered by squamous epithelium with a granular layer, while the distal end of the glans lacks this granular layer [29]. Furthermore, the dermis beneath the glans epithelium differs from the dermis found in other areas of the shaft. It is composed of dense connective tissue. The connective tissue within the papillary layer of the glans dermis merges with the dense connective tissue surrounding the corpus cavernosum of the penis. This arrangement separates the vascular sinus of the corpus cavernosum, which contains abundant elastic fibers, nerves, and blood vessels, within the dermis.

Moon et al. demonstrated the potential space to hold the injected HA gel in lamina propria of glans penis [30] (Fig. 2.6).

2.4.3 The Glans Contains a Large Number of Special Receptors

The glans penis possesses a densely populated surface with numerous receptors, akin to the clitoral glans [31]. Halata and Munger [29] confirmed that the dermal papillary layer of the glans, as well as scattered regions within the deep dermis, contains abundant free nerve endings (FNEs). These FNEs are characterized by Schwann cells, irregularly dispersed nerve fibers, neurotubules, corpuscles of various sizes, and diverse inclusions. Multiple receptor corpuscles are layered on the surface of the glans, including simple corpuscles, Ruffini's corpuscles, and Meissner's corpuscles. While simple corpuscles function as rapidly adapting receptors in the animal penis [32], their role in the human glans remains uncertain. Ruffini's corpuscles are considered type II slowly adapting traction receptors that respond to skin stimuli caused by pulling [33]. Meissner's corpuscles, found in the dermal papillae layer beneath the basal layer of hairless skin (such as fingertips, soles, nipples, and male and female external genitalia), are believed to

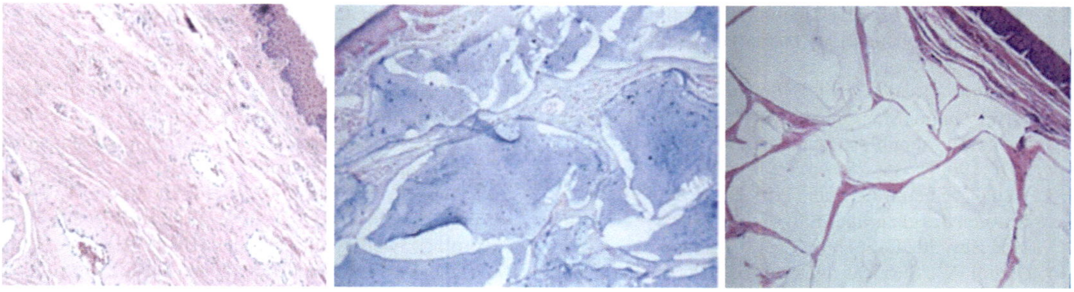

Fig. 2.6 Histological section of the canine glans penis at 6 months postinjection of hyaluronic acid gel. The image demonstrates basophilic, amorphous material retained within the lamina propria, indicating long-term filler residence. Surrounding tissue shows no signs of inflammation, confirming the biocompatibility and stability of the injected gel

respond to low-frequency vibrations and light touch [31]. Although Merkel cells, acting as slow-adapting receptors facilitating receptive and conductive sensory functions, are present in the skin of all primates [34], they are not found within the human glans. This further emphasizes the marked differences in receptors between the glans and other anatomical sites. The nerve fiber bundles within the glans also differ from those in the penile shaft, predominantly consisting of small-diameter Aδ or C-class nerve fibers. The unique receptors in the glans contribute to its insensitivity to light touch, heat, cold [13, 29], and even pinpricks [35].

2.5 Conclusion

A comprehensive understanding of penile anatomy is essential for safe and effective penile augmentation procedures. By respecting anatomical boundaries and focusing on key structures such as Buck's and Dartos fascia, practitioners can optimize outcomes while minimizing complications. The interplay of macro- and microanatomy, vascular supply, and innervation ensures procedural success and preserves penile function. A thorough understanding of the glans anatomy, with its uniqueness and differences from the penis shaft, is the basis for safe and effective management of glans penis augmentation in esthetical or functional request of the patients.

References

1. Wein A. Campbell-Walsh Urología. Ed. Médica Panamericana; 2008.
2. Dwyer ME, Salgado CJ, Lightner DJ, editors. Normal penile, scrotal, and perineal anatomy with reconstructive considerations. Seminars in Plastic Surgery; © Thieme Medical Publishers; 2011.
3. Kozacioglu Z, Kiray A, Ergur I, Zeybek G, Degirmenci T, Gunlusoy B. Anatomy of the dorsal nerve of the penis, clinical implications. Urology. 2014;83(1):121–5.
4. Cold CJ, Taylor JR. The prepuce. BJU Int. 1999;83(S1):34–44.
5. Awad A, Alsaid B, Bessede T, Droupy S, Benoît G. Evolution in the concept of erection anatomy. Surg Radiol Anat. 2011;33:301–12.
6. Hsieh C-H, Liu S-P, Hsu G-L, Chen H-S, Molodysky E, Chen Y-H, et al. Advances in understanding of mammalian penile evolution, human penile anatomy and human erection physiology: clinical implications for physicians and surgeons. Med Sci Monit. 2012;18(7):RA118.
7. Ahn ST, Shim JS, Bae WJ, Kim SW, Kim JJ, Moon DG. Efficacy and safety of penile girth enhancement using hyaluronic acid filler and the clinical impact on ejaculation: a multi-center, patient/evaluator-blinded, randomized active-controlled trial. World J Men Health. 2021;40(2):299.
8. Drake R, Vogl AW, Mitchell AW. Gray's anatomy for students E-book. Elsevier Health Sciences; 2009.
9. Hoznek A, Rahmouni A, Abbou C, Delmas V, Colombel M. The suspensory ligament of the penis: an anatomic and radiologic description. Surg Radiol Anat. 1999;20:413–7.
10. Hinman F. Atlas of urosurgical anatomy. (No Title); 1993.
11. Lue T. In: Sanez de Tejada I, et al., editors. Sexual medicine: sexual dysfunctions in men and women.

Physiology of erectile function and pathophysiology of erectile dysfunction. Paris: Health Publications; 2004.
12. Ottenhof SR, de Graaf P, Soeterik TF, Neeter LM, Zilverschoon M, Spinder M, et al. Architecture of the corpus spongiosum: an anatomical study. J Urol. 2016;196(3):919–25.
13. Wei L, Zheng L, Jiang H, Jiang T. Differences between the glans and shaft of the penis: a review. Sex Med Rev. 2024;12(4):659–63.
14. Hadidi AT. Surgical anatomy of the penis and urethra. In: Hypospadias surgery: an illustrated textbook. Springer; 2022. p. 105–26.
15. Tanagho EA. Anatomy of the genitourinary tract. Smith's General Urology, ed. 2008;14:1–16.
16. Park K. Penis anatomy. In: Penile augmentation. Springer; 2016. p. 27–31.
17. Long LY, Qiang PF, Ling T, Wei ZY, Long ZY, Shan M, et al. A new technique to map the lymphatic distribution and alignment of the penis. Anat Rec. 2015;298(8):1465–71.
18. Vossough A, Pretorius E, Siegelman E, Ramchandani P, Banner M. Magnetic resonance imaging of the penis. Abdominal Radiol. 2002;27(6):640.
19. Costa W, Chagas M, Babi M. Structural and stereological analysis of elastic fibers in the glans penis of young men. Rom J Morphol Embryol. 2012;53(2):393–6.
20. Moon DG, Kwak TI. Penile girth enhancement with injectable HA gel. In: Penile Augmentation; 2016. p. 99–104.
21. Yang J, Chen J, Wu X-f, Song N-j, Xu X-y, Li Q, et al. Glans preservation contributes to postoperative restoration of male sexual function: a multicenter clinical study of glans preserving surgery. J Urol. 2014;192(5):1410–7.
22. Kureel SN, Gupta A, Sunil K, Dheer Y, Kumar M, Tomar VK. Surgical anatomy of the penis in hypospadias: magnetic resonance imaging study of the tissue planes, vessels, and collaterals. Urology. 2015;85(5):1173–8.
23. Özbey H, Kumbasar A. Glans wings are separated ventrally by the septum glandis and frenulum penis: MRI documentation and surgical implications. Turk J Urol. 2017;43(4):525.
24. Moon DG, Kwak TI, Kim JJ. Glans penis augmentation using hyaluronic acid gel as an injectable filler. World J Men Health. 2015;33(2):50.
25. Lee SH, Ha TJ, Koh KS, Song WC. Ligamentous structures in human glans penis. J Anat. 2019;234(1):83–8.
26. Campbell MF, Walsh PC, Wein AJ, Kolon TF, Partin AW, Dmochowski RR, et al. Campbell-Walsh-Wein urology twelfth edition review. (No Title).
27. Yang B. Neuroanatomy of the penile portion of the human dorsal nerve of the penis. Br J Urol. 1998;82(1):109–13.
28. Gairdner D. The fate of the foreskin: a study of circumcision. Obstet Gynecol Surv. 1950;5(5):699.
29. Halata Z, Munger BL. The neuroanatomical basis for the protopathic sensibility of the human glans penis. Brain Res. 1986;371(2):205–30.
30. Moon D, Kwak T, Cho H, Bae J, Park H, Kim J. Augmentation of glans penis using injectable hyaluronic acid gel. Int J Impot Res. 2003;15(6):456–60.
31. Martín-Alguacil N, Cooper RS, Aardsma N, Mayoglou L, Pfaff D, Schober J. Terminal innervation of the male genitalia, cutaneous sensory receptors of the male foreskin. Clin Anat. 2015;28(3):385–91.
32. Pubols JBH, Donovick P, Pubols LM. Opossum trigeminal afferents associated with vibrissa and rhinarial mechanoreceptors. Brain Behav Evol. 1973;7(5):360–81.
33. Chambers MR, Andres K, Mv D, Iggo A. The structure and function of the slowly adapting type II mechanoreceptor in hairy skin. Q J Exp Physiol Cogn Med Sci. 1972;57(4):417–45.
34. Halata Z. The mechanoreceptors of the mammalian skin ultrastructure and morphological classification: ultrastructure and morphological classification. Springer Science & Business Media; 2012.
35. Taylor JR, Lockwood AP, Taylor A. The prepuce: specialized mucosa of the penis and its loss to circumcision. Br J Urol. 1996;77(2):291–5.

Development of Fillers

3

Contents

3.1 Historical Background

The concept of soft tissue fillers dates back to the late nineteenth century, when physicians first explored methods to restore volume loss and correct facial deformities. The earliest documented use of injectable fillers can be attributed to Dr. Franz Neuber in 1893, who introduced autologous fat grafting as a soft tissue augmentation method [1]. This approach, while innovative, had limitations in terms of resorption and unpredictability.

By the early twentieth century, paraffin injections gained popularity as an alternative. Paraffin, a synthetic hydrocarbon, was widely used for cosmetic enhancements. However, complications such as embolization, granuloma formation, and migration led to its eventual abandonment [2].

In the mid-twentieth century, the introduction of injectable silicone marked another pivotal moment in the evolution of dermal fillers. While initially considered a promising material due to its long-lasting effects, silicone injections were eventually restricted by the US Food and Drug Administration (FDA) due to adverse effects such as chronic inflammation, foreign body reactions, and granuloma formation [3]. Despite FDA restrictions, microdroplet injections of silicone remain in off-label use today for certain medical and cosmetic applications [4].

Other synthetic polymers, such as polytetrafluoroethylene (Teflon), were also explored as soft tissue fillers. However, Teflon was abandoned due to its inflammatory properties and injection difficulties [5].

D. G. Moon, *Penile Augmentation with Injectable Hyaluronic Acid*,
https://doi.org/10.1007/978-981-95-5385-3_3

Until the 1980s, none of these early fillers received FDA approval. The first FDA-approved soft tissue filler was Zyderm collagen (Allergan, Inc.), introduced in 1981. This bovine-derived collagen filler became the foundation for modern injectable fillers, leading to increased research and development in the field [6].

Following the approval of Zyderm, a new era of filler technology emerged, leading to the development of hyaluronic acid (HA) derivatives, calcium hydroxylapatite (CaHA), poly-L-lactic acid (PLLA), and polymethylmethacrylate (PMMA), which were once widely used or continue to be widely used today [7]. These advancements revolutionized the field by providing safer, longer-lasting, and biocompatible alternatives to earlier materials.

3.2 Timeline of Filler Development

The evolution of soft tissue fillers over the past century reflects both innovation and lessons learned from early complications. In 1893, Dr. Franz Neuber pioneered autologous fat grafting for facial defects. The early 1900s saw paraffin injections gain popularity, but severe complications such as paraffinomas soon led to their abandonment. Silicone injections emerged in the 1950s and 1960s but were later restricted due to chronic inflammatory responses and migration issues. A significant milestone occurred in 1981 when Zyderm collagen became the first FDA-approved filler, marking the beginning of regulated soft tissue augmentation. The 1990s introduced hyaluronic acid (HA) fillers like Restylane, offering a safer and more biocompatible alternative. The 2000s saw the development of newer materials, including calcium hydroxylapatite (CaHA), poly-L-lactic acid (PLLA), and polymethylmethacrylate (PMMA). In the 2010s and 2020s, HA fillers were further refined and their applications expanded beyond aesthetics into urology, particularly in penile augmentation.

Timeline of Filler Development

1893: Dr. Franz Neuber introduces autologous fat grafting.
1900s: Paraffin injections gain popularity but lead to complications.
1950s–1960s: Silicone injections are introduced but face restrictions.
1981: Zyderm collagen becomes the first FDA-approved filler.
1990s: Introduction of HA-based fillers like Restylane.
2000s: Advances in CaHA, PLLA, and PMMA fillers.

3.3 Synthetic Fillers

With the FDA approval of Zyderm collagen (Allergan, Inc.) in 1981, the field of soft tissue augmentation rapidly expanded. The limitations of collagen fillers, such as short duration and the risk of hypersensitivity reactions, fueled the search for more durable and biocompatible alternatives [8].

Calcium hydroxylapatite (CaHA) fillers emerged as a solution, offering both immediate volumization and collagen stimulation. Radiesse (BioForm Medical, now Merz Aesthetics), approved in 2006, introduced CaHA microspheres suspended in a gel carrier, making it suitable for deep tissue augmentation, including jawline contouring and volume restoration in patients with lipoatrophy [9, 10]. CaHA fillers are FDA-approved for deep facial wrinkles and volume restoration. However, complications such as nodules, hypersensitivity reactions, and potential vascular occlusion have been reported [11]. Proper injection techniques and patient screening are critical to minimize risks. Radiesse is contraindicated in patients with severe allergies or bleeding disorders [12].

Another notable synthetic filler is poly-L-lactic acid (PLLA), which differs from HA and CaHA fillers by stimulating fibroblast activity rather than providing immediate volume. Sculptra (Dermik Laboratories, later acquired by Galderma), approved in 2004, has become widely used for gradual volume restoration, particularly for midface volume loss and HIV-associated lipoatrophy [13]. PLLA fillers are FDA-approved for facial volume loss but require multiple treatment sessions for optimal results. Risks include delayed-onset nodules, asymmetry, and foreign body reactions. Proper dilution and deep subcutaneous injection techniques can mitigate complications [3, 14].

Polymethylmethacrylate (PMMA) fillers represent another category of synthetic fillers that offer permanent structural support. Bellafill (previously ArteFill, Suneva Medical), approved in 2006, contains PMMA microspheres suspended in a collagen matrix. Unlike absorbable fillers, PMMA remains in place, making it suitable for deep nasolabial folds and acne scar correction [15]. PMMA fillers are FDA-approved for nasolabial folds and acne scars but carry the highest risk of permanent complications. Improper placement can result in granulomas, fibrosis, and chronic inflammation. Due to its permanence, careful patient selection and experienced injectors are essential [15].

3.4 Hyaluronic Acid Derivatives

The introduction of hyaluronic acid (HA)-based fillers in the late 1990s revolutionized aesthetic medicine. HA is a naturally occurring glycosaminoglycan that provides hydration and volume to the skin. Its biocompatibility, reversibility with hyaluronidase, and long-lasting effects made it the gold standard for dermal fillers [16].

Popular HA fillers include Restylane (1996, Medicis) and Juvederm (2006, Allergan), both of which have undergone continuous advancements in cross-linking technologies to improve longevity and integration [17]. Newer technologies, such as Vycross® (Allergan) and RHA® (Revance), have improved the elasticity and durability of HA fillers, reducing the risk of adverse effects [18].

HA fillers are widely considered the safest class of fillers due to their reversibility with hyaluronidase. However, risks such as vascular occlusion, delayed hypersensitivity reactions, and biofilm formation exist. The FDA has approved multiple HA products for various indications, including lip augmentation and midface volumization [19].

Ongoing research into bioengineered HA derivatives aims to enhance filler longevity while maintaining a natural feel. The development of hybrid fillers combining HA with other active ingredients, such as collagen stimulators or antioxidants, represents the next frontier in filler technology [20] (Table 3.1).

Table 3.1 Comparison of key fillers: the properties, indications, and risks of commonly used fillers

Filler type	Composition	FDA approval	Primary indications	Longevity	Risks
Zyderm collagen	Bovine collagen	1981	Facial wrinkles	3–6 months	Hypersensitivity reactions
Calcium hydroxylapatite (CaHA)	CaHA microspheres	2006	Deep wrinkles, volume restoration	12–18 months	Nodules, vascular occlusion
Poly-L-lactic acid (PLLA)	Biodegradable polymer	2004	Facial volume loss	2–3 years	Nodules, foreign body reactions
Polymethylmethacrylate (PMMA)	PMMA microspheres	2006	Nasolabial folds, acne scars	Permanent	Granulomas, chronic inflammation
Hyaluronic acid (HA)	Glycosaminoglycan	1996	Lip augmentation, facial volume	6–18 months	Reversible vascular occlusion, biofilm

References

1. Neuber F. Fat grafting. Cuir Kongr Verh Dtsch Otsum Ges Chir. 1893;20:66.
2. Ersek RA, Beisang AA. Bioplastique TM: a new biphasic polymer for minimally invasive injection implantation. Aesth Plast Surg. 1992;16:59–65.
3. Kontis TC. Contemporary review of injectable facial fillers. JAMA Facial Plastic Surgery. 2013;15(1):58–64.
4. Benedetto AV, Lewis AT. Injecting 1000 centistoke liquid silicone with ease and precision. Dermatologic Surg. 2003;29(3):211–4.
5. Landman MD, Strahan RW, Ward PH. Chin augmentation with polytef paste injection. Arch Otolaryngol. 1972;95(1):72–5.
6. Miller P, Levine J, Ahn M, Maas C, Constantinides M. Softform for facial rejuvenation: historical review, operative techniques, and recent advances. Facial Plast Surg. 2000;16(1):23–8.
7. Statistics P. American society of plastic surgeons. 2018 Plastic surgery statistics report. Plast Surg. 2017;25:7–8.
8. Baumann L. Collagen-containing fillers: alone and in combination. Clin Plast Surg. 2006;33(4):587–96.
9. Berlin AL, Hussain M, Goldberg DJ. Calcium hydroxylapatite filler for facial rejuvenation: a histologic and immunohistochemical analysis. Dermatologic Surg. 2008;34:S64–S7.
10. Jacovella PF. Use of calcium hydroxylapatite (Radiesse®) for facial augmentation. Clin Interv Aging. 2008;3(1):161–74.
11. Tansavatdi K, Mangat DS. Calcium hydroxyapatite fillers. Facial Plast Surg. 2011;27(06):510–6.
12. Jacovella PF. Calcium hydroxylapatite facial filler (Radiesse™): indications, technique, and results. Clin Plast Surg. 2006;33(4):511–23.
13. Kates LC, Fitzgerald R. Poly-L-lactic acid injection for HIV-associated facial lipoatrophy: treatment principles, case studies, and literature review. Aesthet Surg J. 2008;28(4):397–403.
14. Lowe NJ, Maxwell CA, Lowe P, Shah A, Patnaik R. Injectable poly-l-lactic acid: 3 years of aesthetic experience. Dermatologic Surg. 2009;35:344–9.
15. Solomon P, Ng CL, Kerzner J, Rival R. Facial soft tissue augmentation with bellafill: a review of 4 years of clinical experience in 212 patients. Plastic Surgery. 2021;29(2):98–102.
16. Betemps JB, Marchetti F, Lim T, Hadjab B, Micheels P, Salomon D, et al. Projection capacity assessment of hyaluronic acid fillers. Plast Aesthet Res. 2018;5(19):10.20517.
17. Kablik J, Monheit GD, Yu L, Chang G, Gershkovich J. Comparative physical properties of hyaluronic acid dermal fillers. Dermatologic Surg. 2009;35:302–12.
18. Wongprasert P, Dreiss CA, Murray G. Evaluating hyaluronic acid dermal fillers: a critique of current characterization methods. Dermatol Ther. 2022;35(6):e15453.
19. Rao V, Chi S, Woodward J. Reversing facial fillers: interactions between hyaluronidase and commercially available hyaluronic-acid based fillers. J Drug Dermatol. 2014;13(9):1053–6.
20. Fakih-Gomez N, Kadouch J. Combining calcium hydroxylapatite and hyaluronic acid fillers for aesthetic indications: efficacy of an innovative hybrid filler. Aesth Plast Surg. 2022;46(1):373–9.

4 Current Hyaluronic Acid Gel

Contents

4.1 Hyaluronic Acid Filler Market Overview

The global dermal filler market has witnessed significant growth, driven by increasing demand for nonsurgical aesthetic enhancements. According to the American Society of Plastic Surgeons (ASPS) 2023 Procedural Statistics Report, a total of 5,294,603 HA filler procedures were performed, making up approximately 85% of all soft tissue augmentation treatments. In contrast, non-hyaluronic acid fillers accounted for 924,549 procedures, reinforcing the dominance of HA-based products in the market [1].

The US dermal filler industry was valued at $1.4 billion in 2023 and is projected to grow at a CAGR of 8.4%, reaching $3.4 billion by 2034 [2]. This growth is attributed to enhanced product longevity, safety advancements, and increased consumer awareness of minimally invasive procedures. Furthermore, HA fillers remain a preferred choice due to their biocompatibility, reversibility with hyaluronidase, and wide application across multiple aesthetic indications [3].

4.2 Properties of Hyaluronic Acid Gel

4.2.1 Cross-Linking

Hyaluronic acid is a naturally occurring glycosaminoglycan with excellent hydrophilic properties, making it an ideal candidate for dermal fillers. However, in its unmodified form, HA has a short half-life of 24–48 h, necessitating chemical modifications to enhance its durability and efficacy [4]. To overcome the short half-life of

D. G. Moon, *Penile Augmentation with Injectable Hyaluronic Acid*,
https://doi.org/10.1007/978-981-95-5385-3_4

free HA polymers, manufacturers cross-link HA units using 1,4-butanediol diglycidyl ether (BDDE), divinyl sulfone, or 2,7,8-diepoxyoctane (DEO), stabilizing the HA superstructure through intermolecular bonds and slowing enzymatic and free radical degradation [5]. Non-cross-linked HA exists as a liquid, whereas cross-linking provides structure and adhesive stick, creating a gel-like consistency [4]. BDDE, the most commonly used cross-linking agent, is considered safe and nonreactive, with residual amounts minimized through purification processes. In Allergan's HA filler range, unreacted BDDE levels are reported at less than two parts per million, and residual BDDE undergoes hydrolysis over time [6]. Despite safety assurances, controversy remains regarding potential toxicity from cross-linking agents, prompting research into alternative cross-linkers such as urea [7]. Higher degrees of cross-linking create stiffer gels resistant to deformation, prolonging filler longevity while reducing hydrophilicity, which may impact tissue integration and increase the risk of foreign body reactions, especially when combined with increased longevity from cross-linking [8].

4.2.2 Particle Sizing

Although cross-linking is essential for creating a lasting HA product, the process effectively results in a large gel-like mass that must be sized to pass through a needle [5]. Sizing is performed using sieves or homogenization, producing biphasic and monophasic gels [9]. Biphasic HA gels consist of cross-linked particles suspended in free HA, enhancing injection ease while maintaining firmness, whereas monophasic HA gels undergo homogenization, yielding smooth, polydensified formulations with a broader particle size distribution [9, 10]. Larger particles are used for deeper injections, exhibiting higher stiffness and longevity, while smaller particles ensure smoother integration for superficial injections [8].

Rheology plays a significant role in HA filler performance. The *complex modulus (G)** represents the total energy required to deform a gel, calculated as the sum of elastic modulus (G′) and viscous modulus (G″). The elastic modulus (G′) determines the gel's ability to recover its shape after deformation and is closely linked to product firmness. Fillers with higher G′ values exhibit greater resistance to mechanical forces, making them ideal for areas requiring structural support, such as the nasolabial folds and marionette lines [11, 12]. However, excessive G′ may lead to palpable nodules and increase the risk of Tyndall effect when injected too superficially [13]. Lower G′ fillers, in contrast, are softer, better suited for dynamic areas like the lips, and provide smoother integration within superficial tissues [4].

4.2.3 HA Concentration

The HA concentration within a filler affects its viscosity, elasticity, and hydrophilic properties. Higher HA concentrations increase viscosity and elasticity, contributing to longer-lasting volume enhancement and improved tissue integration [7]. Fillers with high cohesivity are better suited for volumizing larger areas, as they maintain shape more effectively and provide increased support within the tissue matrix [13]. However, high HA concentrations also attract more water, leading to greater postinjection swelling, which may require clinical consideration when planning treatments.

Cohesivity refers to the tendency of the gel to hold its shape under mechanical stress and is directly correlated with both cross-linking density and HA concentration. Highly cohesive fillers maintain their shape better, preventing migration, and are often preferred for volumizing large areas. In contrast, low-cohesivity fillers spread more evenly, making them ideal for fine lines and superficial wrinkles [13]. The Gavard–Sundaram Cohesivity Scale classifies HA fillers into high cohesivity groups (e.g., Belotero Balance), medium-high cohesivity (e.g., Juvederm Ultra XC), and low cohesivity (e.g., Restylane Lyft) [11].

4.3 Current FDA-Approved Hyaluronic Acid Fillers

Currently available HA fillers exhibit varying properties depending on their formulation [14]. Restylane and Perlane (Galderma, Ft. Worth, TX) are biphasic gels containing particles suspended in a liquid carrier. Restylane, introduced in 1996, is a non-animal-stabilized HA filler with 20 mg/mL HA concentration and an average particle size of 400 μm. Perlane, a similar product, has a larger particle size (750–1000 μm), making it more suitable for deeper injections. Due to its coarser consistency, Perlane requires a 27-gauge needle, compared to the 30-gauge needle used for Restylane (Table 4.1) [15, 16].

Juvederm XC and Juvederm Voluma (Allergan, Irvine, CA) are monophasic gels that do not contain discrete particles but instead consist of cohesive cross-linked HA molecules. Juvederm XC, with 24 mg/mL HA concentration, has a lower G′ and viscosity, making it ideal for areas requiring soft contouring, such as the lips and superficial wrinkles. Juvederm Voluma, approved in 2013, was specifically designed for midface volumization, incorporating both low- and high-molecular-weight HA to enhance cross-linking and increase elastic modulus (G′), resulting in long-term deep soft tissue restoration with effects lasting up to 2 years (Table 4.1) [17].

Belotero Balance (Merz North America, Greensboro, NC) is a polydensified HA filler with nonuniform cross-linking, yielding a low viscosity and the lowest G′ among available HA fillers [18]. This makes it highly suitable for superficial injection in areas requiring seamless integration, such as fine lines, vermillion border definition, and tear trough correction (Table 4.1) [19].

4.4 KFDA-Approved Hyaluronic Acid Fillers for Penile Girth Enhancement

The use of hyaluronic acid (HA) fillers for penile girth enhancement (PGE) originated in South Korea, where researchers first explored the feasibility of injectable fillers for nonsurgical penile augmentation. The earliest reported clinical study on HA-based penile augmentation was conducted using Restylane Sub-Q® (Q-med, Uppsala, Sweden) and demonstrated significant girth enhancement and patient satisfaction over an 18-month follow-up period [20].

Following the success of HA-based augmentation, other fillers such as polymethyl methacrylate (PMMA) and cross-linked dextran (Lipen-10; Chungwha Medipower Corporation, Seoul, Korea) and polylactic acid (PowerFill; REGEN Biotech, Inc., Seoul, Korea) were developed for penile enhancement [21, 22]. However, these products failed to gain widespread acceptance due to complications such as granuloma formation, long-term irregularities, and lack of consistent volume retention [23]. As a result, the demand for biodegradable, biocompatible, and reversible penile fillers led to the development of

Table 4.1 Properties of FDA-approved hyaluronic acid fillers

Product name	HA concentration (mg/mL)	Particle size (μm); mono vs. biphasic	Cross-linker type	Duration (months)	Cohesivity score	G' (PA)
Juvederm Voluma XC	20	n/a; Monophasic	BDDE	18–24	Low-medium	146
Juvederm Ultra XC	24	n/a; Monophasic	BDDE	9–12	Medium-high	110
Restylane Lyft (previous Perlane)	20	750–1000 μm; biphasic	BDDE	12–18	Medium	747
Belotero balance	22.5	(-); Biphasic	BDDE	6–12	High	41
Restylane silk	20	(-); Biphasic	BDDE	6–12	Low	517
Restylane Refyne/Defyne	20	(-); Biphasic	BDDE	12	Medium-high	(-)

(−), information not available

Table 4.2 Properties of KFDA-approved hyaluronic acid fillers for penile girth enhancement

Product name (manufacturer, country)	HA conc. (mg/mL)	Particle size; mono vs. biphasic	Cross-linking; degree	Complex viscosity
Potenfill (Medytox, Korea)	20	≈ 700 μm; mono	BDDE; 10%	No record
Doublofill (Humedix, Korea)	23	≈ 700 μm; mono	BDDE; 12%	200–600 Pa.s
HyaFilia impact (CHA Meditech, Korea)	20	≈ 500 μm; mono	BDDE; 6%	100–600 Pa.s
THE CHAEUM; shape 10 (Hugel bio., Korea)	20	≈ 600 μm/a; mono	BDDE; no record	400 ~ 700 Pa.s

HA-based fillers, which were subsequently approved by the Korean Food and Drug Administration (KFDA).

Extensive clinical research efforts led to the approval of four dedicated HA fillers for penile girth enhancement, including Potenfill (Medytox, Korea), HyaFilia Impact (CHA Meditech, Korea), THE CHAEUM Shape 10 (Hugel Bio, Korea), and Doublofill (Humedix, Korea). These products were evaluated through multicenter, randomized, and comparative trials, demonstrating superior safety and efficacy profiles [24–27]. Studies have reported significant increases in penile girth, with patient and partner satisfaction scores remaining high over an 18-month follow-up period.

Clinical evaluations of penile girth enhancement using hyaluronic acid (HA) fillers have demonstrated consistent and promising outcomes across multiple studies. The mean increase in penile girth reported ranged from 19.1 mm to 22.7 mm, reflecting a substantial augmentation effect achievable through this minimally invasive approach. Importantly, patient-reported satisfaction was notably high, with over 85% of participants rating their outcomes as satisfactory or highly satisfactory.

In terms of safety, no significant cases of granuloma formation, persistent nodules, or vascular complications were documented during follow-up periods. Adverse effects were minimal and predominantly self-limiting, consisting mainly of transient swelling and mild discomfort within the initial post-procedural phase. These findings underscore the favorable safety and efficacy profile of HA-based fillers for penile augmentation.

Among these, Potenfill was shown to be a highly effective filler with a favorable safety profile compared to polylactic acid-based alternatives, while HyaFilia Impact confirmed long-term stability and effectiveness over 18 months [26, 27]. THE CHAEUM Shape 10 exhibited excellent volume retention with minimal adverse effects, and Doublofill was associated with the highest penile girth increase (22.7 mm on average) while maintaining a low incidence of inflammatory complications [24, 25]. These fillers vary in cross-linking degree, HA concentration, and rheological properties, affecting their longevity, tissue integration, and risk of foreign body reactions (Table 4.2).

Doublofill contains the highest degree of cross-linking (12%) and HA concentration (23 mg/mL), which theoretically increases its viscosity, longevity, and structural stability (Table 4.2). However, higher cross-linking degrees may also elevate the risk of foreign body reactions and granuloma formation. Interestingly, clinical trials have reported no significant increase in inflammatory adverse effects with Doublofill compared to other HA fillers [25]. The favorable safety profile and predictable outcomes have positioned HA fillers as the leading choice for penile augmentation procedures in Korea, with ongoing research focusing on improving filler rheology and longevity.

References

1. Statistics P. American society of plastic surgeons. 2018 Plastic surgery statistics report. Plast Surg. 2017;25:7–8.

2. Market LM. Transparency market research. Transparency Market Reasearch [Online] Available from: https://www.transparencymarketresearch.com/cellulose-acetatephthalatemarkethtml#:~:text=Cellulose%20acetate%20phthalate%20is%20derived%20from%20plant-based%20raw,capsules%20or%20as%20an%20enteric%20film%20coating%20material.2020.
3. Betemps JB, Marchetti F, Lim T, Hadjab B, Micheels P, Salomon D, et al. Projection capacity assessment of hyaluronic acid fillers. Plast Aesthet Res. 2018;5(19):10.20517.
4. Kablik J, Monheit GD, Yu L, Chang G, Gershkovich J. Comparative physical properties of hyaluronic acid dermal fillers. Dermatologic Surg. 2009;35:302–12.
5. Tezel A, Fredrickson GH. The science of hyaluronic acid dermal fillers. J Cosmet Laser Ther. 2008;10(1):35–42.
6. De Boulle K, Glogau R, Kono T, Nathan M, Tezel A, Roca-Martinez J-X, et al. A review of the metabolism of 1, 4-butanediol diglycidyl ether-crosslinked hyaluronic acid dermal fillers. Dermatologic Surg. 2013;39(12):1758–66.
7. Fallacara A, Manfredini S, Durini E, Vertuani S. Hyaluronic acid fillers in soft tissue regeneration. Facial Plast Surg. 2017;33(01):087–96.
8. Bentkover SH. The biology of facial fillers. Facial Plast Surg. 2009;25(02):073–85.
9. Beasley KL, Weiss MA, Weiss RA. Hyaluronic acid fillers: a comprehensive review. Facial Plast Surg. 2009;25(02):086–94.
10. Flynn TC, Sarazin D, Bezzola A, Terrani C, Micheels P. Comparative histology of intradermal implantation of mono and biphasic hyaluronic acid fillers. Dermatologic Surg. 2011;37(5):637–43.
11. Sundaram H, Rohrich RJ, Liew S, Sattler G, Talarico S, Trévidic P, et al. Cohesivity of hyaluronic acid fillers: development and clinical implications of a novel assay, pilot validation with a five-point grading scale, and evaluation of six US Food and Drug Administration–approved fillers. Plast Reconstr Surg. 2015;136(4):678–86.
12. Moers-Carpi M, Vogt S, Santos BM, Planas J, Vallve SR, Howell DJ. A multicenter, randomized trial comparing calcium hydroxylapatite to two hyaluronic acids for treatment of nasolabial folds. Dermatologic Surg. 2007;33:S144–S51.
13. Fabi SG, Champagne JP, Nettar KD, Maas CS, Goldman MP. Efficacy and safety of and patient satisfaction with injectable hyaluronic acid with 0.3% lidocaine hydrochloride for the treatment of superficial perioral lines or superficial lateral canthal lines. Dermatologic Surg. 2013;39(11):1613–20.
14. Pierre S, Liew S, Bernardin A. Basics of dermal filler rheology. Dermatologic Surg. 2015;41:S120–S6.
15. Maas CS, Bapna S. Pins and needles: minimally invasive office techniques for facial rejuvenation. Facial Plast Surg. 2009;25(04):260–9.
16. Ali MJ, Ende K, Maas CS. Perioral rejuvenation and lip augmentation. Facial Plast Surg Clin North Am. 2007;15(4):491–500.
17. Callan P, Goodman GJ, Carlisle I, Liew S, Muzikants P, Scamp T, et al. Efficacy and safety of a hyaluronic acid filler in subjects treated for correction of midface volume deficiency: a 24 month study. Clin Cosmet Investig Dermatol. 2013:81–9.
18. Hevia O, Cohen BH, Howell DJ. Safety and efficacy of a cohesive polydensified matrix hyaluronic acid for the correction of infraorbital hollow: an observational study with results at 40 weeks. J Drug Dermatol. 2014;13(9):1030–6.
19. Lorenc ZP, Fagien S, Flynn TC, Waldorf HA. Clinical application and assessment of Belotero: a roundtable discussion. Plast Reconstr Surg. 2013;132(4S-2):69S–76S.
20. Kwak TI, Oh M, Kim JJ, Moon DG. The effects of penile girth enhancement using injectable hyaluronic acid gel, a filler. J Sex Med. 2011;8(12):3407–13.
21. Kim MT, Ko K, Lee WK, Kim SC, Yang DY. Long-term safety and longevity of a mixture of polymethyl methacrylate and cross-linked dextran (Lipen-10®) after penile augmentation: extension study from six to 18 months of follow-up. World J Men Health. 2015;33(3):202–8.
22. Yang D, Ko K, Lee S, Moon D, Kim J, Lee W. Efficacy and safety of a newly developed polylactic acid microsphere as an injectable bulking agent for penile augmentation: 18-months follow-up. Int J Impot Res. 2017;29(4):135–41.
23. Ahn ST, Il Kwak T, Park KS, Kim JJ, Moon DG. Complications of glans penis augmentation. Int J Impot Res. 2019;31(4):245–55.
24. Yang DY, Jeong HC, Ahn ST, Bae WJ, Moon DG, Kim SW, et al. A comparison between hyaluronic acid and polylactic acid filler injections for temporary penile augmentation in patients with small penis syndrome: a multicenter, patient/evaluator-blind, comparative, randomized trial. J Sex Med. 2020;17(1):133–41.
25. Ahn ST, Shim JS, Bae WJ, Kim SW, Kim JJ, Moon DG. Efficacy and safety of penile girth enhancement using hyaluronic acid filler and the clinical impact on ejaculation: a multi-center, patient/evaluator-blinded, randomized active-controlled trial. World J Men Health. 2021;40(2):299.
26. Yang DY, Jeong HC, Ko K, Lee SH, Lee YG, Lee WK. Comparison of clinical outcomes between hyaluronic and polylactic acid filler injections for penile augmentation in men reporting a small penis: a multicenter, patient-blinded/evaluator-blinded, non-inferiority, randomized comparative trial with 18 months of follow-up. J Clin Med. 2020;9(4):1024.
27. Yang DY, Ko K, Lee SH, Lee WK. A comparison of the efficacy and safety between hyaluronic acid and polylactic acid filler injection in penile augmentation: a multicenter, patient/evaluator-blinded, randomized trial. J Sex Med. 2019;16(4):577–85.

Current Guideline of Penile Augmentation

5

Contents

Penile augmentation procedures have garnered increasing attention in both medical and cosmetic fields, yet their safety, efficacy, and ethical considerations remain subjects of ongoing debate. As demand for these procedures rises, professional medical organizations have sought to provide evidence-based recommendations to guide clinical practice. The European Association of Urology (EAU), the Sexual Medicine Society of North America (SMSNA), and the International SOciety for Sexual Medicine (ISSM) have each published guidelines and position statements addressing the indications, risks, and ethical considerations associated with penile enlargement interventions [1–3].

The European Association of Urology (EAU) and the Sexual Medicine Society of North America (SMSNA) have published guideline documents and position statements addressing penile size concerns, penile dysmorphic disorder, and cosmetic penile enhancement procedures, emphasizing psychological screening, cautious patient selection, and the limited evidence supporting many augmentation techniques [1, 2]. Both the EAU and SMSNA emphasize the importance of distinguishing men with true anatomical abnormalities—such as micropenis or adult-acquired buried penis—from those with penile dysmorphic disorder (PDD), a condition characterized by persistent preoccupation with perceived penile inadequacy despite normal measurements [1, 2]. Patients with PDD are at increased risk of dissatisfaction, repeated procedures, and psychological harm following aesthetic interventions. The ICSM 2024 consensus reinforces and expands upon this stance by providing explicit recommendations on psychological screening in the context of penile augmentation. ICSM highlights that an in-depth assessment should include accurate penile measurements, evaluation of sexual function, assessment of patient motivation, and screening for body dysmorphic disorder and related psychopathology (ICSM Recommendations 1–5) [3].

Non-surgical options for penile augmentation Non-surgical approaches are commonly requested by men seeking penile augmentation, particularly those reluctant to undergo operative intervention or those requiring initial conservative management. These options include penile traction therapy, vacuum erection devices, hormonal therapy, and injectable fillers. Overall, the

D. G. Moon, *Penile Augmentation with Injectable Hyaluronic Acid*,
https://doi.org/10.1007/978-981-95-5385-3_5

evidence supporting durable penile enlargement with non-surgical modalities remains limited, and patient counseling regarding realistic outcomes is essential.

Among the nonsurgical treatment options, penile traction therapy (PTT) has been identified as a low-risk intervention with modest effects on stretched penile length [4–8]. Several prospective and observational studies have demonstrated modest increases in flaccid and stretched penile length, typically averaging up to approximately 2 cm following a minimum of 3–6 months of consistent daily use. Gains in erect penile length are less consistent, and treatment success is highly dependent on patient compliance and duration of therapy. Both the EAU and SMSNA acknowledge that PTT may offer limited length improvement in selected patients but emphasize the need for prolonged use and appropriate patient expectations [1, 2]. Penile traction therapy may be offered to selected patients seeking penile lengthening, with counseling that expected gains are modest and require sustained, compliant use (Strong Recommendation, Moderate Quality of Evidence) (ICSM Recommendation 6) [3].

Vacuum erection devices (VEDs), although widely marketed, have not been shown to produce substantial or lasting elongation [9]. Vacuum erection devices generate negative pressure around the penis, resulting in increased penile blood flow and temporary engorgement. Although VEDs are well established in erectile rehabilitation, particularly following radical prostatectomy, evidence supporting their use for permanent penile length or girth augmentation is lacking. Any perceived increase in penile size is typically transient and related to vascular congestion rather than structural tissue change. VEDs are not recommended as a definitive method for penile augmentation due to insufficient evidence demonstrating sustained changes in penile size (Expert Opinion)(ICSM 2024).

Hormonal therapy, on the other hand, is only indicated in patients with documented endocrinological deficiencies that affect penile growth [10]. Penile development is androgen-dependent during fetal life and early childhood. Testosterone or gonadotropin therapy has demonstrated efficacy in increasing penile size in prepubertal boys with confirmed micropenis or disorders of sex development. However, there is no evidence supporting penile enlargement following hormonal therapy in post-pubertal males or in men with normal penile anatomy, including those with penile dysmorphic disorder or adult-acquired buried penis. Hormonal therapy should be restricted to prepubertal patients with micropenis or disorders of sex development and should not be used to increase penile size after puberty (Strong Recommendation, High Quality of Evidence) (ICSM Recommendation 7) [3].

Surgical options for penile augmentation Surgical penile augmentation represents the most invasive category of interventions and should be considered only after comprehensive clinical, psychological, and sexual assessment, and following failure or rejection of conservative and minimally invasive options. Given the irreversible nature of many surgical procedures and the potential for significant functional and aesthetic complications, careful patient selection and informed consent are paramount. ICSM 2024 overarching surgical principle The ICSM 2024 consensus emphasizes that penile augmentation surgery should not be approached as a purely cosmetic procedure. Instead, it should be framed within a reconstructive and functional paradigm, prioritizing patient safety, realistic expectations, and long-term outcomes. Surgical intervention is appropriate only when; Psychological stability is established, Indications are clearly defined, Expected benefits outweigh foreseeable risks, and The surgeon possesses appropriate reconstructive expertise. (ICSM Recommendations 9–13).

Suspensory ligament release (SLR) is designed to increase the apparent flaccid penile length by allowing greater externalization of the penile shaft. It does not increase true corporal length or erect penile size. The procedure is frequently combined with V-Y plasty, suprapubic fat reduction, or postoperative traction therapy to optimize cosmetic outcomes. Furthermore, suspensory ligament division is associated with complications such as penile instability, altered angulation, and sensory disturbances. ICSM acknowledges that SLR may improve flaccid appearance only and stresses that patients must be explicitly counseled regarding; Lack of erect length gain, Risk of penile instability during erection, Scar contracture and re-adhesion, and Potential need for revision surgery. (ICSM Recommendation 14 – Expert Opinion) Other surgical techniques, including grafting and flap procedures, are not currently recommended for routine use due to high complication rates and a lack of long-term efficacy data [1].

Injectable fillers for penile augmentation Injectable fillers are among the most commonly requested minimally invasive options for penile girth enhancement. These techniques involve the placement of filler materials into the subdartos plane to increase penile circumference without altering corporal anatomy. Historically, a wide variety of substances have been injected for penile augmentation, with markedly different safety profiles. The use of non-medical and non-resorbable materials, including paraffin, petroleum jelly (Vaseline), silicone oil, and industrial fillers, is associated with severe complications such as foreign body granulomas, chronic inflammation, tissue necrosis, infection, penile deformity, and, in extreme cases, Fournier's gangrene. These materials should be strictly prohibited. The use of autologous fat grafting, hyaluronic acid fillers, and other injectable materials for girth enhancement is addressed cautiously, as these approaches may yield temporary volume increase but also pose risks of migration, granuloma formation, and resorption over time [1]. For the first time, the ICSM 2024 provides explicit guidance on injectable fillers for aesthetic penile augmentation [3]. The consensus panel states that; Unsafe materials, including paraffin, silicone oil, and other non-medical substances, must not be used for penile augmentation. Biodegradable fillers, particularly hyaluronic acid (HA), and autologous fat injection are considered relatively safe options when performed by experienced clinicians using appropriate techniques. Patients must be counseled that repeat treatments are likely required over time, as resorption and volume loss are expected. This position is reflected in ICSM Recommendations 16 and 17, which emphasize safety, reversibility, and informed consent (Weak Recommendation, Low Quality of Evidence). HA fillers are favored due to their biocompatibility, reversibility, and favorable short-term safety profile. Autologous fat injection avoids foreign material implantation but is associated with variable resorption rates, asymmetry, and the potential need for repeat procedures. Silicone penile implants, such as the Penuma device, remain experimental, and the EAU advises that further clinical studies are necessary to establish their long-term safety and effectiveness [1]. Silicone sleeve implants represent a distinct category between fillers and reconstructive surgery, intended to provide permanent girth enhancement. ICSM 2024 classifies subcutaneous penile implants as experimental, recommending that they; Be offered only by experienced reconstructive surgeons, Be accompanied by detailed counseling regarding infection, extrusion, deformity, and explantation risks, Not be promoted as routine cosmetic procedures. (ICSM Recommendation 18 – Expert Opinion).

The SMSNA, in its position statement on cosmetic penile enhancement procedures, echoes similar concerns regarding the lack of robust long-term safety data for many available interventions [2]. The society acknowledges the increasing demand for penile augmentation but highlights the importance of patient counseling and informed consent. According to the SMSNA, injectable fillers such as hyaluronic acid (HA) and poly-L-lactic acid (PLA) may offer a temporary increase in penile girth with relatively low risks, but longitudinal studies are required to assess their durability and safety over extended periods. The SMSNA explicitly discourages the use of permanent fillers such as silicone, paraffin, or polymethyl methacrylate (PMMA) due to the high incidence of complications, including fibrosis, chronic inflammation, and nodular formations [2].

The surgical approaches addressed in the SMSNA statement include suspensory ligament release, grafting, and silicone sleeve implants. The society notes that while suspensory ligament release may yield an increase in flaccid penile length, it is often accompanied by a loss of penile stability and other functional complications [2, 11]. Grafting and flap-based augmentation procedures are classified as experimental techniques that should only be performed in highly specialized centers under rigorous clinical evaluation. Regarding silicone sleeve implants such as Penuma, the SMSNA highlights that these devices remain investigational and should only be performed under institutional review board (IRB) oversight. Patients considering such interventions must be fully informed of potential complications, including infection, extrusion, and device-related deformities. Techniques such as sliding and slicing penile lengthening procedures remain highly experimental, with insufficient evidence to recommend their routine use [12].

Given the available evidence and the concerns raised by leading medical societies, clinicians should adhere to best practices when addressing patients seeking penile augmentation. The process should begin with a comprehensive patient assessment, including a detailed medical and psychosexual history, objective penile measurements, and psychological screening when indicated. Patients must be counseled on the realistic outcomes and potential risks associated with both surgical and nonsurgical augmentation techniques.

While advances in surgical techniques and injectable materials have expanded the options available for penile augmentation, the ICSM 2024 consensus underscores that patient safety, psychological well-being, and ethical practice must remain central to clinical decision-making. Aesthetic penile procedures, particularly injectable fillers and surgical interventions, may offer short-term cosmetic improvement but are associated with variable durability and a non-negligible risk of complications, including altered sensation, erectile dysfunction, penile deformity, and the need for revision surgery.

Overall, the field of penile augmentation remains an evolving area of study with limited high-quality evidence supporting most interventions. While the use of HA fillers for penile girth enlargement has gained popularity for its effectiveness and safety, procedures aimed at increasing penile length remain controversial due to inconsistent results and high complication rates. As such, clinicians should exercise caution when considering these procedures, prioritizing patient safety, ethical considerations, and evidence-based practice.

The European Association of Urology (EAU), the Sexual Medicine Society of North America (SMSNA), and the International Society for Sexual Medicine (ISSM, ICSM 2024) have each provided guidelines and position statements on penile augmentation procedures. While there is consensus on several aspects, notable differences exist in their recommendations and emphasis. The Fifth International Consultation on Sexual Medicine represents the first global consensus to explicitly address aesthetic penile augmentation, integrating psychological screening, non-surgical options, and surgical interventions within a unified evidence-based framework. By reinforcing strict contraindications for unsafe materials, recognizing the relative safety—but limited durability—of biodegradable fillers and autologous fat, and discouraging invasive surgery in men with normal penile anatomy, the ICSM 2024 provides clinicians with clear guidance to balance patient expectations with medical responsibility. Despite these advances, substantial gaps in high-quality evidence persist, particularly regarding long-term outcomes and patient-reported satisfaction. Continued prospective studies and standardized outcome reporting are essential to refine best practices and ensure that penile augmentation procedures are performed ethically, safely, and in the best interests of patients. (Table 5.1).

Table 5.1 Comparison of current guidelines for premature ejaculation

Aspect	EAU guidelines	SMSNA position	ICSM 2024
Psychological evaluation	Strongly recommends psychological screening for body dysmorphic disorder (BDD) in patients with normal penile dimensions seeking augmentation. Advises psychological counseling before any intervention in such cases.	Emphasizes the importance of patient counseling and informed consent. Recommends psychological assessment before procedures like suspensory ligament division.	Mandatory distinction between normal variation, PDD, micropenis, and buried penis; psychiatric referral advised when PDD suspected (Rec 1, 5 – Expert Opinion).
Nonsurgical interventions	Identifies penile traction therapy (PTT) as a low-risk option with modest effects on stretched penile length. Notes that vacuum erection devices (VEDs) have not shown substantial or lasting elongation.	Acknowledges that injectable fillers like hyaluronic acid (HA) and poly-L-lactic acid (PLA) may offer temporary girth enhancement with relatively low risks but calls for more longitudinal studies. Strongly discourages permanent fillers such as silicone or paraffin due to severe complications.	PTT can be offered for lengthening; average gain 2 cm after ≥3 months; requires compliance (Moderate, Evidence B) Considered HA gel injection relatively safe and reversible; re-injection likely over time (Moderate, Evidence C) Considered Autologous fat injection relatively safe; high variability and need for repeat procedures (Rec 16 – Moderate, Evidence C) Unsafe injectable materials (silicone, paraffin, oils) must not be used due to severe complications (Strong, Evidence B).
Surgical interventions	Notes weak evidence supporting suspensory ligament release (SLR) and associates it with complications like penile instability. Does not recommend grafting and flap procedures due to high complication rates and lack of long-term efficacy data. Considers the use of autologous fat grafting, HA fillers, and other injectables cautiously, citing risks of migration and granuloma formation.	Finds SLR reasonable when offered by experienced surgeons to select patients who are properly informed about potential risks. Advises against graft-and-flap procedures outside of research settings due to limited data. Recommends silicone sleeve implants be performed only under investigational protocols with research oversight.	SLR may restore genital appearance in AABP; improves flaccid length only; risks must be emphasized (Expert Opinion).

References

1. Falcone M, Bettocchi C, Carvalho J, Ricou M, Boeri L, Capogrosso P, et al. European association of urology guidelines on penile size abnormalities and dysmorphophobia: summary of the 2023 guidelines. Eur Urol Focus. 2024;10:432–41.
2. Trost L, Watter DN, Carrier S, Khera M, Yafi FA, Bernie HL, et al. Cosmetic penile enhancement procedures: an SMSNA position statement. J Sex Med. 2024;21:573–8.
3. Chung E, Jenkins L, Moon DG, Ziegelmann M, Deveci S, Lin HC, et al. Penile augmentation and cosmetic surgery: recommendations from the Fifth International Consultation on Sexual Medicine (ICSM 2024). Sex Med Rev. 2025 Dec 4:qeaf067. https://doi.org/10.1093/sxmrev/qeaf067. Online ahead of print.
4. García Gómez B, Alonso Isa M, García Rojo E, Fiorillo A, Romero OJ. Penile length augmentation surgical and non-surgical approaches for aesthetical purposes. Int J Impot Res. 2022;34:332–6.
5. Colpi G, Martini P, Scroppo F, Mancini M, Castiglioni F. Efficacy of the daily penis-stretching technique to elongate the 'small penis'. Int J Imp Res. 2001;13:47.
6. Gontero P, Di Marco M, Giubilei G, Bartoletti R, Pappagallo G, Tizzani A, et al. A pilot phase-II prospective study to test the 'efficacy' and tolerability of a penile-extender device in the treatment of 'short penis'. BJU Int. 2009;103:793–7.
7. Nikoobakht M, Shahnazari A, Rezaeidanesh M, Mehrsai A, Pourmand G. Effect of penile-extender device in increasing penile size in men with shortened penis: preliminary results. J Sex Med. 2011;8:3188–92.
8. Nowroozi MR, Amini E, Ayati M, Jamshidian H, Radkhah K, Amini S. Applying extender devices in patients with penile dysmorphophobia: assessment of tolerability, efficacy, and impact on erectile function. J Sex Med. 2015;12:1242–7.
9. Aghamir MK, Hosseini R, Alizadeh F. A vacuum device for penile elongation: fact or fiction? BJU Int. 2006;97:777–8.
10. Main KM, Schmidt IM, Toppari J, Skakkebaek NE. Early postnatal treatment of hypogonadotropic hypogonadism with recombinant human FSH and LH. Eur J Endocrinol. 2002;146:75–9.
11. Aboul Fotouh El Gharably M, Ghoneima W, Lotfi MA, AbdelWahab M, Elkady A, Abdel-Rassoul MA. The efficacy of suspensory ligament release and pubic lipectomy via penopubic Z Plasty during penile prosthesis implantation in improving sexual satisfaction: a prospective randomized controlled trial. J Sex Med. 2022;19:852–63.
12. Barham D, Barnard J, Gelman J. (102) complications of the Penuma penile implant for genital enhancement. J Sex Med. 2023;20(qdad060):97.

Part II

Penile Girth Enhancement

6 Historical Development of Penile Girth Enhancement (PGE)

Contents

D. G. Moon, *Penile Augmentation with Injectable Hyaluronic Acid*,
https://doi.org/10.1007/978-981-95-5385-3_6

6.1 Introduction

Penile girth enhancement (PGE) has become an increasingly prominent topic in aesthetic and functional urology, reflecting the cultural, psychological, and personal dimensions of male sexual health. While true micropenis—defined as a stretched penile length less than 2.5 standard deviations below the mean—is a medically recognized indication for surgical intervention [1, 2], the majority of men seeking PGE have normal penile dimensions and are motivated by perceived aesthetic inadequacies or the desire for enhanced sexual confidence [3].

Over the past century, methods for increasing penile girth have evolved dramatically. Early approaches were characterized by the subcutaneous injection of non-biocompatible materials such as paraffin, petroleum jelly, mineral oil, and even metallic mercury, often performed by untrained individuals [4–7]. These hazardous practices frequently resulted in severe complications, including foreign body granulomas, paraffinomas, penile deformity, and tissue necrosis, which necessitated complex reconstructive surgeries [8, 9].

The medicalization of PGE began with the introduction of structured surgical techniques such as autologous fat transfer and dermofat grafting. While these methods provided a more controlled and biocompatible solution, they were associated with variable outcomes due to issues like graft resorption, contour irregularities, and donor site morbidity [10–12].

In recent decades, the development of acellular dermal matrices (allografts) and porcine-derived xenografts further expanded surgical options. These biologic materials aimed to overcome the limitations of autologous tissue harvesting, although technical challenges and graft-related complications persisted [13, 14].

The advent of injectable hyaluronic acid (HA) fillers marked a paradigm shift in PGE. These minimally invasive procedures offer biocompatibility, reversibility, and high patient satisfaction, transforming the field and setting new standards for safety and efficacy [15].

This chapter reviews the historical development of PGE and examines current surgical and nonsurgical techniques. Special attention is given to dermofat grafting, autologous fat transfer, biologic grafts, and HA fillers, highlighting their technical considerations, clinical outcomes, and complications.

6.2 Evolution of Penile Girth Enhancement (PGE)

The evolution of penile girth enhancement is a story of trial, error, and refinement spanning more than a century. Early methods reflected cultural perceptions of masculinity and were often driven by psychological and aesthetic motivations rather than clear medical indications [3].

6.2.1 Early Materials and Techniques

In the early twentieth century, subcutaneous injections of paraffin, petroleum jelly, mineral oil, and metallic mercury became popular among men seeking penile enlargement [4–7]. Performed without medical oversight, these interventions led to devastating complications such as paraffinomas, chronic inflammation, necrosis, and deformity, requiring complex reconstructive procedures [8, 9].

The introduction of liquid silicone in the 1970s was initially heralded as an improvement. However, long-term follow-up revealed serious adverse effects including granuloma formation, migration, vascular embolization, sensory loss, and significant distortion of penile anatomy [16, 17]. These complications underscored the need for safer, medically supervised interventions.

Autologous Fat Grafting Autologous fat grafting marked a significant step forward. Fat harvested via liposuction was injected between the tunica albuginea and Buck's fascia to enhance girth. While initial results were promising, resorption rates of 50–70% resulted in volume loss, asymmetry, and nodular formation [18, 19]. Panfilov reported variable satisfaction, with a subset of patients requiring revision surgeries for contour irregularities [10].

Dermal-Fat Grafts To address these shortcomings, dermal-fat grafts were introduced. These composite grafts combined dermis and subcutaneous fat, offering improved volume stability and structural support. They were positioned between the dartos fascia and Buck's fascia to achieve more durable outcomes. Despite these advantages, partial graft loss, fibrosis, and resorption continued to limit success [11].

Allografts and Xenografts The next refinement involved acellular dermal matrices (AlloDerm) and xenografts (MegaDerm), designed to eliminate donor site morbidity. These materials facilitated host cell infiltration and neovascularization but posed technical challenges during implantation and sometimes suffered from graft detachment [13, 14].

Surgical Innovations Advanced surgical techniques such as Austoni's saphenous vein graft [20] and Shaeer's superficial circumflex iliac artery island flap [21] offered substantial girth gains but involved complex operations and carried risks of scarring and functional compromise.

Hyaluronic Acid Fillers The modern shift hyaluronic acid (HA) fillers revolutionized PGE by introducing a minimally invasive, outpatient-based procedure. With high biocompatibility, reversibility, and patient satisfaction, HA injections became the preferred method worldwide. Studies report penile circumference increases from 7.48 cm to 11.26 cm, sustained over 12–18 months with minimal complications [22].

6.2.2 Summary

The evolution of PGE illustrates a progression from hazardous experimental approaches to refined, patient-centered techniques. While surgical grafting methods represented incremental improvements, the emergence of HA fillers has redefined patient expectations and clinical practice. Future research should aim to standardize techniques and evaluate long-term outcomes to further enhance safety and efficacy.

6.3 Penile Girth Enhancement with Dermofat Graft

Autologous dermofat grafting has been widely adopted as a surgical technique for penile girth enhancement (PGE), especially in regions where surgical approaches remain popular. Initially developed to overcome the limitations of autologous fat transfer, dermofat grafting provides improved volume stability and aesthetic outcomes for properly selected patients.

6.3.1 Introduction

The procedure involves transplanting a composite graft consisting of dermis and subcutaneous fat into the penile shaft to increase circumference. Positioned between the dartos fascia and Buck's fascia, the graft offers structural support and enhanced volume retention. This technique has gained recognition for its relatively high graft survival rates and its ability to maintain penile contour with minimal fat resorption compared to fat-only injections [11].

6.3.2 Mechanism of Graft Survival

The survival of dermofat grafts has been explained by two primary theories. The host cell replacement theory proposes that transplanted adipose cells degenerate over time, releasing fat that is gradually resorbed while new adipocytes form from host-derived precursors. Alternatively, the cell survival theory suggests that a proportion of the transplanted adipose cells survive by establishing early revascularization from the subdermal vascular network, with neovascularization initiating around Day 4 post-transplant and stabilizing within 6–8 months [12, 13]. The dartos fascia, being richly vascularized, serves as an ideal recipient bed for the graft. When survival fails, the result is often fibrotic scar tissue formation within a year [15].

6.3.3 Surgical Technique (Figs. 6.1 and 6.2)

Dermofat grafting begins with harvesting tissue from donor sites such as the buttocks, lower abdomen, inner thigh, or medial upper arm. Surgeons typically harvest 20–30% more tissue than estimated requirements to compensate for the predictable postoperative absorption of graft material [14]. The epidermis is removed using a split-thickness grafting technique, and the dermofat layer is carefully dissected. This tissue must be handled with great care to prevent fat necrosis. Closure of the donor site is performed in layers and covered with antibiotic-soaked dressings to minimize the risk of infection.

Following graft preparation, a subdermal pocket is created on the penis by making either a circular or longitudinal skin incision, usually positioned just below the coronal sulcus. The graft is placed longitudinally along the penile shaft and secured at multiple points with absorbable sutures to prevent migration. A meticulous multilayered closure of the penile skin reduces tension on the wound and promotes optimal healing [18].

Postoperatively, patients are closely monitored for signs of infection, edema, or wound complications. The urinary catheter is typically removed on the first postoperative day once the patient is stable and voiding independently. Prophylactic antibiotics are administered for 5 to 7 days to reduce the risk of infection, and patients are advised to avoid vigorous physical or sexual activity during the initial recovery phase to promote graft integration and stability. Regular follow-up visits are crucial for evaluating girth retention and identifying any early complications.

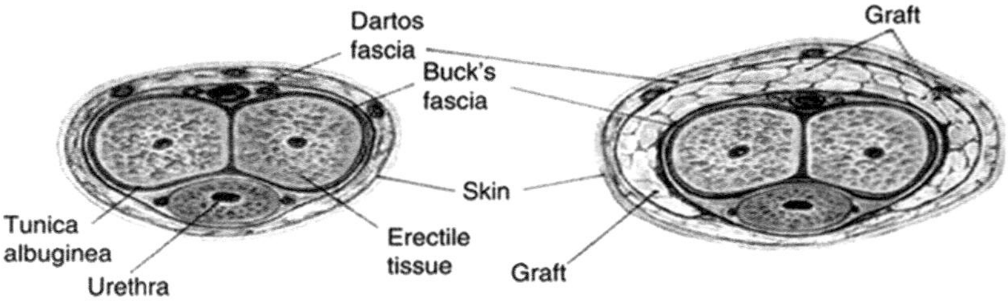

Fig. 6.1 Schematic diagram of dermofat graft for penile augmentation

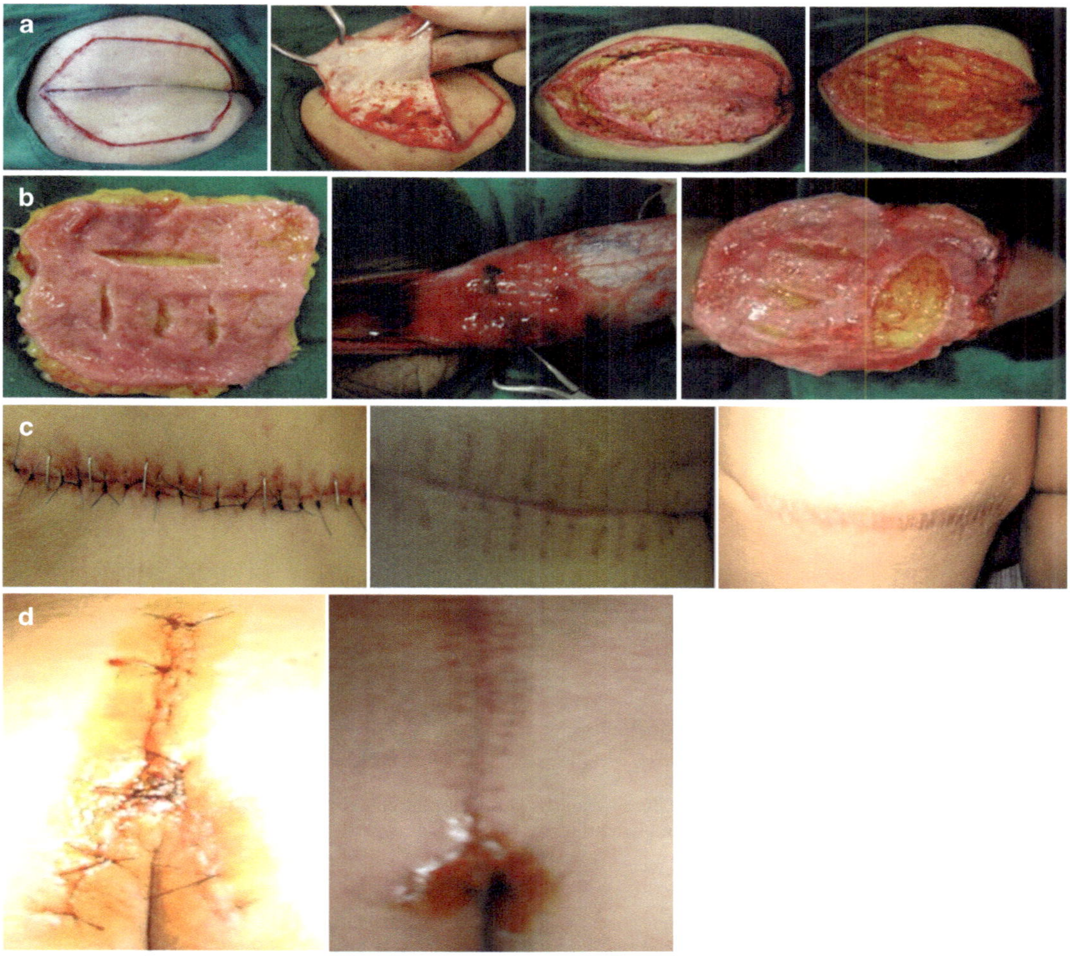

Fig. 6.2 Autologous dermofat graft. (**a**) Dissection of epidermis at selected donor site, (**b**) Preparation, fixation of dermal fat graft, wound repair, (**c**) Donor site closure postoperative donor site scar, (**d**) Other kind of donor site scar at lower back

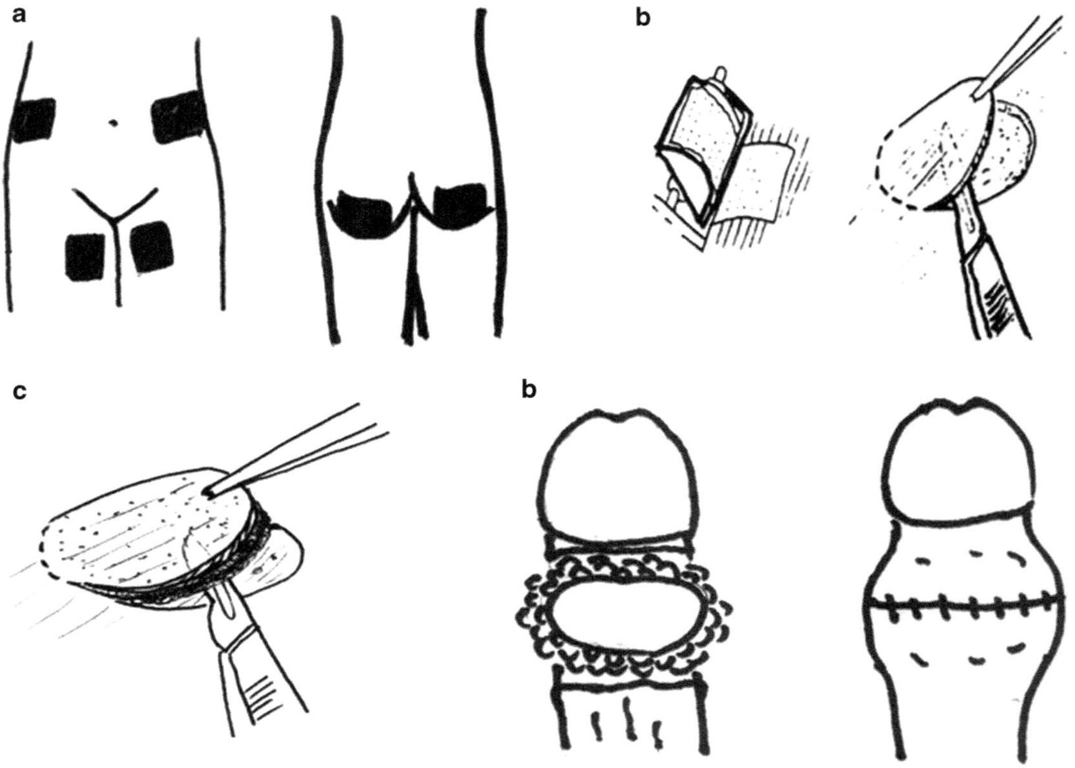

Autologous dermofat graft. (**a**) Selection of donor site. (**b**) Dissection of epidermis. (**c**) Splitting dermofat graft from donor site. (**d**) Fixation of dermal fat graft and wound repair

6.3.4 Clinical Outcomes

Dermofat grafting has demonstrated promising outcomes in clinical studies. Reported penile girth increases range between 65.7% and 80.0%, while penile length gains vary from 14.3% to 70.1% depending on individual factors and surgical technique [10, 11]. Patient satisfaction is generally high, with immediate postoperative satisfaction rates of 88.9% among patients and 66.7% among their partners. Over longer follow-up periods, satisfaction slightly decreases due to issues such as scar formation (16.7%) and gradual reduction of graft volume (11.1%) [11].

6.3.5 Complications and Management

Complications associated with dermofat grafting are relatively uncommon but require prompt recognition and management when they occur. Early postoperative findings such as edema and ecchymosis are generally self-limiting and respond well to compression dressings. Infections, although rare, are minimized through adherence to aseptic techniques and timely administration of prophylactic antibiotics; severe cases may necessitate graft removal and secondary reconstruction after the infection has resolved. Skin necrosis and wound dehiscence can result from

Table 6.1 Cause and management of complications after dermofat graft

Complication	Cause and management
Edema and ecchymosis	Common early post-op. Resolves with *compression dressings*. Severe cases may require *aspiration*
Infection	Prevented with *sterile techniques* and *early grafting*. If severe, *graft removal and revision after 3 months*
Skin necrosis and wound rupture	Due to *high tension* or *poor circulation*. *Debridement and resuturing* may be required
Penile curvature	Caused by *asymmetric graft placement*. Severe cases may require *revision surgery*
Epidermal cysts	Develop from *residual sebaceous glands* Most resolve *spontaneously or by aspiration*
Seroma	Accumulation of *fat fluid and exudate*. Small amounts absorb naturally; larger ones require *needle aspiration*
Graft absorption	*Fat: 50%, Dermofat: 20–30%, dermis: 15–20%*. Larger graft *reduces absorption*
Calcification	Rare. Caused by *hydrolyzed fat deposits* detected in *X-rays*

excessive tension or compromised vascularity at the graft site, necessitating debridement and meticulous resuturing.

Other complications include penile curvature, often caused by asymmetric graft placement, which may require corrective surgery, and seroma formation due to the accumulation of fluid or fat exudate. While small seromas typically resolve spontaneously, larger collections may require aspiration. Graft absorption rates vary across tissue types, with approximate resorption of 50% in fat, 20–30% in dermofat, and 15–20% in dermis. Calcification is a rare complication, detectable on radiographic imaging as hydrolyzed fat deposits [11]. These complications, along with their causes and management strategies, are summarized in Table 6.1, serving as a practical reference for clinicians performing this procedure.

6.3.6 Long-Term Results

Studies with mean follow-up durations of 34.8 months (range: 3–57 months) report sustained improvements in penile girth, with an immediate postoperative increase of 24.3% and a retained gain of 18% at long-term follow-up. Penile length enhancements have also been observed, with increases of 43% immediately postoperatively and 7.9% maintained over time [10].

6.3.7 Summary

Autologous dermofat grafting remains a viable surgical technique for penile girth enhancement. Its success depends on meticulous surgical technique, proper patient selection, and attentive postoperative care. While the emergence of minimally invasive methods such as hyaluronic acid fillers has shifted global trends toward nonsurgical solutions, dermofat grafting continues to hold relevance in aesthetic urology for patients seeking a more permanent augmentation option.

6.4 Penile Girth Enhancement with Autologous Fat Transfer (AFT)

6.4.1 Introduction

Autologous fat transfer (AFT) emerged as one of the first minimally invasive methods for penile girth enhancement (PGE). The procedure involves harvesting adipose tissue from donor sites using liposuction, purifying the fat, and reinjecting it into the penile shaft. While conceptually simple and initially attractive for its autologous nature and avoidance of foreign materials, AFT has shown inconsistent results due to variable fat survival rates and technical challenges [18].

Penile augmentation using autologous fat gained popularity in the late twentieth century as part of augmentative phalloplasty. Procedures aimed at penile lengthening and girth enhancement were often performed in combination, including suspensory ligament release, skin flap construction, and fat injection [19]. In PGE specifically, AFT involves transferring fat harvested from the patient's own body into the penile dartos layer. Early studies reported average girth increases of approximately 2.6 cm, with injection volumes ranging between 23 and 49 mL depending on patient anatomy and desired outcomes [10]. However, despite these promising initial results, long-term follow-up has revealed significant limitations, including unpredictable absorption and postoperative deformities [11].

6.4.2 Technique for AFT

The AFT procedure begins with fat harvesting from donor sites such as the lower abdomen or bilateral thighs. A tumescent solution containing lidocaine, epinephrine, and bicarbonate is first infiltrated into the subcutaneous tissue to facilitate liposuction and reduce bleeding. Fat is then extracted using a 4-mm harvesting cannula and processed through centrifugation at 3000 rpm for 3 minutes to separate viable adipocytes from oil, blood, and other debris [19].

Purified fat is reinjected into the penile shaft at the dartos level (Colles' fascia layer) using a blunt-tip 18-gauge cannula. Multiple puncture sites are created at 11, 1, 3, and 9 o'clock positions to ensure even distribution of fat across the shaft's circumference. Care is taken to avoid the urethral region between 5 and 7 o'clock to minimize the risk of complications. Small aliquots of fat are deposited in the superficial, middle, and deep layers of Colles' fascia using a retrograde threading technique, with the cannula moved back and forth to achieve uniformity and reduce the likelihood of nodularity. Any remaining fat is stored aseptically for possible touch-up sessions within weeks or months [19].

6.4.3 Complications and Management

Autologous fat transfer (AFT) presents several notable complications due to the inherent unpredictability of fat survival and the unique dynamics of penile tissue. Early postoperative challenges such as fat absorption and atrophy are common, reflecting the limited vascular support for larger fat deposits. These larger volumes often succumb to central liquefaction and necrosis, leading to cyst formation and progressive loss of volume over time [11].

Fat migration and asymmetry frequently result from the mobility of loose fascial planes within the penis, and such complications are often exacerbated by sexual activity. Irregular nodules and contour deformities arise from uneven fat resorption, leaving visible and palpable irregularities that may require surgical correction.

Rarely, foreign body granulomas develop when autologous fat is inadvertently mixed with synthetic materials, inciting an inflammatory reaction and subsequent granuloma formation. Severe complications such as erectile dysfunction and sensory loss, although uncommon, can occur secondary to vascular compromise or extensive fibrosis, with significant functional implications [11, 15].

A summarized overview of these complications and their management strategies is presented in Table 6.2. This table serves as a practical reference for clinicians and highlights the importance of preventive measures, such as using small-volume fat deposits and ensuring even distribution, to reduce postoperative morbidity.

6.4.4 Long-Term Outcomes

Long-term studies of AFT have reported high absorption rates, ranging from 50% to 70%, resulting in significant volume loss over time. Repeated fat injections often fail to achieve durable results, and the risk of fat migration, asymmetry, and palpable nodules remains high [11]. These limitations have shifted clinical preference toward alternative techniques such as

Table 6.2 Cause and management of complications after autologous fat transfer

Complication	Cause and management
Fat absorption and atrophy	Unpredictable resorption due to poor vascularization; larger deposits risk liquefaction and cysts.
Fat migration and asymmetry	Caused by loose fascial planes; exacerbated by sexual activity, leading to proximal/distal displacement.
Irregular fat nodules and deformities	Uneven resorption results in lumps; revision surgery may be required for correction.
Foreign body granuloma formation	Occurs when fat mixes with synthetic fillers, causing inflammatory granulomatous reactions.
Erectile dysfunction and sensory loss	Rare; results from vascular injury or fibrosis; may lead to functional impairment.

dermofat grafts and hyaluronic acid fillers, which offer greater predictability and patient satisfaction [15].

6.4.5 Summary

While autologous fat transfer is conceptually appealing due to its simplicity and use of autologous tissue, its clinical application in penile girth enhancement is limited by high resorption rates and postoperative complications. The technique requires meticulous surgical execution and careful patient counseling about potential outcomes and the likelihood of revision surgery. With the advent of more reliable options such as dermofat grafting and hyaluronic acid fillers, AFT has become a less favored choice for permanent penile augmentation.

6.5 Penile Girth Enhancement with Biograft (Allograft, Xenograft)

6.5.1 Introduction

Biologic grafts have become an important adjunct in penile girth enhancement (PGE), offering a less invasive alternative to autologous grafts with the added benefit of avoiding donor-site morbidity. These grafts are derived from mammalian tissues, including human, bovine, and porcine sources, and are processed through decellularization, cross-linking, and sterilization to preserve their extracellular matrix (ECM). The preserved ECM facilitates host-cell integration and remodeling, supporting stable augmentation of the penile shaft [13].

Allografts, such as acellular dermal matrices (ADM), are derived from cadaveric human skin. Products like AlloDerm® (LifeCell Inc., USA) have been extensively utilized in reconstructive surgery and burn care due to their biocompatibility and support for tissue regeneration [13, 23]. Xenografts, obtained from animal tissues such as porcine dermis or bovine pericardium, include widely used products like MegaDerm Ultra® (L&C BIO Inc., Korea) and Lyoplant® (B. Braun, Germany). These materials are designed to elicit minimal immune response while promoting rapid host-cell infiltration and neovascularization [24, 25].

In PGE, these biologic grafts provide consistent cosmetic results, enhanced penile symmetry, and improved durability compared with autologous dermofat grafting. However, their use is not without challenges, including risks of fibrosis, infection, and graft resorption [26, 27].

6.5.2 Surgical Technique

Biografts are prepared by hydrating them in antibiotic-infused saline for at least 20 min before implantation. The surgeon identifies Buck's fascia-facing side of the graft by applying blood, ensuring correct orientation. Grafts are tailored to match penile dimensions, with strategic mesh incisions or punctures added to enhance flexibility and encourage tissue integration [27].

Two main surgical approaches are utilized. The infrapubic incision, preferred for its direct access, involves creating transverse, Z-plasty, or inverted V-Y incisions to expose the dartos fascia while avoiding damage to vascular and lymphatic structures. The graft is positioned between the dartos fascia and Buck's fascia and anchored at multiple points with absorbable sutures to ensure stability and prevent migration. The alternative circumcision incision allows similar placement but carries a higher risk of suture line disruption in uncircumcised patients [25].

Postoperatively, compression dressings are maintained for 5 days, with prophylactic intravenous antibiotics given for 2 days followed by oral therapy for an additional week. Patients are advised to avoid sexual activity for 4 weeks and abstain from smoking or alcohol use during the critical healing phase to optimize graft survival (Fig. 6.3).

6.5.3 Clinical Outcomes

In a clinical series involving 24 patients with a mean follow-up of 2 years, biografting achieved a penile girth increase of 2.2 cm and length gain of 2.4 cm. The overall success rate was 83%, with most patients reporting satisfactory cosmetic and functional results. However, complications such as graft resorption (8.3%), skin necrosis (4.2%), and infection (4.2%) were observed [12, 13].

Histological studies confirm rapid fibroblast infiltration, neovascularization, and collagen remodeling within xenografts. The highly porous

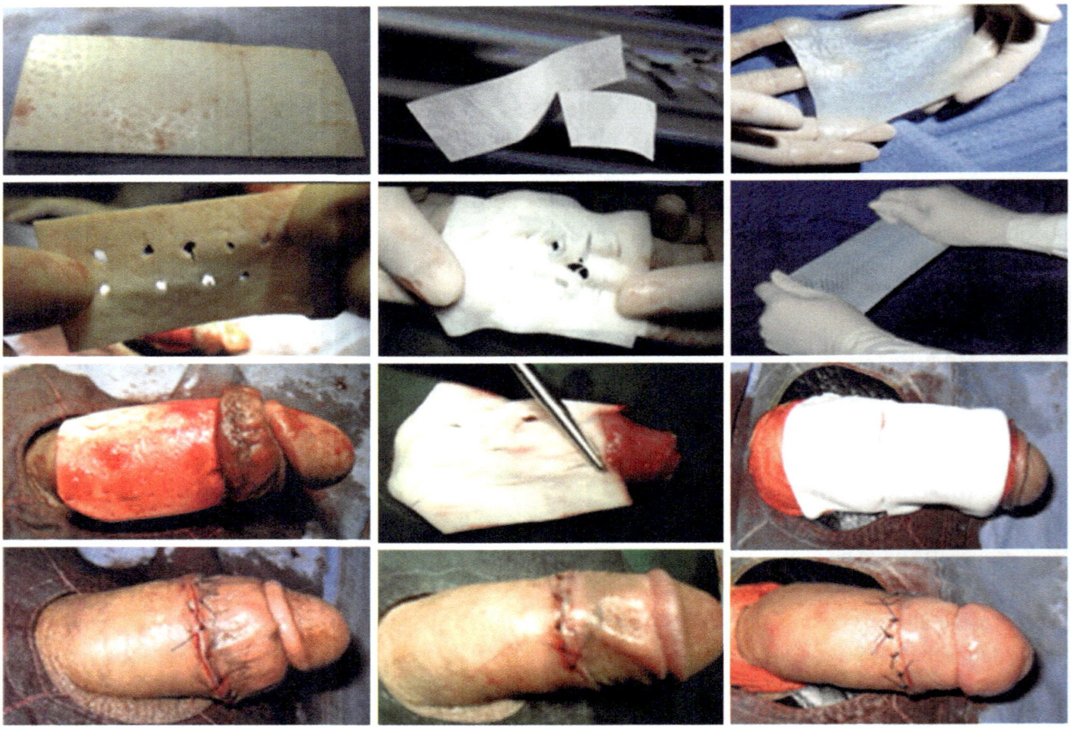

Fig. 6.3 Representative pictures of PGE with Alloderm, Lyoplant, and Matriderm

architecture of these materials supports host-cell migration and vascularization, ensuring long-term graft survival [27].

6.5.4 Complications and Management

Despite their promising potential, biografts carry a specific set of complications related to graft integration and host response. Early issues such as penile edema, skin discoloration, and bruising are typically self-limiting. More severe complications include wound dehiscence, hematoma, and infection, often associated with inadequate surgical technique or poor postoperative compliance [26].

Skin necrosis may result from impaired vascularization, particularly in patients with preexisting comorbidities or smokers, and requires immediate debridement and potential graft removal (Fig. 6.4). Fibrosis and graft resorption remain significant concerns, leading to penile shortening, rigidity, or deformity. Proper graft fixation and size customization are essential to minimize these risks [13].

An overview of these complications and their management is summarized in Table 6.3.

6.5.5 Late Complication

While biologic grafts are valued for their ability to produce a natural penile contour, late complications have been reported in a subset of patients. Some individuals experience sensory changes, including decreased penile sensation, ejaculatory difficulties, and even painful erections. These symptoms are often attributed to the thickness or rigidity of the dermal graft [25]. In severe cases, patients have requested graft removal to alleviate discomfort during sexual activity [28] (Fig. 6.5).

Clinically, fibrotic encircling masses may restrict expansion of the corpora cavernosa during erection, resulting in pain and functional impairment. However, graft removal is technically challenging due to extensive fibrosis and integration of the material within host tissues. Histological examination of excised grafts often reveals dense collagen bundles and fibroblast proliferation, consistent with chronic foreign body response [28].

In a patient of previous PGE and indirect glans penis augmentation (GPA) with ACDM, hard encircled mass along corporal body and cavernosal tip beneath the corpus spongiosum of glans penis are seen on sonography. After removal thick hard mass, plenty of pinkish thick collagen bundle and fibrosis with spindle shaped fibroblast are seen (H& E, x200).

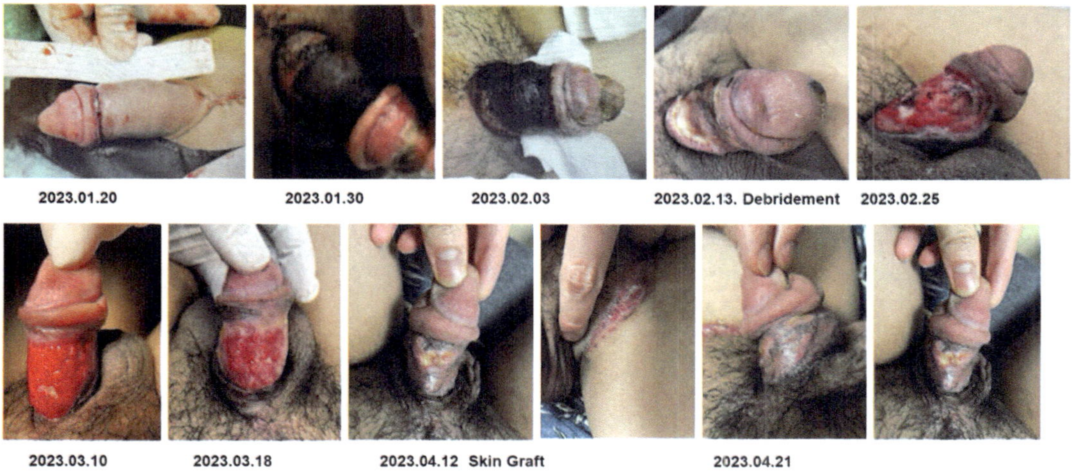

Fig. 6.4 A case of serious complication of PGE with ACDM. The most common complication of ACDM, 3–5 days after skin discoloration for poor blood supply; skin necrosis 2 weeks later; debridement 3 weeks later and skin graft 3 months later. When penile skin necrosis and infection are found, allograft must be removed as soon as possible

Table 6.3 Complications and management of biograft (allograft/xenograft) for PGE

Complication	Cause and management
Penile edema	Usually resolves with compression dressings; large transudate accumulation may require aspiration.
Skin discoloration and bruising	Temporary, resolves within 2–3 weeks.
Wound dehiscence and hematoma	Avoided with tension-free closure; treated with debridement and careful resuturing if present.
Skin necrosis and infection	Common cause: *Staphylococcus epidermidis*. Prevention: Pre-op skin preparation; sterile techniques, antibiotic irrigation, and limited OR traffic. Treatment: Immediate graft removal if necrosis/infection develops.
Suture line disruption	More common in circumcision incision cases. Prevented by meticulous suturing and postoperative care.
Fibrosis and graft resorption	Leads to penile shortening and rigidity; requires careful surgical planning and long-term follow-up.
Penile curvature and deformity	Proper graft fixation and size customization reduce risk.

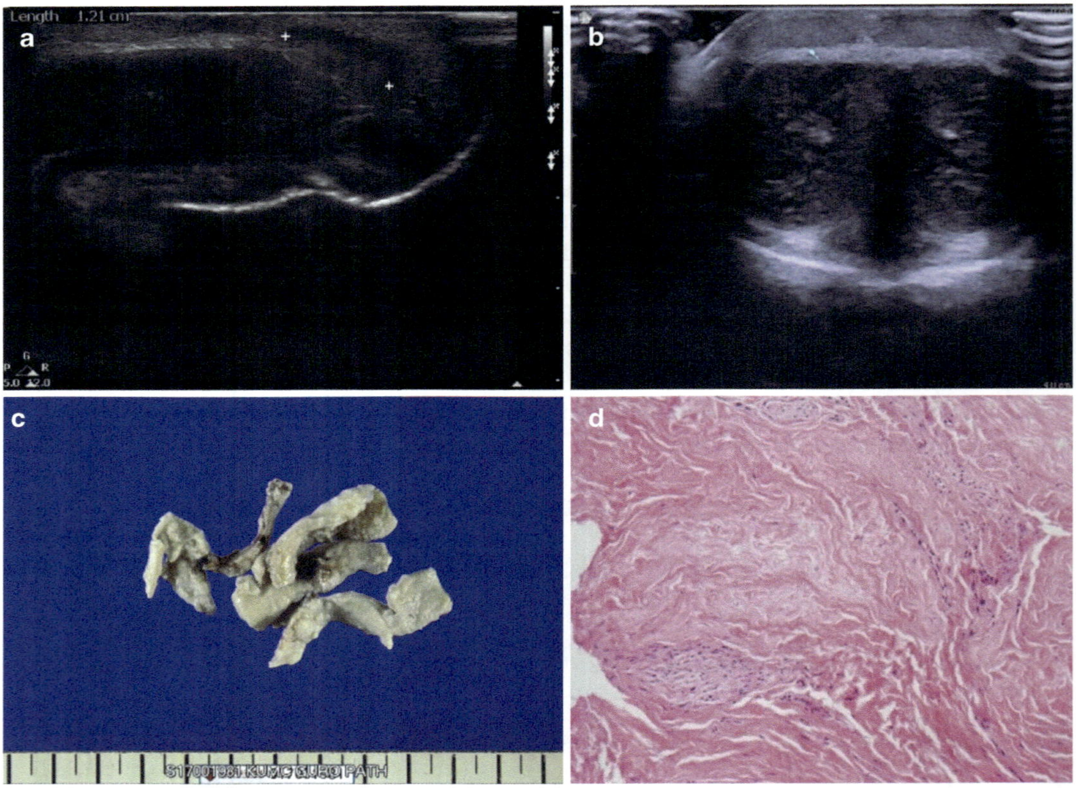

Fig. 6.5 Late complication of PGE with ACDM

6.5.6 Summary and Future Directions

Biografts have emerged as a promising alternative to autologous grafts in penile girth enhancement (PGE), offering advantages such as reduced donor-site morbidity, consistent cosmetic outcomes, and favorable biocompatibility. Both allografts and xenografts facilitate host-tissue integration and remodeling, providing stable augmentation results. However, challenges such as fibrosis, partial graft resorption, and late-onset complications, including sensory changes and painful erections, remain areas of concern. The

Table 6.4 Key takeaways from PGE techniques

	Advantages	Disadvantages	Remarks
Autologous fat transfer (AFT)	Readily available, minimally invasive, and low rejection risk	High resorption rates (50–70%), unpredictable volume retention, fat migration, and asymmetry	Less reliable for long-term augmentation; often requires multiple sessions or revision surgery.
Dermofat grafting	Better volume retention (20–30% resorption), structural support	Donor site morbidity, technical demands, fibrosis risk	Viable for patients seeking semi-permanent results but requires meticulous technique.
Allograft (acellular dermal matrix)	No donor-site morbidity, good graft survival, better symmetry and durability	Risk of fibrosis, necrosis, and resorption; limited long-term data	Promising alternative; success depends on graft handling and patient selection.
Xenograft (porcine/bovine dermis and pericardium)	Minimal immune response, stable results in some series	Limited long-term data, potential for rejection, fibrosis	Emerging option; further studies needed to confirm durability and safety.
Injectable hyaluronic acid (HA) fillers	Minimally invasive, reversible, high biocompatibility, excellent patient satisfaction.	Temporary effect (12–24 months), touch-ups needed	Currently the most popular option due to safety, simplicity, and effectiveness.

success of biografts depends largely on meticulous surgical technique, patient selection, and rigorous postoperative monitoring [13, 27] (Table 6.4). Future innovations in biomaterial design and long-term outcome studies are needed to establish their role as a mainstream option in aesthetic urology.

6.6 Hyaluronic Acid Fillers: The Modern Shift (Expanded Narrative)

The introduction of hyaluronic acid (HA) fillers has marked a paradigm shift in penile girth enhancement (PGE), offering a minimally invasive, outpatient procedure that aligns with modern aesthetic and functional expectations. HA fillers are composed of a naturally occurring glycosaminoglycan, which provides excellent biocompatibility, biodegradability, and reversibility. Initially developed for facial rejuvenation, HA-based products rapidly gained global acceptance for soft-tissue augmentation and are now the most widely used injectable material for penile augmentation [15].

Clinical studies consistently demonstrate significant increases in penile circumference following HA injection, with mean gains ranging from 2.4 cm to 3.8 cm (approximately 35–50% over baseline) [15]. The longevity of these effects varies according to the HA formulation, degree of cross-linking, and injection technique, with most studies reporting sustained augmentation for 12–18 months and some documenting residual volume beyond 24 months [15, 18]. Notably, touch-up sessions can extend the aesthetic outcomes and allow for fine adjustments to contour and symmetry.

Safety remains a cornerstone advantage of HA fillers. Unlike permanent grafts or silicone implants, HA is gradually metabolized by endogenous enzymes and can be rapidly reversed by hyaluronidase in cases of overcorrection or complications. The overall complication rate is low, with most adverse events limited to mild, self-limiting issues such as edema, bruising, and transient irregularities. Serious complications like vascular compromise or nodularity are exceedingly rare and are further mitigated by proper patient selection and advanced injection techniques [15].

From a patient-centered perspective, HA fillers meet the growing demand for minimally invasive interventions with short recovery times and high satisfaction rates. Surveys reveal that over 85% of men report improved self-confidence and sexual satisfaction following HA-based PGE, with partner satisfaction rates similarly high [15, 18]. These outcomes reflect not only physical changes but also improvements in psychological well-being and body image.

Emerging innovations in HA technology promise to enhance its utility further. Cross-linked HA gels with higher viscoelasticity offer improved longevity, while hybrid formulations incorporating bioactive molecules (e.g., peptides, growth factors) are under investigation for their regenerative potential. Future directions may include combining HA fillers with autologous biologics such as platelet-rich plasma (PRP) or adipose-derived stem cells to enhance tissue integration and reduce reabsorption.

Collectively, these attributes position HA fillers as the gold standard for penile girth enhancement in contemporary practice. As surgical options continue to evolve, the minimally invasive nature, safety profile, and reversibility of HA fillers ensure their place at the forefront of aesthetic urology.

6.6.1 Conclusion: Penile Girth Enhancement Techniques

The evolution of penile girth enhancement (PGE) reflects a century-long journey from rudimentary, high-risk interventions to advanced, patient-centered techniques. Autologous fat transfer (AFT) and dermofat grafting offered early solutions for penile augmentation but were limited by high resorption rates and technical complexities. The introduction of biologic grafts—both allografts and xenografts—addressed some limitations by eliminating donor-site morbidity and improving structural support, yet these approaches remain technically demanding and carry inherent risks such as fibrosis and partial graft resorption [13, 15, 27].

By contrast, hyaluronic acid (HA) fillers have transformed PGE into a minimally invasive, outpatient procedure with high patient satisfaction, minimal downtime, and a favorable safety profile. Their reversibility and adaptability make them the preferred option in contemporary aesthetic urology.

6.7 Future Outlook

As aesthetic and functional urology advances, the future of PGE will likely focus on optimizing minimally invasive techniques and integrating regenerative medicine. Emerging innovations include cross-linked HA formulations for enhanced longevity, stem cell-enriched gels, and hybrid approaches combining fillers with autologous biologics such as platelet-rich plasma (PRP). Multimodal treatments could offer synergistic effects, improving volume retention and tissue integration.

Rigorous multicenter clinical trials and long-term follow-up studies are necessary to establish standardized protocols, refine patient selection criteria, and evaluate safety profiles. With these developments, PGE techniques are expected to become increasingly tailored, safe, and durable.

6.8 Final Recommendation

For most men seeking penile girth enhancement, hyaluronic acid fillers offer the optimal balance of safety, efficacy, and reversibility. They align with modern patient preferences for minimally invasive procedures and rapid recovery. Surgical techniques—including dermofat grafting and biologic grafts—remain viable for select patients seeking more permanent augmentation, but they require thorough preoperative counseling and careful technical execution. Continued innovation in biomaterials and regenerative strategies promises to expand the therapeutic landscape and enhance outcomes in the years ahead.

References

1. Mondaini N, Ponchietti R, Gontero P, Muir G, Natali A, Caldarera E, et al. Penile length is normal in most men seeking penile lengthening procedures. Int J Impot Res. 2002;14(4):283–6.
2. Wessells H, Lue TF, McAninch JW. Penile length in the flaccid and erect states: guidelines for penile augmentation. J Urol. 1996;156(3):995–7.
3. Vardi Y, Lowenstein L. Penile enlargement surgery—fact or illusion? Nat Clin Pract Urol. 2005;2(3):114–5.

4. Cohen JL, Keoleian CM, Krull EA. Penile paraffinoma: self-injection with mineral oil. J Am Acad Dermatol. 2001;45(6):S222–S4.
5. Oh KJ, Park K, Kang TW, Kwon DD, Ryu SB. Subcutaneous metallic mercury injection for penile augmentation. Urology. 2007;69(1):185.e3–4.
6. Santucci RA, Zehring RD, McClure D. Petroleum jelly lipogranuloma of the penis treated with excision and native skin coverage. Urology. 2000;56(2):331.
7. Nyirády P, Kelemen Z, Kiss A, Bánfi G, Borka K, Romics I. Treatment and outcome of vaseline-induced sclerosing lipogranuloma of the penis. Urology. 2008;71(6):1132–7.
8. Du Geon Moon JWY, Bae JH, Han CS, Kim YK, Kim JJ. Sexual function and psychological characteristics of penile paraffinoma. Asian J Androl. 2003;5:191–4.
9. Akkus E, Iscimen A, Tasli L, Hattat H. Paraffinoma and ulcer of the external genitalia after self-injection of Vaseline. J Sex Med. 2006;3(1):170–2.
10. Panfilov DE. Augmentative phalloplasty. Aesth Plast Surg. 2006;30:183–97.
11. Park NC. Penile girth enhancement with Dermofat Graft. Penile Augmentation; 2016. p. 57–63.
12. Kim JY. Penile girth enhancement with xenograft. In: Penile Augmentation. Springer; 2016. p. 93–8.
13. Jung G-w. Penile girth enhancement with allograft. In: Penile Augmentation. Springer; 2016. p. 83–92.
14. Kim J-Y, Jean HS, Kim BJ, Song KY. 948: clinical safety, histologic findings and surgical methods in complex Phalloplasty using type I collagen. J Urol. 2007;177(4S):314.
15. Moon DG, Kwak TI. Penile girth enhancement with injectable HA gel. In: Penile Augmentation; 2016. p. 99–104.
16. Colombo F, Casarico A. Penile enlargement. Curr Opin Urol. 2008;18(6):583–8.
17. Vardi Y, Harshai Y, Gil T, Gruenwald I. A critical analysis of penile enhancement procedures for patients with normal penile size: surgical techniques, success, and complications. Eur Urol. 2008;54(5):1042–50.
18. Lee SW, Lee WH. Penile girth enhancement with autologous fat transfer. In: Penile Augmentation; 2016. p. 65–9.
19. Coleman WP, Hendry SL II. Principles of liposuction. Semin Cutan Med Surg. 2006;25:138.
20. Austoni E, Guarneri A, Cazzaniga A. A new technique for augmentation phalloplasty: albugineal surgery with bilateral saphenous grafts—three years of experience. Eur Urol. 2002;42(3):245–53.
21. Shaeer O. Girth augmentation of the penis using flaps "shaeer's augmentation phalloplasty": the superficial circumflex iliac flap. J Sex Med. 2014;11(7):1856–62.
22. Ahn ST, Shim JS, Bae WJ, Kim SW, Kim JJ, Moon DG. Efficacy and safety of penile girth enhancement using hyaluronic acid filler and the clinical impact on ejaculation: a multi-center, patient/evaluator-blinded, randomized active-controlled trial. World J Men Health. 2021;40(2):299.
23. Pannucci CJ, Antony AK, Wilkins EG. The impact of acellular dermal matrix on tissue expander/implant loss in breast reconstruction: an analysis of the tracking outcomes and operations in plastic surgery database. Plast Reconstr Surg. 2013;132(1):1–10.
24. Kim H, Bruen K, Vargo D. Acellular dermal matrix in the management of high-risk abdominal wall defects. Am J Surg. 2006;192(6):705–9.
25. James Bruno J, I, Senderoff DM, Fracchia JA, Armenakas NA. Reconstruction of penile wounds following complications of AlloDerm-based augmentation phalloplasty. Plast Reconstr Surg. 2007;119(1):1e–4e.
26. Vrankovic D, Mrcela T, Mursic B, Splavski B, Dmitrovic B, Mrcela M, et al. Physical and histologic properties of substitutes used for the anterior fossa region dural repair. Skull Base Surg. 1999;9(01):9–13.
27. Lee JH, Kim HG, Lee WJ. Characterization and tissue incorporation of cross-linked human acellular dermal matrix. Biomaterials. 2015;44:195–205.
28. Ahn ST, Il Kwak T, Park KS, Kim JJ, Moon DG. Complications of glans penis augmentation. Int J Impot Res. 2019;31(4):245–55.

Current Publications for Penile Girth Enhancement (PGE) with HA Gel

7

Contents

D. G. Moon, *Penile Augmentation with Injectable Hyaluronic Acid*,
https://doi.org/10.1007/978-981-95-5385-3_7

7.1 Historical Evolution of Penile Augmentation: From Dangerous to Safe Techniques

The desire for penile augmentation has a long and complex history, reflecting cultural ideals of masculinity and aesthetic preferences across centuries. Early attempts at penile enhancement were often primitive and fraught with complications. In 1899, Robert Gersuny introduced the use of mineral oil, including paraffin, for soft tissue augmentation after employing it for testicular reconstruction. While this technique gained initial attention, it quickly revealed severe long-term complications such as paraffinomas, tissue necrosis, and gross deformities that frequently required surgical intervention. These disastrous outcomes underscored the critical need for biocompatibility and reversibility in injectable materials [1].

7.2 The Search for Effective and Safe Penile Enhancement

Throughout the twentieth century, surgical approaches emerged as alternatives to injectable substances. Techniques such as dermal-fat grafting, PMMA and silicone injections, and suspensory ligamentolysis became widely practiced. However, they also carried significant risks, including unpredictable aesthetic results, granuloma formation, fibrosis, and psychological dissatisfaction among patients [2]. These experiences highlighted the limitations of earlier methods and set the stage for the pursuit of safer, less invasive techniques capable of delivering consistent outcomes.

7.3 Modern Advances: The Role of Injectable Fillers

The introduction of hyaluronic acid (HA)-based soft tissue fillers has revolutionized aesthetic medicine and created new opportunities for penile girth enhancement (PGE). Building on lessons learned from earlier materials, HA fillers offer a minimally invasive, biocompatible, and reversible option with a favorable safety profile. Their use in PGE represents a significant advancement, particularly in response to growing patient demand for safer alternatives to traditional surgical methods.

The first comprehensive clinical review on penile girth enhancement strategies classified augmentation techniques into three broad categories: medical approaches, injectable fillers, and prosthetic implants with reconstructive techniques [3]. Among these, injectable fillers—particularly HA gel—emerged as the most promising due to their nonpermanent nature, minimal downtime, and adaptability to patient needs.

Despite this progress, complications related to penile augmentation remain underreported in the literature, and standardized clinical guidelines are still lacking. This highlights the necessity for expert-driven protocols and consensus recommendations to ensure patient safety and optimize outcomes in the use of injectable fillers for penile augmentation.

7.4 The First Clinical Study on PGE with HA Gel: Kwak et al. [4]

7.4.1 Background and Justification

By the early 2010s, the demand for penile girth enhancement was increasing steadily, driven by both aesthetic and functional concerns among patients. However, existing methods such as autologous fat grafting, dermal-fat grafts, and synthetic fillers presented unpredictable results and significant risks. Recognizing the need for a minimally invasive, reversible, and biocompatible alternative, Kwak et al. (2011) pioneered the use of hyaluronic acid (HA) gel for penile girth enhancement [4].

7.4.2 Study Design and Methodology

This prospective clinical study enrolled 50 men who reported subjective concerns regarding small penile size. The procedure utilized Restylane Sub-Q (Q-Med, Sweden), an HA-based filler with established safety in facial aesthetics. Injections were performed using a 21-gauge cannula and the "back-and-forth" technique to ensure uniform distribution. A roller was employed postinjection to homogenize the filler placement and avoid lump formation. Follow-up evaluations extended to 18 months, with 41 participants completing the full study period.

Outcome measures included penile girth changes (measured at the midshaft), patient and partner satisfaction scores, and the incidence of adverse events or complications.

7.4.3 Results and Clinical Findings

The outcomes of this prospective study demonstrated a significant and durable enhancement in penile girth following hyaluronic acid (HA) gel injection. At baseline, the mean penile circumference was recorded as 7.48 ± 0.35 cm, representing the pre-procedural measurement across the enrolled cohort. Post-procedure assessments revealed a substantial increase, with the mean girth rising to 11.41 ± 0.34 cm at 1 month. This change was highly significant ($p < 0.0001$), underscoring the immediate volumizing effect achieved through HA gel implantation.

Importantly, this augmentation effect exhibited excellent persistence over time. At 18 months postinjection, the mean penile circumference remained largely stable at 11.26 ± 0.33 cm. The minimal reduction from the 1-month measurement suggests a favorable longevity of the filler material and its integration within penile tissues, supporting the role of HA as a reliable and biocompatible agent for penile girth enhancement.

Patient-reported outcomes further reinforced the efficacy of the intervention. On a standardized 4-point satisfaction scale, patients expressed high levels of contentment, with mean scores of 3.71 ± 0.46 at the 1-month follow-up. Although there was a slight decline at 18 months, satisfaction scores remained robust at 3.34 ± 0.53, reflecting enduring aesthetic and functional benefits. Partner satisfaction scores mirrored these findings, highlighting the broader relational and psychosexual impact of the procedure.

Adverse events were infrequent and clinically insignificant. Two patients reported minor focal depressions at the 1-month evaluation, which did not require additional intervention and resolved spontaneously over time. Crucially, no inflammatory reactions, nodular formations, granulomas, or serious complications were observed during the entire follow-up period. These findings affirm the high safety profile of HA-based penile augmentation when performed using meticulous technique and appropriate patient selection.

7.4.4 Impact and Clinical Significance

This study marked a paradigm shift in PGE by establishing HA gel as a safe and effective alternative to traditional augmentation techniques. It provided the first prospective clinical evidence supporting the feasibility of HA-based PGE, laying the groundwork for subsequent research and adoption of this method worldwide. The findings emphasized the advantages of HA fillers, including their biocompatibility, reversibility, and ability to maintain results over extended periods with minimal risk.

7.5 Key Clinical Studies on PGE with HA (2011 Onward)

7.5.1 Key Clinical Studies on PGE with HA Gel

Following the landmark 2011 study by Kwak et al., a growing body of clinical evidence has reinforced the efficacy and safety of hyaluronic acid (HA) gel in penile girth enhancement. These studies include randomized controlled trials (RCTs), comparative analyses, and meta-analyses, collectively validating HA fillers as a preferred method for PGE.

7.5.2 Pioneering Research and Clinical Evidence

Yang and colleagues conducted a series of multicenter RCTs between 2017 and 2020 to compare HA with polylactic acid (PLA) fillers. Their findings consistently demonstrated superior initial girth enhancement with HA fillers and a more favorable safety profile. In a 2017 study, Yang et al. reported a mean increase of +2.7 cm with PLA that was sustained over 18 months, highlighting PLA's durability but also noting delayed complications such as mild transient nodules [5].

Subsequent studies, including a 2019 trial published in *The Journal of Sexual Medicine*, compared HA and PLA directly. HA achieved larger girth gains at early follow-up (16.95 mm vs. 13.49 mm at 48 weeks), although no significant difference was observed between the two fillers by the study's end [6]. In 2020, a further study demonstrated HA's superior early results (mean increase: +2.1 cm for HA vs. +1.6 cm for PLA, $p = 0.031$) with fewer adverse events (5.1% for HA vs. 14.3% for PLA) [7].

Ahn et al. expanded the clinical scope by examining the impact of PGE on ejaculatory function [8]. Their multicenter, patient- and evaluator-blinded, randomized controlled trial showed that HA fillers not only achieved significant girth increases (+22.74 mm) but also improved premature ejaculation parameters, including prolonged intravaginal ejaculation latency time (IELT) and improved Premature Ejaculation Profile (PEP) scores [9] (Table 7.1).

7.5.3 Comparative and Meta-Analytical Studies

Kusumaputra et al. conducted a meta-analysis comparing HA and PLA fillers for PGE. The analysis concluded that HA provided superior outcomes in both penile girth augmentation and post-procedure sexual satisfaction. Moreover, HA's reversibility and biocompatibility further reinforced its preference over PLA [13].

Le Penske et al. reviewed outcomes and complications across multiple filler types, emphasizing the variability in results and the necessity of injector expertise. Their findings underscored HA's favorable safety profile and adaptability compared to more permanent or semipermanent fillers [14] (Table 7.2).

7.5.4 Safety and Complications

While earlier reports highlighted significant complications with non-HA fillers, studies involving HA fillers have consistently shown low rates of adverse events. Shaeer et al. (2009) and Ono et al. (2010) documented delayed granuloma formation, migration, and chronic inflammation with PMMA and polyacrylamide hydrogel injections [19, 20]. In contrast, HA's reversibility through hyaluronidase provides a critical safety advantage, allowing for prompt management of any overcorrection or nodularity [21] (Tables 7.3 and 7.4).

Table 7.1 Summary of PGE clinical studies of HA and other fillers

Study	Sample size	Follow-up duration	Filler type	Penile girth increase	Satisfaction scores	Adverse events	Key findings
Kwak et al. (2011) [4]	50 (41 completed)	18 months	HA (Restylane sub-Q)	7.48 cm to 11.26 cm (sustained)	High (3.34/4 at 18 months)	Mild, no major complications	First clinical study proving HA effectiveness and safety
Zhang et al. (2022) [10]	38 (HA only)	12 months	HA only	Flaccid: +2.44 cm, erect: +0.80 cm	Significant improvements in IMGI, IIEF, and BPAS	Low complication rate	HA led to psychological benefits and erectile improvements
Kim et al. (2015) [11]	20 (PMMA & Dextran)	18 months	PMMA & Dextran	Sustained at 18 months	Sustained high satisfaction	No systemic migration detected	PMMA and dextran durable with no migration
Yang et al. (2017) [5]	23 (PLA only)	18 months	PLA only	PLA: +2.7 cm (sustained 18 months)	VAS improved from 51.6 to 74.3	Six mild transient cases, no serious AEs	PLA safe and effective for long-term augmentation
Yang et al. (2019) [6]	72 (HA = 36, PLA = 36)	48 weeks	HA vs. PLA	HA: +16.95 mm, PLA: +13.49 mm (48 wks)	No significant difference between HA & PLA	Mild & transient, HA [1], PLA [3] cases	HA better initial gains, but equal at 48 weeks
Yang et al. (2020) [7]	74 (HA = 39, PLA = 35)	24 weeks	HA vs. PLA	HA: +2.1 cm, PLA: +1.6 cm ($p = 0.031$)	HA: +1.8, PLA: +1.6 (VAS)	HA (5.1%), PLA (14.3%), no serious AEs	HA > PLA for initial girth, no difference in satisfaction
Yang et al. (2020) [9]	67 (HA = 33, PLA = 34)	18 months	HA vs. PLA	Significant in both HA & PLA ($p < 0.001$)	Significantly increased for both HA & PLA	HA (9.1%), PLA (5.9%), no serious AEs	HA & PLA comparable for efficacy & safety
Ahn et al. (2021) [8]	64 (HA = 32, PLA = 32)	24 weeks	HA vs. PLA	HA: +22.74 mm, PLA: +20.23 mm	Both groups had significant increases	No serious AEs reported	PGE improved ejaculation parameters (PEP, IELT)
Kim et al. (2025) [12]	301 (HA = 125, PLA = 134, PMA = 42)	24 weeks	HA vs. PLA vs. PMA	PMA > HA > PLA (statistically significant)	Smaller satisfaction gain in PMA group	No serious/systemic AEs, local AEs: HA (7.2%), PLA (11.9%), PMA (14.3%)	PMA had greatest girth increase, but lowest satisfaction

Table 7.2 Review articles on penile augmentation, summarizing key findings, focus areas, and clinical implications

Review article	Focus area	Key findings	Clinical implications
Falagario et al. (2024)—Medicina [15]	Surgical and minimally invasive penile augmentation outcomes, complications, Qo	Various surgical and minimally invasive options exist; complications and risks must be considered	Surgical and minimally invasive PA require individualized patient counseling
Le Penske et al. (2024)—Urology [14]	Injectable penile fillers, risks, biocompatibility, complication management	Penile fillers have unpredictable outcomes due to different materials and biocompatibility	More studies are needed on filler longevity, risks, and complication management
Kusumaputra et al. (2023)—Ann Med Surg [13]	Systematic review and meta-analysis of HA vs. PLA efficacy and safety	HA is superior in girth enhancement and post-augmentation sexual satisfaction vs. PLA	HA is a more effective PA filler, but long-term safety and reinjection data are needed
Xing et al. (2022)—Curr Urol Rep [16]	Comprehensive review of aesthetic PA procedures, psychological impact	Minimally invasive fillers (HA, PLA, PMMA) are growing in popularity; more research needed	Growing demand for aesthetic PA, but there is no ideal injectable filler yet
Salloum et al. (2021)—Dermatol Surg [17]	Systematic review of nonsurgical penile augmentation methods	No standardized approach; HA fillers appear to be the safest and most effective option	Further randomized trials are necessary to establish clinical guidelines
Abo-Hedibah et al. (2021)—Abdom Radiol	Imaging and inflammatory complications of penile girth augmentation	Inflammatory complications, granulomas, and infections can be serious but are rare	Early imaging can help detect complications and improve treatment strategies
Romero-Otero et al. (2021)—BJU Int [18]	Systematic review of surgical & noninvasive penile enhancement	Quality of studies is low, preventing strong evidence-based recommendations	Standardized criteria for assessing PA outcomes and safety are lacking
Trost et al. (2024)—SMSNA Position Statement [22]	Cosmetic penile enhancement procedures, guidelines, and safety concerns	HA and PLA fillers provide temporary girth enhancement with acceptable safety; permanent fillers (silicone, paraffin) strongly discouraged due to severe complications	Clinicians should use IRB-approved research protocols; further studies needed to standardize injectable therapies and assess long-term outcomes

Table 7.3 Complications of HA and other fillers in PGE

Filler type	Common complications	Reversibility	Long-term safety
Hyaluronic acid (HA)	Mild edema, transient lumpiness, occasional overcorrection, minor asymmetry, rare infection	High (hyaluronidase can dissolve HA)	Good (requires maintenance injections)
Polylactic acid (PLA)	Granuloma formation, delayed nodules, mild inflammation	Limited (no specific enzyme for dissolution)	Moderate (granulomas possible, but overall safe)
Polymethyl methacrylate (PMMA)	Foreign body reaction, fibrosis, hard nodules, risk of migration	Irreversible (requires surgical excision if complications arise)	Poor (permanent material, potential long-term complications)
Silicone	Severe granulomas, migration, chronic inflammation, high complication rates	Irreversible (removal is difficult and can cause severe scarring)	Very poor (high chronic inflammation risk)
Paraffin/Vaseline	Severe paraffinomas, tissue necrosis, chronic inflammation, permanent disfigurement	Irreversible (high risk of permanent damage)	Extremely poor (historically disastrous outcomes)
Autologous fat grafting	High absorption rate, uneven absorption leading to asymmetry, fat necrosis, infection risk	Partially reversible (fat reabsorption occurs unpredictably)	Moderate (risk of asymmetry and volume loss over time)
Hyaluronic acid (HA)—self-injection [21]	Acute hypersensitivity reaction, inflammation	High if treated with hyaluronidase, but self-injection risk	Risky with improper technique (self-injection cases)
Synthetic fillers—unknown [19]	Delayed granuloma formation, filler migration, resorption	Variable, may require surgical removal	Poor (delayed complications can appear beyond follow-up period)
Polyacrylamide hydrogel [20]	Severe foreign body granulomas, migration, chronic inflammation, difficult removal	Irreversible, surgical excision often needed	Very poor (increasing cases in Asia, complications difficult to treat)

Table 7.4 KFDA approval studies of Korean HA gel [8]

Trade name (manufacturer, country)	Study design	Sample size	Mean penile Girth increase at 24 wks, mm	Complications	Injection dosage, mL (mean±SD)	HA conc., mg/mL	Particle size, μm	Cross-linking, degree	Complex viscosity
Potenfill (Medytox, Korea)	Prospective, patient/evaluator-blinded, randomized, multicenter trial	65 (HA: 33, PLA: 32)	21	Injection site deformation: 1; injection site inflammation: 1	20.8±1.5	20	~700	BDDE, 10%	No record
HyaFilia Impact (CHA Meditech, Korea)	Prospective, patient/evaluator-blinded, randomized, multicenter trial	62 (HA: 30, PLA: 32)	19.1	Injection site inflammation: 1; injection site pain: 2	16.4±2.7	20	~500	BDDE, 6%	200–600 Pa.s
THE CHAEUM; Shape 10 (Hugel Bio, Korea)	Prospective, patient/evaluator-blinded, randomized, multicenter trial	59 (HA: 30, PLA: 29)	20.6	Injection site induration: 1	19.1±1.4	20	~600	BDDE, no record	100–600 Pa.s
Doublofill (Humedix, Korea)[a]	Prospective, patient/evaluator-blinded, randomized, multicenter trial	64 (HA: 32, PLA: 32)	22.7	Injection site inflammation: 2	19.7±0.7	23	~700	BDDE, 12%	400~700 Pa.s

HA hyaluronic acid, *PLA* polylactic acid, *BDDE* 1,4-butanediol diglycidyl ether
[a]Current study

7.6 Guidelines and International Perspectives on PGE

The increasing global interest in penile girth enhancement (PGE) using injectable fillers has prompted professional societies to issue position statements and guidelines to ensure safe and ethical practice. Among these, the Sexual Medicine Society of North America (SMSNA) and the International Consultation on Sexual Medicine (ICSM) have played pivotal roles in shaping clinical recommendations.

7.6.1 Sexual Medicine Society of North America (SMSNA) Position Statement (2024)

The SMSNA's 2024 position statement on cosmetic penile enhancement procedures provides an authoritative perspective on the use of injectable fillers for PGE [22]. The document emphasizes the importance of a comprehensive patient evaluation, including psychological assessment, before proceeding with any penile augmentation intervention. Recognizing that many men seeking these procedures may have normal penile dimensions, the SMSNA recommends offering psychological counseling and setting realistic expectations.

Regarding injectable fillers, the SMSNA acknowledges the role of biodegradable materials such as hyaluronic acid (HA) and polylactic acid (PLA) for temporary girth enhancement. The position statement specifically discourages the use of permanent fillers like silicone, paraffin, and PMMA due to the high incidence of severe long-term complications including granulomas, migration, and chronic inflammation. The SMSNA advises that absorbable fillers be administered only by qualified medical professionals in appropriately equipped clinical settings under strict aseptic conditions.

Furthermore, the SMSNA highlights the need for standardized injection techniques and long-term follow-up studies to establish robust safety and efficacy data. By advocating for cautious and evidence-based application of injectable fillers, the SMSNA underscores its commitment to patient safety and ethical clinical practice.

7.6.2 International Consultation on Sexual Medicine (ICSM) 2025 Guideline (Pre-publication)

The upcoming 2025 ICSM guideline on penile augmentation, approved for publication at the ISSM meeting in Madrid, further reinforces the role of HA fillers in modern PGE. The guideline states:

> Biodegradable biopolymer fillers (such as hyaluronic acid) and autologous fat injections are considered relatively safe; however, additional procedures will likely be required over time (Moderate Recommendation, Evidence Strength C). The use of silicone, paraffin, and oil-based fillers for penile girth enhancement is strongly discouraged due to significant risks of adverse events (Strong Recommendation, Evidence Strength B).

This position aligns closely with the SMSNA's recommendations and reflects a growing international consensus that HA fillers represent the most favorable balance of safety, efficacy, and reversibility for penile augmentation.

The ICSM guideline also calls for future research to focus on refining injection techniques, optimizing filler properties, and standardizing outcome measures for PGE. These recommendations are particularly significant given the elective and aesthetic nature of the procedure, where patient expectations and safety must be carefully balanced.

7.7 Conclusion and Future Perspectives

Penile girth enhancement (PGE) using hyaluronic acid (HA) gel represents a major advancement in the field of sexual medicine and aesthetic urology. Over the past decade, numerous prospective studies, randomized controlled trials, and meta-analyses have validated the efficacy, safety, and patient satisfaction associated with

HA-based augmentation. Unlike earlier materials, HA gel offers biocompatibility, reversibility, and adaptability to individual patient needs, making it the preferred filler for modern penile augmentation procedures.

Global endorsements from professional societies such as the Sexual Medicine Society of North America (SMSNA) and the International Consultation on Sexual Medicine (ICSM) further strengthen the case for HA fillers as the standard of care. These organizations highlight the importance of ethical practice, standardized injection techniques, and ongoing monitoring to ensure optimal outcomes and minimize complications.

Despite these advances, certain challenges remain. The field still lacks standardized protocols for injection techniques, reinjection strategies, and long-term management. Additionally, the need for high-quality, large-scale clinical trials persists to provide stronger evidence for guideline development. Addressing these gaps will require international collaboration among clinicians, researchers, and regulatory bodies.

7.8 Future Directions in HA-Based PGE May Include

Development of HA formulations tailored specifically for penile augmentation.

Expanded indications beyond aesthetic enhancement, such as treatment for premature ejaculation and penile reconstruction.

Establishment of global registries to track outcomes and complications in real-world clinical settings.

By integrating scientific evidence, practical injector experience, and patient-centered care, HA-based penile augmentation continues to evolve as a safe, effective, and ethical solution to meet the growing demand for male genital enhancement.

References

1. Kontis TC, Rivkin A. The history of injectable facial fillers. Facial Plast Surg. 2009;25(02):067–72.
2. Foster H. What comes after farce?: art and criticism at a time of debacle: Verso Books; 2024.
3. Hehemann MC, Towe M, Huynh LM, El-Khatib FM, Yafi FA. Penile girth enlargement strategies: what's the evidence? Sexual Med Rev. 2019;7(3):535–47.
4. Kwak TI, Oh M, Kim JJ, Moon DG. The effects of penile girth enhancement using injectable hyaluronic acid gel, a filler. J Sex Med. 2011;8(12):3407–13.
5. Yang D, Ko K, Lee S, Moon D, Kim J, Lee W. Efficacy and safety of a newly developed polylactic acid microsphere as an injectable bulking agent for penile augmentation: 18-months follow-up. Int J Impot Res. 2017;29(4):136–41.
6. Yang DY, Ko K, Lee SH, Lee WK. A comparison of the efficacy and safety between hyaluronic acid and polylactic acid filler injection in penile augmentation: a multicenter, patient/evaluator-blinded, randomized trial. J Sex Med. 2019;16(4):577–85.
7. Yang DY, Jeong HC, Ahn ST, Bae WJ, Moon DG, Kim SW, et al. A comparison between hyaluronic acid and polylactic acid filler injections for temporary penile augmentation in patients with small penis syndrome: a multicenter, patient/evaluator-blind, comparative, randomized trial. J Sex Med. 2020;17(1):133–41.
8. Ahn ST, Shim JS, Bae WJ, Kim SW, Kim JJ, Moon DG. Efficacy and safety of penile girth enhancement using hyaluronic acid filler and the clinical impact on ejaculation: a multi-center, patient/evaluator-blinded, randomized active-controlled trial. World J Men Health. 2021;40(2):299.
9. Yang DY, Jeong HC, Ko K, Lee SH, Lee YG, Lee WK. Comparison of clinical outcomes between hyaluronic and polylactic acid filler injections for penile augmentation in men reporting a small penis: a multicenter, patient-blinded/evaluator-blinded, non-inferiority, randomized comparative trial with 18 months of follow-up. J Clin Med. 2020;9(4):1024.
10. Zhang CL, Quan Y, Li H, Li Q, Bai WJ, Xu T, Zhang XW. Penile augmentation with injectable hyaluronic acid gel: an alternative choice for small penis syndrome. Asian J Androl. 2022;24(6):601–606. https://doi.org/10.4103/aja20223.
11. Kim MT, Ko K, Lee WK, Kim SC, Yang DY. Long-Term safety and longevity of a mixture of polymethyl methacrylate and cross-linked dextran (Lipen-10®) after penile augmentation: Extension study from six to 18 months of follow-up. World J Mens Health. 2015;33(3):202–8. https://doi.org/10.5534/wjmh.2015.33.3.202. Epub 2015 Dec 23.

12. Kim DW, Jeong HC, Ko K, Yang DY, Kim JK, Lee SH, et. al. Which dermal filler is better for penile augmentation for aesthetic purposes? A prospective, single-surgeon study based on real-world experience. World J Mens Health. 2025;43(2):428–436. https://doi.org/10.5534/wjmh.240105. Epub 2024 Jul 31.
13. Kusumaputra A, Setiawan MR, Soebadi MA, Wirjopranoto S. Efficacy and complications of hyaluronic acid and polylactic acid for penile augmentation: a systematic review and meta-analysis. Ann Med Surg. 2023;85(9):4531–8.
14. Le Penske W, Leslie DC, Latini JM, Lerner LB. Injectable penile enhancement procedures: a review of agents, risks, and complications. Urology. 2024;189:126.
15. Falagario UG, Piramide F, Pang KH, Durukan E, Tzelves L, Ricapito A, et al. Techniques for penile augmentation surgery: a systematic review of surgical outcomes, complications, and quality of life. Medicina (B Aires). 2024;60(5):758.
16. Xing MH, Hou SW, Raheem OA. Aesthetic penile augmentation procedures: a comprehensive and current perspective. Curr Urol Rep. 2022;23(12):355–61.
17. Salloum A, Bazzi N, Haber R. Nonsurgical methods for penile augmentation: a systematic review. Dermatologic Surg. 2021;47(3):e81–e5.
18. Romero-Otero J, Manfredi C, Ralph D, Osmonov D, Verze P, Castiglione F, et al. Non-invasive and surgical penile enhancement interventions for aesthetic or therapeutic purposes: a systematic review. BJU Int. 2021;127(3):269–91.
19. Shaeer O, Shaeer K. Delayed complications of gel injection for penile girth augmentation. J Sex Med. 2009;6(7):2072–8.
20. Ono S, Ogawa R, Hyakusoku H. Complications after polyacrylamide hydrogel injection for soft-tissue augmentation. Plast Reconstr Surg. 2010;126(4):1349–57.
21. Coskuner ER, Canter HI. Desire for penile girth enhancement and the effects of the self-injection of hyaluronic acid gel. J Cutan Aesthet Surg. 2012;5(3):198–200.
22. Trost L, Watter DN, Carrier S, Khera M, Yafi FA, Bernie HL, et al. Cosmetic penile enhancement procedures: an SMSNA position statement. J Sex Med. 2024;21(6):573–8.

Development and Principles of Penile Girth Enhancement using Injectable Hyaluronic Acid Gel

8

Contents

8.1 Introduction: The Birth of a New Paradigm

Penile girth enhancement (PGE) has long been a topic of interest in aesthetic and functional urology, reflecting male patients' desire for improved self-esteem and sexual confidence. Traditional surgical methods—including autologous fat grafting, dermofat implants, and silicone injections—offered initial promise but were often complicated by high rates of asymmetry, fat reabsorption, fibrosis, and even necrosis [1–3].

The emergence of soft tissue fillers, particularly hyaluronic acid (HA), transformed this landscape. HA, a naturally occurring glycosaminoglycan, had already demonstrated its utility in facial aesthetics

D. G. Moon, *Penile Augmentation with Injectable Hyaluronic Acid*,
https://doi.org/10.1007/978-981-95-5385-3_8

due to its biocompatibility, reversibility, and predictable biodegradability [4, 5]. These properties, combined with the minimally invasive nature of injection-based procedures, made HA fillers an attractive candidate for penile augmentation.

This chapter integrates the historical development of HA-based PGE and its clinical refinement into a practical, evidence-based approach for contemporary practice.

8.2 Development and Initial Clinical Evaluation of HA-Based PGE

The application of hyaluronic acid (HA) fillers in penile girth enhancement (PGE) began as a natural extension of their success in facial aesthetics and glans penis augmentation [6, 7]. Building on prior experience with glans augmentation for premature ejaculation, the authors initiated a prospective clinical study between 2006 and 2008 to evaluate the feasibility, efficacy, and safety of HA-based PGE.

8.2.1 Study Design and Patient Cohort

The study enrolled 50 men (mean age: 42.5 years; range: 27–61 years) dissatisfied with their penile girth despite normal anatomical dimensions. After exclusion of individuals with severe phimosis, concealed penis, or psychiatric disorders such as body dysmorphic disorder, 41 patients were followed for up to 18 months. Comprehensive counseling emphasized realistic expectations, potential complications, and postoperative care [8].

8.2.2 Injection Technique and Procedural Details

The procedure utilized Restylane Sub-Q® (Q-med, Sweden), a cross-linked HA filler chosen for its viscoelasticity and proven safety profile in soft tissue augmentation [4, 5]. Under local anesthesia with EMLA® cream, the filler was injected into the subcutaneous plane between Buck's fascia and dartos fascia using a 21G cannula.

Cannula entry points were selected either just above the penopubic junction or below the coronal sulcus at the 10–11 o'clock and 1–2 o'clock positions to avoid vascular injury. A "back-and-forth" threading technique ensured even filler distribution along the shaft, while a roller was used postinjection to homogenize the material and correct minor irregularities.

Figure 8.1 illustrates the cross-sectional anatomy and optimal injection plane, while Figs. 8.2 and 8.3 shows the procedural steps and immediate postoperative results.

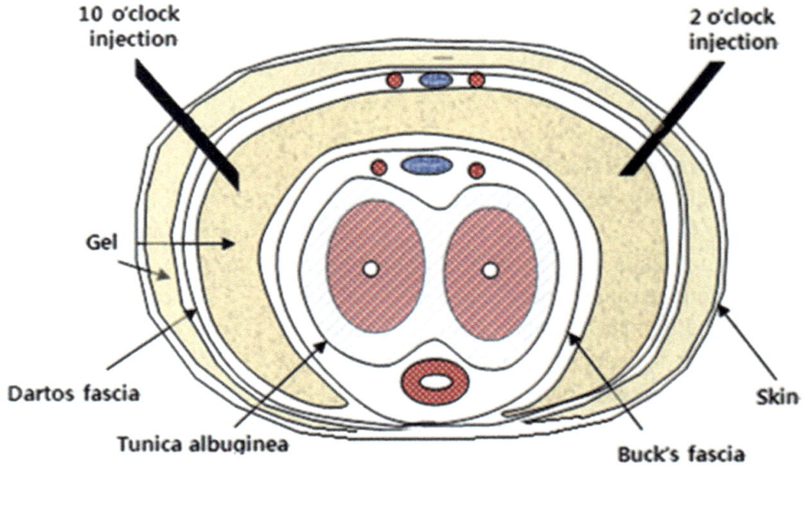

Fig. 8.1 Cross-sectional view of anatomical diagram showing planes of HA gel injection. The hyaluronic acid (HA) gel was injected in the subcutaneous layer, just "deep to" the dartos fascia just below the coronary sulcus and just above the penopubic junction

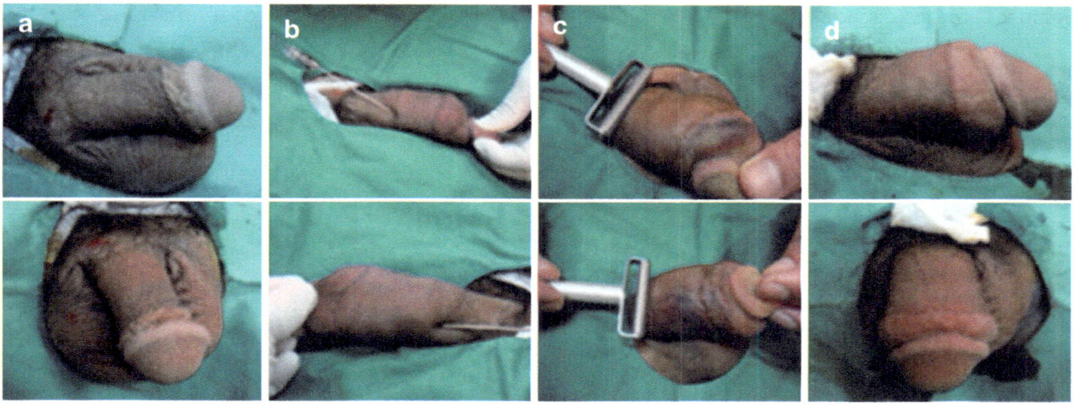

Fig. 8.2 Representative figure of penile girth enhancement using injectable hyaluronic acid gel. (**a**) Preoperative figure of penile girth. (**b**) Filler was injected into the fascial layer of penile body using 21G cannula with the "back-and-forth technique." For the ease of injection into the whole length of the penis, cannula was inserted just above penopubic junction or just below the coronal sulcus at 10–11 o'clock and 1–2 o'clock to avoid dorsal pedicle injury. (**c**) Initial uneven distribution can be manipulated with roller. (**d**) Immediate postoperative figure of penis

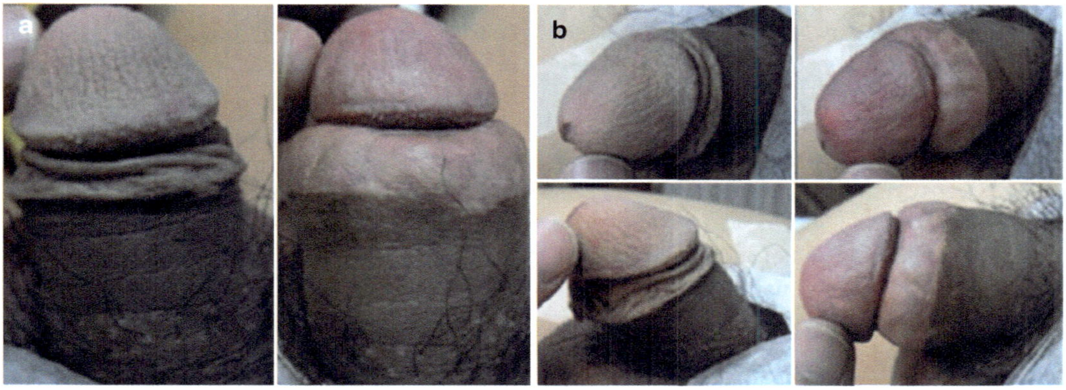

Fig. 8.3 (**a**) Dorsal view of the representative figure for penile girth enhancement. (**b**) Lateral view with glans penis augmentation using injectable hyaluronic acid (HA) gel at 18 months. The injected HA gel effectively enhanced penile girth and the implants are well maintained without asymmetry until 18 months. In the augmented penis, the girth and glans are looking good esthetically

8.2.3 Outcomes and Long-Term Results

The mean volume of injected HA gel was 20.56 cc (range: 18–22 cc). Penile midshaft circumference increased significantly from a baseline of 7.48 ± 0.35 cm to 11.41 ± 0.34 cm at 1 month ($P < 0.0001$). This gain was well maintained at 18 months, with a mean circumference of 11.26 ± 0.33 cm.

Patient satisfaction remained high throughout follow-up, with scores averaging 3.71 ± 0.46 at 1 month and 3.34 ± 0.53 at 18 months on a 4-point scale. Partner satisfaction closely mirrored these findings. Minor complications were limited to two cases of focal depression due to early resumption of sexual activity; both were corrected with superficial reinjections.

Table 8.1 Changes of penile girth and patient and partner's satisfaction after penile girth enhancement

	Preoperative	1 month	18 months
Maximum circumference (cm)	7.48 ± 0.35	11.41 ± 0.34*	11.26 ± 0.33[a]
Patient's satisfaction		3.71 ± 0.46	3.34 ± 0.53
Partner's satisfaction		3.65 ± 0.48	3.38 ± 0.49
Patient's visual estimation (Gr)	0	0	0
0			
1		0	0
2		0	0
3		2	0
4		39	41

Data are expressed as mean ± standard deviation
Maximal circumference: measured at midshaft by tapeline
Residual volume estimated the visual analogue scale from Gr 0 to Gr 4: Gr 0, no residual volume; Gr 1, less than 25% of initial volume; Gr 2, less than 50%; Gr 3, less than 75%; and Gr 4, more than 75% or nearly same as initial volume
Satisfaction (5 Gr): Gr 0, very dissatisfied; Gr 1, moderately dissatisfied; Gr 2, about equally satisfied and dissatisfied; Gr 3, moderately satisfied; Gr 4, very satisfied
Gr = grade
[a]$P < 0.001$

Table 8.1 summarizes key clinical outcomes, including girth changes, satisfaction scores, and complications.

8.2.4 Clinical Significance and Early Lessons

This pioneering study demonstrated that HA fillers could provide a minimally invasive, reversible, and well-tolerated option for PGE. The isovolumic degradation property of cross-linked HA allowed stable girth maintenance over 18 months. Importantly, no cases of granuloma formation, delayed hypersensitivity, or serious adverse events were observed.

These findings established HA-based PGE as a viable alternative to more invasive techniques, laying the foundation for subsequent refinements in technique and filler technology.

8.3 General Principles for Successful PGE

The evolution of hyaluronic acid (HA) filler use in penile girth enhancement (PGE) has refined not only the choice of materials but also the procedural techniques and perioperative protocols. Achieving optimal outcomes requires a comprehensive understanding of patient selection, injection strategies, and postoperative management.

8.3.1 Patient Selection and Preoperative Planning

Success in PGE begins with selecting appropriate candidates. Ideal patients are healthy men aged 20–65 years who desire cosmetic enhancement and maintain realistic expectations. Exclusion criteria include anatomical abnormalities such as micropenis, severe phimosis, or Peyronie's disease, as well as psychiatric conditions like body dysmorphic disorder [9].

Preoperative counseling plays a critical role in aligning patient expectations with achievable results. Patients are informed of the procedure's minimally invasive nature, the potential need for maintenance injections, and the importance of postoperative compliance.

Local anesthesia with EMLA® cream suffices for most cases, though a dorsal penile nerve block can be considered in sensitive patients. Prophylactic oral antibiotics are recommended pre- and post-procedure to minimize infection risk.

8.3.2 Injection Techniques and Advanced Refinements

8.3.2.1 Retrograde and Anterograde Injection Technique

The technique of injecting filler while withdrawing the needle or cannula is known as the retrograde injection technique, whereas injecting filler while advancing the needle or cannula is referred to as the antegrade injection technique (Fig. 8.4). Retrograde injection, wherein filler is deposited as the cannula is withdrawn, has become the preferred approach in PGE. This technique offers improved control and safety by facilitating negative pressure during withdrawal, allowing early detection of intravascular entry. Additionally, retrograde delivery ensures even filler distribution and provides tactile feedback on tissue resistance, enabling adjustments in real time [10].

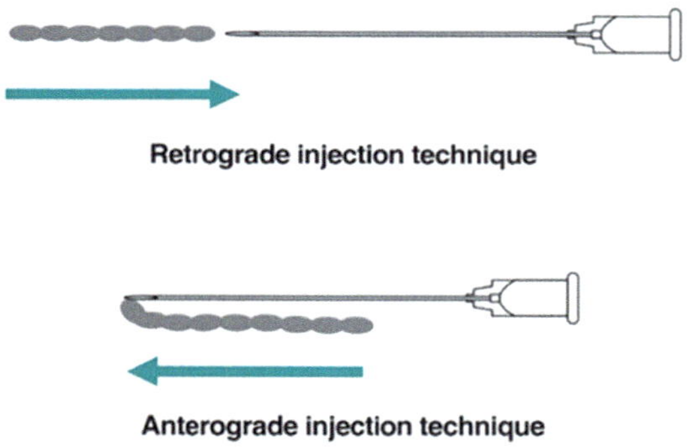

Fig. 8.4 Retrograde and anterograde injection technique

When combined with fanning and cross-hatching patterns, retrograde injection minimizes the number of entry points while achieving comprehensive coverage. In contrast, anterograde injection is reserved for specific scenarios but carries a slightly higher risk of uneven deposition.

8.3.2.2 Adaptation of Facial Aesthetic Techniques to Penile Augmentation

Advanced injection techniques from facial aesthetics have been successfully adapted for PGE to enhance precision and aesthetic harmony [4, 11] (Fig. 8.5).

The serial puncture technique involves placing small, consistent deposits at regular intervals, making it particularly useful for localized corrections and precise volumization. Linear threading allows for continuous filler deposition along the cannula track, creating uniform thickness and smooth contours throughout the shaft. Fanning extends coverage from a single entry point by employing multiple retrograde passes in different directions, thus minimizing trauma and reducing the number of puncture sites. Cross-hatching uti-

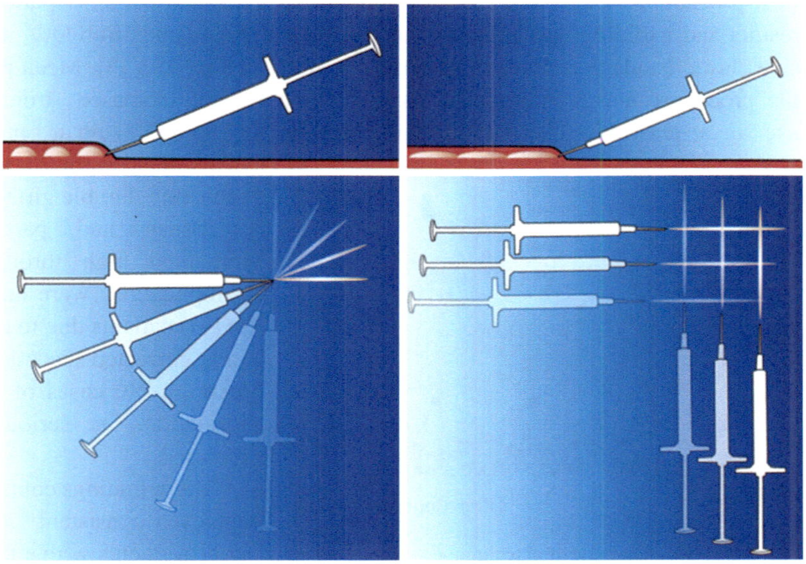

Fig. 8.5 Illustrations of advanced dermal filler techniques adapted for PGE: (above, left) serial puncture; (above, right) linear threading; (below, left) fanning; (below, right) cross-hatching

lizes a lattice-like pattern of overlapping filler placement, enhancing structural support and minimizing the risk of asymmetry or surface irregularities. Together, these techniques provide injectors with versatile options to tailor the augmentation to individual anatomical variations while optimizing safety and aesthetic outcomes.

8.3.2.3 The Dual-Plane Concept for Volume and Contour Harmony

The dual-plane technique represents a sophisticated approach to PGE (Fig. 8.6). A firm, highly cross-linked HA filler is first deposited in the deep subcutaneous layer between Buck's fascia and dartos fascia to establish robust girth. A softer filler is then introduced into the superficial subdermal plane to refine contours and create a natural tactile quality.

This method distributes filler loads across two planes, reducing the risk of overfilling, vascular compression, and migration. Clinical experience suggests that the dual-plane strategy reduces surface undulations and enhances the long-term aesthetic stability of the augmented penis.

8.3.3 Postoperative Management and Long-Term Care

Post-procedural care is vital to maintaining results and avoiding complications. A compressive elastic bandage is applied immediately after the procedure and recommended for nighttime use for at least 4 weeks. Patients must abstain from sexual activity and strenuous exercise during this period to prevent filler displacement.

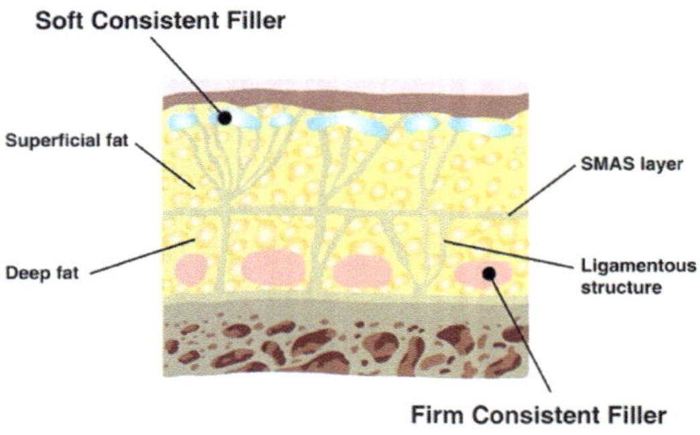

Fig. 8.6 Dual-plane injection technique

Follow-up visits at 1, 2, 4, 12, 24, and 48 weeks allow for monitoring of girth retention and early identification of issues such as minor asymmetry or nodularity. In such cases, superficial reinjection or hyaluronidase may be employed to correct irregularities [12].

This section establishes a solid framework for clinicians, blending technical mastery with patient-centered care to ensure safe and predictable outcomes in HA-based PGE.

8.4 Clinical Outcomes and Lessons Learned

The integration of hyaluronic acid (HA) fillers into penile girth enhancement (PGE) has been supported by a growing body of clinical evidence. Early studies established its feasibility and safety, while subsequent trials and real-world experience have provided critical insights into optimizing outcomes and managing challenges.

8.4.1 Long-Term Outcomes from Early Clinical Studies

In the original prospective study conducted from 2006 to 2008, 41 patients underwent PGE using Restylane Sub-Q® and were followed for 18 months [8]. Mean penile midshaft circumference increased from 7.48 ± 0.35 cm to 11.41 ± 0.34 cm at 1 month ($P < 0.0001$) and was maintained at 11.26 ± 0.33 cm at 18 months, reflecting durable girth augmentation.

Patient and partner satisfaction scores remained high throughout follow-up. Minor complications were limited to focal depressions in two patients due to early sexual activity; these were corrected successfully with superficial reinjections. No cases of inflammation, granuloma formation, or serious adverse events were reported.

These findings confirmed that HA fillers could achieve consistent aesthetic and functional improvements with a favorable safety profile.

8.4.2 Insights from the Phase III Multicenter Trial

A pivotal multicenter, randomized, active-controlled trial in 2021 further validated the safety and efficacy of HA-based PGE [13]. This study demonstrated significant and sustained improvements in penile girth and patient satisfaction, with a mean injected volume of 15–22 mL.

Notably, the trial also observed a significant increase in intravaginal ejaculatory latency time (IELT), rising from 5.36 min at baseline to 7.86 min posttreatment ($p = 0.0001$). This secondary effect suggests that HA fillers may reduce penile shaft sensitivity, providing additional benefits in patients with premature ejaculation. Importantly, no adverse impact on erectile function or sexual satisfaction was noted.

8.4.3 Lessons Learned in Clinical Practice

Over nearly two decades of clinical experience with HA-based PGE, several critical lessons have emerged that continue to refine patient outcomes. One of the most important factors is postoperative compliance. Adherence to guidelines, particularly abstaining from sexual activity for at least 1 month, has proven essential to prevent filler migration and asymmetry.

Equally significant is the mastery of injection techniques. The adoption of advanced methods, including dual-plane delivery and retrograde injection, has substantially reduced complications while improving aesthetic and tactile results. These refinements allow for more even filler distribution, minimize vascular compression, and enhance long-term volume retention.

Anatomical considerations must also guide clinical decision-making. Patients presenting with redundant prepuce or obesity-related concealed penis often require adjunctive procedures such as circumcision or penile elongation to achieve optimal outcomes. These preemptive interventions help prevent filler displacement and maintain symmetry.

Finally, clinicians should recognize that HA-based PGE, while durable, is subject to gradual resorption over time. Periodic touch-up injections may therefore be necessary to maintain desired penile girth, and patients should be counseled accordingly during preoperative consultations.

This growing body of evidence and clinical experience reinforces HA-based PGE as a safe, effective, and patient-centered option for penile augmentation.

8.5 Future Perspectives and Expanded Indications

Hyaluronic acid (HA)-based penile girth enhancement (PGE) has now reached a pivotal stage in its evolution. Initially developed as a minimally invasive alternative to surgical augmentation, HA fillers have established a new paradigm in aesthetic urology. As clinical experience accumulates and patient demand grows, the scope of HA-based PGE is expanding, both geographically and in its potential therapeutic applications.

8.5.1 Expanding Global Adoption and Regulatory Approvals

The widespread use of HA fillers in facial and body contouring procedures has paved the way for their acceptance in penile augmentation. Countries in Asia and Europe have been at the forefront of this trend, driven by cultural factors and a preference for minimally invasive interventions [13].

The Korean Ministry of Food and Drug Safety (KMFDS) was among the first regulatory bodies to approve HA fillers for PGE based on robust clinical evidence. This approval, supported by results from multicenter trials demonstrating efficacy and safety [13], has catalyzed broader interest among international urologic and aesthetic communities.

As more countries recognize the legitimacy of HA-based PGE, the need for standardized training and consensus guidelines becomes critical. International organizations such as the International Society for Sexual Medicine (ISSM) and Asia Pacific Society for Sexual Medicine (APSSM) are well-positioned to lead the development of evidence-based recommendations.

8.5.2 Secondary Benefits: Potential Role in Premature Ejaculation Management

An intriguing observation from clinical studies is the secondary benefit of HA-based PGE in managing premature ejaculation (PE). The Phase III trial demonstrated a significant increase in intravaginal ejaculatory latency time (IELT), from 5.36 min at baseline to 7.86 min posttreatment ($p = 0.0001$) [13].

This effect is thought to arise from the filler's barrier function, which reduces penile shaft sensitivity by physically increasing the distance between external stimuli and sensory nerve endings in the penile skin. While this phenomenon was not the primary endpoint of the trial, it suggests a promising adjunctive role for HA-based PGE in patients with PE, particularly those resistant to pharmacological therapies. Further research is warranted to explore this application and optimize treatment protocols.

8.5.3 Innovations in Filler Technology

The next frontier in HA-based PGE lies in the development of advanced filler formulations. Newer products such as highly cross-linked HA gels with enhanced viscoelastic properties offer improved volume retention and reduced degradation rates. Innovations in delivery systems, including cannula designs that minimize trauma and allow for more precise placement, are also contributing to safer and more predictable outcomes.

Moreover, the dual-plane injection strategy has shown promise in addressing the limitations of single-plane delivery, offering greater contour control and aesthetic refinement. Future research may also explore bioengineered fillers with regenerative properties to stimulate collagen production and further enhance longevity.

8.5.4 Addressing Challenges and Building Consensus

Despite its success, HA-based PGE continues to face challenges. Variability in techniques, lack of standardized outcome measures, and disparities in practitioner training highlight the need for consensus guidelines. Long-term safety studies, particularly beyond 5 years, remain limited and are crucial for further establishing the procedure's place in clinical practice.

Ongoing efforts by international expert panels and guideline committees aim to address these gaps. As these initiatives mature, they are expected to solidify HA-based PGE as an accepted and standardized treatment option within sexual medicine.

This section underscores the dynamic trajectory of HA-based PGE—from a novel alternative to invasive surgery to a versatile tool with both aesthetic and functional benefits.

8.6 Conclusion: Establishing HA Fillers as the Standard of Care

The evolution of penile girth enhancement (PGE) reflects a broader shift in aesthetic and functional urology toward minimally invasive, patient-centered approaches. Traditional surgical methods, though effective in selected cases, have been hindered by significant risks, long recovery times, and frequent complications. Hyaluronic acid (HA)-based PGE, in contrast, offers a biocompatible, reversible, and well-tolerated alternative that aligns with modern demands for safety and predictability.

Pioneering studies and nearly two decades of clinical experience have demonstrated that HA fillers can achieve substantial and durable increases in penile girth, with high patient and partner satisfaction. Advanced techniques such as retrograde injection, dual-plane delivery, and adaptations from facial aesthetics have further refined outcomes, allowing clinicians to tailor treatments to individual anatomical variations and patient goals.

Beyond cosmetic enhancement, emerging evidence suggests a potential therapeutic role for HA-based PGE in managing premature ejaculation, expanding its relevance within sexual medicine. Regulatory approvals and growing international acceptance underscore its viability as a mainstream option.

As innovation in filler technology continues and consensus guidelines are developed, HA-based PGE is poised to become a cornerstone of contemporary male aesthetic practice. By mastering its principles and adhering to evidence-based protocols, clinicians can offer patients a safe, effective, and satisfying solution to penile augmentation that meets both aesthetic and functional aspirations.

This closes the chapter with authority and clarity, echoing the narrative style Springer favors for surgical and aesthetic textbooks.

References

1. Wessells H, Lue TF, McAninch JW. Penile length in the flaccid and erect states: guidelines for penile augmentation. J Urol. 1996;156(3):995–7.
2. Alter G, Jordan G. Penile elongation and girth enhancement. AUA Update Series. 2007;26:229–37.
3. Vardi Y, Harshai Y, Gil T, Gruenwald I. A critical analysis of penile enhancement procedures for patients with normal penile size: surgical techniques, success, and complications. Eur Urol. 2008;54(5):1042–50.
4. Rohrich RJ, Ghavami A, Crosby MA. The role of hyaluronic acid fillers (Restylane) in facial cosmetic surgery: review and technical considerations. Plast Reconstr Surg. 2007;120(6S):41S–54S.
5. Kovach BT, Sengelmann RD. Soft tissue augmentation. Adv Dermatol. 2007;23:1–31.
6. Moon D, Kwak T, Cho H, Bae J, Park H, Kim J. Augmentation of glans penis using injectable hyaluronic acid gel. Int J Impot Res. 2003;15(6):456–60.
7. Kim J, Kwak T, Jeon B. Cheon J, Moon D. Human glans penis augmentation using injectable hyaluronic acid gel. Int J Impot Res. 2003;15(6):439–43.
8. Kwak TI, Oh M, Kim JJ, Moon DG. The effects of penile girth enhancement using injectable hyaluronic acid gel, a filler. J Sex Med. 2011;8(12):3407–13.
9. Moon DG, Kwak TI, Kim JJ. Glans penis augmentation using hyaluronic acid gel as an injectable filler. World J Men Health. 2015;33(2):50.
10. Hong G-W, Kim S-B, Yoon SE, Wan J, Felice F, Velthuis PJ, et al. Injection Techniques for Filler Procedures With Illustration: Narrative Review. J Craniofac Surg. 2025;10(1097)
11. Littara A, Palmieri B, Rottigni V, Iannitti T. A clinical study to assess the effectiveness of a hyaluronic acid-based procedure for treatment of premature ejaculation. Int J Impot Res. 2013;25(3):117–20.
12. Hirsch RJ, Brody HJ, Carruthers JD. Hyaluronidase in the office: a necessity for every dermasurgeon that injects hyaluronic acid. J Cosmet Laser Ther. 2007;9(3):182–5.
13. Ahn ST, Shim JS, Bae WJ, Kim SW, Kim JJ, Moon DG. Efficacy and safety of penile girth enhancement using hyaluronic acid filler and the clinical impact on ejaculation: a multi-center, patient/evaluator-blinded, randomized active-controlled trial. World J Men Health. 2021;40(2):299.

9 Tips and Tricks for Penile Girth Enhancement (PGE) with Hyaluronic Acid (HA)

Contents

9.1 Introduction

Penile girth enhancement (PGE) has long been a subject of interest for both patients and clinicians, reflecting broader concerns about penile size, sexual confidence, and aesthetic harmony. Traditional surgical techniques such as dermofat grafting, autologous fat transfer (AFT), and synthetic implants have been used with varying degrees of success. However, these methods often entail significant drawbacks including scarring, asymmetry, granuloma formation, and the risk of permanent deformities, necessitating complex surgical revisions in some cases [1, 2].

The introduction of injectable fillers, particularly hyaluronic acid (HA), has fundamentally altered the landscape of PGE. Initially developed for facial aesthetics, HA fillers have gained global popularity due to their biocompatibility, biodegradability, and reversibility. These properties make HA an ideal material for soft-tissue augmentation, offering a safer and more predictable alternative to earlier permanent fillers such as polymethyl methacrylate (PMMA) and poly-L-lactic acid (PLA), which are associated with higher rates of complications and often require surgical removal in adverse cases [3, 4].

D. G. Moon, *Penile Augmentation with Injectable Hyaluronic Acid*,
https://doi.org/10.1007/978-981-95-5385-3_9

Clinical studies have validated the safety and efficacy of HA fillers in PGE, demonstrating significant and sustained increases in penile circumference, high patient satisfaction, and low complication rates. For example, Ahn et al. reported a multicenter randomized trial showing that HA-based PGE resulted in a mean girth increase of over 3 cm with minimal adverse events and durable effects lasting beyond 12 months [5]. Similarly, Yang et al. compared HA with PLA fillers and found HA to offer superior patient satisfaction and a more favorable safety profile [6].

However, success in real-world practice is not determined by product efficacy alone. PGE with HA is a highly technique-dependent procedure where small variations in injection depth, volume distribution, and filler rheology can lead to markedly different outcomes. Common challenges such as uneven filler placement, migration—particularly distal ventral migration in uncircumcised men—and gradual asymmetry due to isovolumic degradation necessitate advanced technical expertise and patient-centered management [7, 8].

This chapter presents practical insights and refined strategies developed over 25 years of clinical experience with HA-based PGE. Drawing on case-based scenarios and hands-on experience, it highlights key principles for optimizing outcomes and minimizing complications. By integrating a deep understanding of filler properties, penile anatomy, and patient expectations, practitioners can achieve consistently safe and satisfying results with HA-based penile girth enhancement.

9.2 Why "Tips and Tricks" Are Essential for PGE with HA

While clinical studies have validated the efficacy and safety of hyaluronic acid (HA) fillers for penile girth enhancement (PGE), translating these findings into real-world success is far from straightforward. HA-based PGE is not a standardized, protocol-driven procedure; rather, it is a highly technique-sensitive intervention where subtle variations in approach can profoundly influence both aesthetic and functional outcomes [1, 2].

One key factor contributing to this variability is the diversity of HA filler formulations. Products differ significantly in terms of rheological properties such as viscosity, elasticity, and cross-linking density. These characteristics directly affect how the filler behaves within penile tissues, including its injectability, spread, and resistance to migration [3, 4]. For instance, a filler with high viscosity and elasticity may offer superior volume retention but could be more challenging to distribute evenly without technical skill, increasing the risk of lumps or asymmetry.

Patient anatomical variability adds another layer of complexity. Differences in penile skin elasticity, subcutaneous tissue thickness, and vascular patterns can influence filler distribution and integration. In some patients, redundant preputial tissue or obesity-related concealed penis may create anatomical "dead spaces" where fillers are prone to accumulate, resulting in irregularities or distal ventral migration. In such cases, adjunctive procedures such as circumcision may be advisable prior to augmentation [5].

Another critical consideration is the dynamic nature of HA within tissues. Unlike permanent implants, HA is gradually degraded by hyaluronidase activity in the body. This isovolumic degradation often preserves relative shape initially but can lead to subtle contour changes over time. Without planned touch-up sessions, these changes may result in asymmetry or patient dissatisfaction, especially in individuals with high aesthetic expectations [6].

The operator's experience and adaptability are therefore central to success. Novice practitioners may rely heavily on published protocols, but these often lack the granularity needed for nuanced decision-making in live cases. For example, understanding how to modulate injection depth in different penile zones, adjust filler volume in areas with preexisting asymmetry, or select cannula gauge appropriate for high-viscosity gels can mean the difference between a natural, harmonious result and a visibly augmented, unnatural appearance [7, 8].

This section underscores that mastery of HA-based PGE lies not merely in understanding the science but in developing a repertoire of practical strategies—"tips and tricks"—that address the unique challenges of each case. By adopting these insights, clinicians can elevate their practice from technically competent to predictably excellent.

9.3 Practical Considerations for Injection-Based PGE

In penile girth enhancement (PGE) with hyaluronic acid (HA) fillers, the pathway to consistent and satisfying results lies in understanding the intricate interplay between filler properties, anatomical variability, and technical execution. The clinician's ability to navigate these factors determines whether the procedure achieves a harmonious augmentation or produces avoidable complications.

One of the foundational decisions involves selecting the appropriate HA filler. The rheological properties of available products—such as viscosity, elasticity, and degree of cross-linking—vary widely among manufacturers and influence their performance in penile tissues. High-viscosity, highly cross-linked HA gels often provide longer-lasting volumizing effects but demand greater technical precision for uniform placement. Without experience, their higher resistance to extrusion can lead to uneven distribution or localized lumps. In contrast, less viscous fillers are easier to inject but may integrate less predictably, increasing the risk of migration, particularly in areas of thin or highly mobile subcutaneous tissue [1, 2].

Augmentation strategy also plays a critical role in determining long-term outcomes. A staged approach—where smaller volumes of filler are administered over multiple sessions—has proven to be superior to single-session, high-volume injections. Incremental augmentation allows penile tissues to adapt naturally, reducing risks such as overstretching, vascular compromise, and surface irregularities. This method also creates opportunities to refine symmetry and address subtle contour imperfections during follow-up visits. Patients often find this gradual enhancement more acceptable and are reassured by the ability to make adjustments along the way [3, 4].

Technical execution requires careful attention to instrument choice and injection technique. For modest volumes, a 27-gauge needle may suffice, offering precise delivery for targeted corrections. However, as augmentation volumes increase, a blunt-tip cannula of larger diameter—such as 21G or 22G—is preferred to minimize trauma, improve patient comfort, and facilitate even filler spread within the subcutaneous plane. In cases involving highly viscous HA gels or large-volume administration, specialized automatic injectors or injection guns can provide significant advantages. These devices deliver filler at a controlled, consistent rate, ensuring smoother distribution and reducing the physical demands on the operator, which in turn lowers the risk of uneven pressure-related tissue trauma [5, 6].

Equally important is the clinician's readiness to manage complications effectively. Hyaluronidase, an enzyme capable of degrading HA, should always be available as part of the procedural armamentarium. Whether addressing overcorrection, nodular formations, or filler migration, the timely and judicious application of hyaluronidase enables resolution of issues without compromising the overall aesthetic result [8].

Lastly, managing patient expectations is crucial. Many patients harbor unrealistic beliefs about the degree of enlargement achievable or the permanence of the augmentation. Clear communication regarding the gradual nature of enhancements, the expected longevity of HA fillers, and the necessity of periodic touch-up sessions fosters trust and aligns expectations with clinical realities [7].

By weaving together these elements—thoughtful product selection, conservative volume planning, refined injection techniques, preparedness for complication management, and proactive patient education—clinicians can elevate PGE with HA from a technical procedure to a highly individualized art form. This experiential approach, honed over decades of practice, underscores the centrality of clinical judgment and adaptability in achieving superior outcomes.

9.4 Differentiating PGE with HA from Other Techniques

Penile girth enhancement (PGE) using hyaluronic acid (HA) fillers occupies a unique position in the spectrum of male genital augmentation. Unlike surgical methods such as dermofat grafting or implantation of synthetic materials, HA-based augmentation offers a minimally invasive, reversible, and highly customizable approach that aligns with the growing preference for nonsurgical aesthetic interventions.

Permanent augmentation techniques—while capable of producing substantial volumetric changes—carry significant risks, including fibrosis, granulomatous reactions, extrusion, and irreversible deformities. Synthetic implants such as polymethyl methacrylate (PMMA) microspheres and poly-L-lactic acid (PLA) have been associated with foreign body reactions and nodular formations that often necessitate complex surgical removal [1, 2]. These complications, coupled with variable aesthetic outcomes, have limited the acceptance of such techniques outside highly specialized surgical settings.

In contrast, HA fillers have demonstrated a favorable safety profile in both clinical trials and long-term observational studies. Their biocompatibility and biodegradability minimize the risk of chronic inflammatory responses, and their reversibility with hyaluronidase provides an added layer of safety in managing unexpected outcomes [3, 4]. The dynamic nature of HA also allows for periodic adjustments—whether to maintain volume, correct asymmetries, or respond to changes in patient preferences over time. This flexibility is particularly valuable given the psychological and aesthetic sensitivities often associated with male genital enhancement [5].

Furthermore, HA fillers integrate more naturally with penile tissues compared to rigid synthetic implants. This integration supports not only aesthetic improvements but also functional considerations such as preserving penile sensation and erectile function. Unlike permanent materials that may impair tissue compliance or create palpable irregularities, properly injected HA maintains the natural elasticity of penile skin, contributing to both a visually harmonious result and patient comfort during sexual activity [6].

Another significant advantage of HA-based PGE is the reduced downtime and lower threshold for patient acceptance. The procedure is performed in an outpatient setting under local anesthesia, with most patients resuming normal activities within days. This contrasts sharply with surgical options, which require general anesthesia, prolong recovery, and carry higher risks of infection and scarring [8].

While HA augmentation is not without its challenges—such as the need for periodic reinjection due to biodegradation or the potential for filler migration—these are manageable with proper technique and follow-up care. When performed by skilled clinicians, HA-based PGE offers a balance of efficacy, safety, and patient satisfaction that has positioned it as the preferred option in many practices worldwide [7].

Ultimately, the success of HA-based PGE lies in its adaptability. By tailoring filler selection, injection technique, and post-procedural management to each patient's unique anatomy and goals, clinicians can achieve outcomes that rival those of more invasive methods while avoiding their inherent risks.

9.5 Positioning "Tips and Tricks" as Essential Knowledge

The true mastery of penile girth enhancement (PGE) using hyaluronic acid (HA) fillers transcends the boundaries of clinical trials and textbook protocols. While randomized controlled studies provide valuable evidence regarding safety and efficacy, they often fail to capture the nuanced challenges and dynamic decision-making required in daily clinical practice. For practitioners engaged in HA-based PGE, the accumulation of hands-on experience becomes the most critical determinant of success.

Over 25 years of clinical experience have revealed that achieving consistently superior outcomes is not merely about selecting the right filler or following a standardized injection technique. It demands a deep understanding of how HA behaves within penile tissues, how anatomical variations influence filler distribution, and how to respond proactively to complications or suboptimal results. This "experiential intelligence" allows clinicians to refine their approach in real time, adapting to the unique requirements of each patient.

For example, understanding the subtle differences in filler rheology can guide the selection of a product that matches not only the desired volume but also the mechanical characteristics of the patient's penile tissues. Recognizing when to switch from needle-based delivery to a blunt-tip cannula, or when to employ an automatic injector for high-viscosity gels, is equally important. These decisions, though seemingly minor, often spell the difference between a natural, harmonious augmentation and a result marred by irregularities or patient dissatisfaction.

Patient management further highlights the value of practical insights. Clear communication about expected outcomes, the necessity of periodic touch-ups, and the importance of post-procedural care helps align patient expectations with clinical realities. Addressing concerns proactively—whether they involve mild asymmetry, initial discomfort, or anxiety over filler resorption—strengthens the therapeutic alliance and supports long-term satisfaction.

This chapter's compilation of "tips and tricks" reflects decades of iterative learning, distilled into practical strategies that address common pitfalls and optimize results. These insights are not intended as rigid rules but as a flexible toolkit to guide clinicians in achieving safe, predictable, and aesthetically pleasing outcomes. By adopting this experiential knowledge, practitioners can elevate HA-based PGE from a technical procedure to a patient-centered art form that restores both confidence and quality of life.

9.6 Key Considerations and Technical Challenges in PGE with HA Fillers

Penile girth enhancement (PGE) using hyaluronic acid (HA) fillers is deceptively straightforward on the surface. However, in clinical reality, it requires the practitioner to navigate a complex interplay of anatomical, technical, and patient-related variables to achieve uniformly satisfactory results. This section delves into the nuanced considerations and technical challenges that are crucial for elevating outcomes from adequate to excellent.

One of the foremost technical challenges lies in achieving symmetry. The cylindrical shape of the penile shaft and its highly mobile subcutaneous tissue layer make even filler distribution particularly challenging. Minor deviations in injection depth or delivery pressure can result in contour irregularities or localized nodules. This is further complicated by natural asymmetries in penile anatomy, which may predispose certain areas to disproportionate filler accumulation. Such outcomes, although often subtle initially, tend to become more noticeable as the filler undergoes isovolumic degradation over time [1].

Distal ventral migration is another well-recognized issue, especially in uncircumcised patients. In these cases, the preputial space provides a potential "dead zone" where filler material can accumulate, leading to undesirable contour changes. For patients with significant preputial redundancy, circumcision prior to augmentation may be advisable to eliminate this anatomical risk factor [2].

The degradation behavior of HA fillers introduces additional complexity. While isovolumic degradation maintains relative volume initially, over time, subtle shifts in contour may emerge as the filler is metabolized. Without planned touch-up sessions, these changes can undermine patient satisfaction. Consequently, adopting a proactive reinjection strategy becomes essential—not merely for volume maintenance but also for preserving symmetry and aesthetic integrity [3].

Measurement of outcomes presents its own set of challenges. Traditional methods such as circumferential tape measurement may lack accuracy, especially in patients with baseline irregularities or obesity-related concealed penis. Visual assessment, performed collaboratively by the clinician and patient, often provides a more practical and meaningful evaluation of success. Digital photography and patient-reported satisfaction scores can complement this approach, offering a multidimensional understanding of results [4].

The evolution of HA filler technology has contributed significantly to addressing these challenges. Earlier collagen-based fillers were limited by hypersensitivity reactions and a brief duration of effect, often requiring frequent reinjections [5]. Modern HA fillers, in contrast, offer improved longevity, enhanced biocompatibility, and superior tissue integration. Their reversibility with hyaluronidase adds a layer of safety unmatched by irreversible fillers like PMMA and PLA, which have been associated with granulomatous reactions and often require surgical excision for correction [6, 8, 9].

Nevertheless, not all HA fillers perform equally in the penile environment. Factors such as gel hardness, particle size, cohesiveness, and HA concentration influence not only volume retention but also injectability and patient comfort. A higher concentration of cross-linked HA, while offering extended persistence, may also demand greater technical skill for even distribution [7]. Careful product selection tailored to patient-specific anatomical and aesthetic considerations is, therefore, indispensable for achieving consistent, natural results.

Complications—though generally mild with HA fillers—remain an ever-present risk. Technical errors, such as excessive volume deposition or uneven depth of injection, can lead to contour deformities, vascular compromise, or inflammatory responses. Fortunately, most adverse events related to HA are self-limiting or amenable to correction with hyaluronidase. In contrast, complications from permanent fillers may manifest years later and often necessitate complex surgical management [5].

By integrating these technical considerations with a deep understanding of penile anatomy and filler behavior, clinicians can develop a comprehensive strategy that anticipates challenges and addresses them proactively. Such an approach ensures that PGE with HA fillers achieves its potential as a safe, reversible, and aesthetically rewarding procedure.

9.7 Key Technical Considerations

The technical execution of penile girth enhancement (PGE) using hyaluronic acid (HA) fillers requires meticulous planning and an intimate understanding of both the tools and techniques involved. While the filler itself plays a critical role, the clinician's choice of instruments, delivery method, and procedural strategy often determines the safety, efficiency, and aesthetic success of the augmentation.

The selection of the injection device—whether needle or cannula—is a pivotal decision (Fig. 9.1). Smaller volumes of filler, typically 1–3 mL, can often be administered effectively with a 27-gauge needle. This approach provides fine control, particularly for targeted corrections or touch-up sessions. However, as the augmentation volume increases, a blunt-tip cannula of larger diameter (21G or 22G) is preferred. Cannulas minimize tissue trauma, reduce the risk of vascular injury, and facilitate more uniform filler distribution within the subcutaneous plane. Their flexibility also allows for smoother navigation around delicate anatomical structures [1] (Fig. 9.2).

In cases requiring the administration of highly viscous HA gels or larger augmentation volumes (5–10 mL), specialized automatic injectors or mechanical injection guns become invaluable (Fig. 9.3). These devices deliver filler at a controlled, consistent rate, ensuring even tissue distribution while reducing operator fatigue. The benefit of such devices is particularly evident during multipass techniques or when treating patients with thicker subcutaneous tissues that offer greater resistance to filler deposition. By automating delivery pressure, injectors mitigate the risk of uneven extrusion forces that can lead to filler clumping or streaking [2, 3].

Syringe size also influences injection feasibility and ergonomics. While 1 mL and 3 mL syringes allow for manual injection with minimal resistance, larger syringes (5 mL and 10 mL) are more challenging to manage. As syringe volume increases, the extrusion force required rises disproportionately, often making manual injection impractical. Automatic injectors overcome this

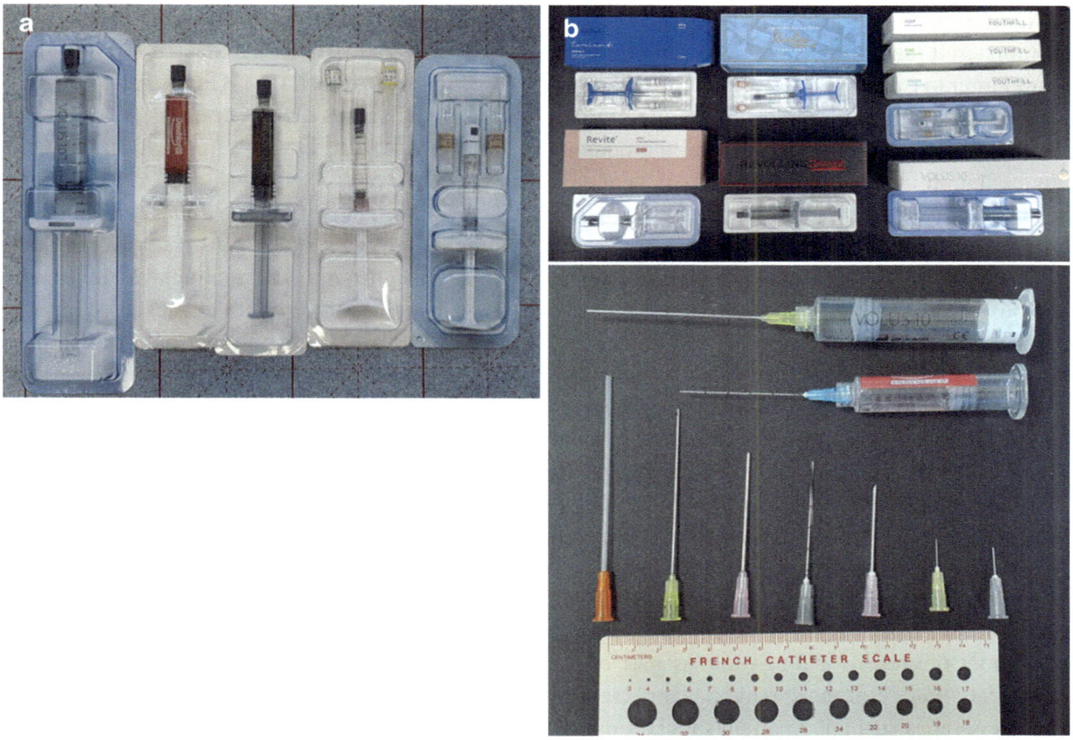

Fig. 9.1 (**a**) Prefilled syringe with hyaluronic acid filler of different volumes (1, 3, 5, and 10 mL), (**b**) 27G and 18G needles, and various cannulas commonly used for penile girth enhancement

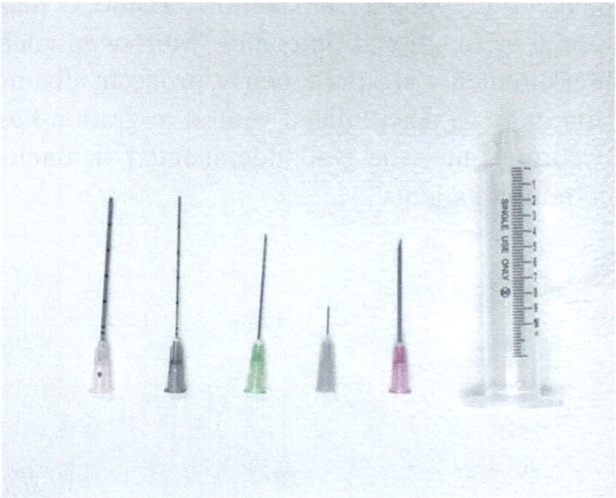

Fig. 9.2 Various calibers of needles and cannulas compared with a 10 mL syringe, illustrating size differences critical for selecting appropriate instruments during penile girth enhancement procedures

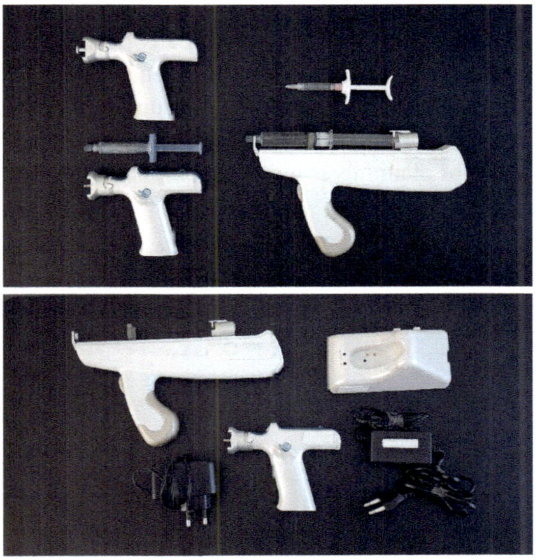

Fig. 9.3 Automatic injector device compatible with prefilled HA syringes, designed to provide consistent injection pressure, reduce operator fatigue, and ensure precise filler distribution during large-volume penile girth enhancement

limitation, enabling high-viscosity gels to be administered smoothly and consistently even from larger syringes [4].

Volume planning deserves equal attention. A conservative approach that favors incremental augmentation over multiple sessions is generally safer and yields more natural results. This strategy minimizes the risk of skin overstretching, vascular compromise, and mechanical stress on subcutaneous tissues. It also allows for adjustments based on how the filler settles in the tissues and how the patient perceives their initial results [5].

Finally, establishing appropriate retouch intervals is vital for maintaining long-term outcomes. As HA fillers undergo gradual biodegradation, periodic reinjections help preserve aesthetic volume and correct minor irregularities. Regular follow-up appointments not only optimize results but also build patient confidence in the procedure's safety and reliability. Clear communication about the need for touch-ups as part of the treatment plan reinforces realistic expectations and encourages sustained patient satisfaction [6].

By paying careful attention to these technical aspects—instrument choice, delivery mechanics, syringe volume, augmentation strategy, and follow-up protocols—clinicians can achieve superior results that are both aesthetically pleasing and functionally sound. These refinements, honed through years of clinical practice, underscore that success in HA-based PGE lies as much in precision and planning as it does in product efficacy.

9.8 Misunderstandings from Publications of PGE: Insights from KFDA Approval Studies and Korean Clinical Data

The evolution of penile girth enhancement (PGE) using hyaluronic acid (HA) fillers in Korea offers unique insights into the realities of this procedure—insights often underrepresented in the global literature. While international publications have focused predominantly on controlled trials and short-term outcomes, long-term real-world experiences in Korea reveal both the strengths and limitations of HA-based PGE.

A critical observation emerges from reviewing Korea's KFDA approval studies. In these trials, regulatory emphasis was placed on objective measures such as residual implant volume and penile circumference at 6 months postinjection. These parameters were essential for demonstrating the filler's longevity and augmentative effect. However, they tell only part of the story. Circumferential measurements at the proximal, mid, and distal shaft levels—even when meticulously recorded—do not fully capture the nuances of patient satisfaction, aesthetic harmony, or functional outcomes. Moreover, such measurements are particularly prone to distortion in cases where distal ventral migration has occurred, an issue well documented in uncircumcised patients [1].

Trade name (manufacturer, country)	Study design	Sample size	Mean penile Girth increase at 24 wks, mm	Complications	Injection dosage, mL (mean±SD)	HA conc., mg/mL	Particle size, μm	Cross-linking, degree	Complex viscosity
Potenfill (Medytox, Korea)	Prospective, patient/evaluator-blinded, randomized, multicenter trial	65 (HA: 33, PLA: 32)	21	Injection site deformation: 1; injection site inflammation: 1	20.8±1.5	20	~700	BDDE, 10%	No record
HyaFilia Impact (CHA Meditech, Korea)	Prospective, patient/evaluator-blinded, randomized, multicenter trial	62 (HA: 30, PLA: 32)	19.1	Injection site inflammation: 1; injection site pain: 2	16.4±2.7	20	~500	BDDE, 6%	200–600 Pa.s
THE CHAEUM; Shape 10 (Hugel Bio, Korea)	Prospective, patient/evaluator-blinded, randomized, multicenter trial	59 (HA: 30, PLA: 29)	20.6	Injection site induration: 1	19.1±1.4	20	~600	BDDE, no record	100–600 Pa.s
Doublofill (Humedix, Korea)[a]	Prospective, patient/evaluator-blinded, randomized, multicenter trial	64 (HA: 32, PLA: 32)	22.7	Injection site inflammation: 2	19.7±0.7	23	~700	BDDE, 12%	400~700 Pa.s

HA hyaluronic acid, *PLA* polylactic acid, *BDDE* 1,4-butanediol diglycidyl ether
[a]Current study

In clinical practice, a single large-volume injection—sometimes referred to colloquially as the "big shot" approach—rarely achieves durable or harmonious results. Instead, the experience of Korean practitioners has consistently supported a staged retouch strategy. Incremental enhancements not only reduce complications such as skin overstretching and irregular filler distribution but also allow for dynamic adjustments based on individual tissue response and patient feedback. This iterative approach has proven indispensable for managing filler behavior over time, including the inevitable biodegradation and potential asymmetries that may develop as HA integrates with surrounding tissues [2, 3].

Recent publications from Korea further support these principles. Yang et al. presented a multicenter retrospective analysis comparing HA, polylactic acid (PLA), and polymethyl methacrylate (PMMA) fillers. Their findings highlighted that while PMMA provided greater initial augmentative effects, it was associated with higher complication rates and lower patient satisfaction. In contrast, HA and PLA offered more favorable safety profiles and higher patient-reported outcomes, underscoring the importance of balancing volumizing potential with procedural reversibility and safety [4, 5].

Perhaps most importantly, the Korean experience reinforces the critical role of hyaluronidase as a safety net in HA-based PGE. Unlike permanent fillers, which can only be corrected through complex surgical intervention, HA-related complications—whether overfilling, nodules, or migration—can be effectively managed with hyaluronidase. This enzyme has not only enabled corrective interventions but also instilled confidence in patients and physicians alike, establishing HA fillers as the gold standard for nonsurgical PGE [5].

These lessons underscore a fundamental shift in perspective: longevity and volumetric enhancement, while desirable, should not be considered the ultimate goals of PGE. Instead, the emphasis must lie on procedural safety, patient-centered outcomes, and the feasibility of long-term maintenance through retouching and refinement. It is this philosophy, developed through decades of Korean clinical practice, that positions HA-based PGE as both a science and an art.

9.8.1 The Role of Uro-Andrologists in PGE

Penile girth enhancement (PGE) using hyaluronic acid (HA) fillers demands more than technical proficiency; it requires a comprehensive understanding of male sexual health, penile anatomy, and patient psychology. Uro-andrologists, with their specialized training and holistic perspective, are uniquely positioned to deliver this complex intervention safely and effectively.

Beyond performing the procedure itself, these specialists play a pivotal role in guiding patients through the often sensitive and emotionally charged decision-making process. Cultural perceptions of masculinity and sexual confidence, particularly in Asian societies, underscore the importance of empathetic communication and ethical practice. Uro-andrologists are entrusted with the responsibility of balancing patient desires for aesthetic enhancement with realistic expectations and medical appropriateness.

In a world where untrained practitioners and nonmedical providers increasingly offer penile augmentation services, the presence of well-trained uro-andrologists serves as a bulwark against unethical practices and preventable harm. Cases of filler misuse, self-injection, and genital mutilation highlight the dangers of leaving such procedures in unqualified hands. By contrast, uro-andrologists ensure procedural safety through evidence-based techniques, vigilant complication management, and long-term follow-up care.

As custodians of male sexual health, these physicians bring an irreplaceable layer of expertise and responsibility to the evolving field of PGE.

9.8.2 The Future of HA Fillers in PGE

Advances in HA filler technology are set to further refine the practice of PGE. Innovations in cross-linking chemistry, rheological optimization, and bioactive filler formulations promise improved volume retention, smoother tissue integration, and reduced biodegradation rates. These developments may extend the duration of augmentative effects while maintaining the reversibility and safety profile that make HA fillers the preferred choice today.

In parallel, the growing body of long-term clinical studies will help define standardized protocols, patient selection criteria, and touch-up strategies tailored to diverse populations. International guidelines are expected to evolve as evidence accumulates, providing clearer pathways for incorporating PGE into mainstream andrological practice.

Perhaps most importantly, the future of HA-based PGE lies in its acceptance not only as a cosmetic procedure but as a legitimate aspect of male sexual wellness. As cultural barriers erode and patient demand rises, well-trained uro-andrologists will be called upon to lead the field, ensuring that innovation does not outpace safety and ethical standards.

9.8.3 Conclusion: The Key to Success in PGE

Penile girth enhancement with hyaluronic acid (HA) fillers represents a milestone in the evolution of male aesthetic and functional interventions. Its success lies in three foundational principles:

1. Precision in technique—mastery of filler properties, anatomical knowledge, and injection skills to achieve even distribution and avoid complications such as migration or asymmetry.
2. Patient-specific approach—tailoring treatment plans to individual anatomy, cultural expectations, and psychological needs.
3. Long-term maintenance and refinement—employing staged retouching, periodic reinjection, and the judicious use of hyaluronidase to sustain aesthetic and functional outcomes.

When performed by skilled uro-andrologists, HA-based PGE is not merely a cosmetic procedure but a transformative intervention that enhances patient confidence and quality of life. The future of this field will depend on continued innovation, ethical practice, and the unwavering commitment of specialists to provide safe, patient-centered care.

References

1. Sundaram H, Voigts B, Beer K, Meland M. Comparison of the rheological properties of viscosity and elasticity in two categories of soft tissue fillers: calcium hydroxylapatite and hyaluronic acid. Dermatologic Surg. 2010;36(Suppl 3):1859–65.
2. Ahn ST, Shim JS, Bae WJ, Kim SW, Kim JJ, Moon DG. Efficacy and safety of penile girth enhancement using hyaluronic acid filler and the clinical impact on ejaculation: a multicenter, patient/evaluator–blinded, randomized active-controlled trial. World J Mens Health. 2022;40(2):299–307.
3. Yang DY, Ko K, Lee SH, Lee WK. A comparison of the efficacy and safety between hyaluronic acid and polylactic acid filler injection in penile augmentation: a multicenter, patient/evaluator–blinded, randomized trial. J Sex Med. 2019;16(4):577–85.
4. Flynn TC, Sarazin D, Bezzola A, Terrani C, Micheels P. Comparative histology of intradermal implantation of monophasic hyaluronic acid filler and polyphasic hyaluronic acid filler. Dermatologic Surg. 2011;37(5):637–43.
5. Christensen L, Breiting V, Janssen M, Vuust J, Høgdall E. Adverse reactions to injectable soft tissue permanent fillers. Aesth Plast Surg. 2005;29(1):34–48.
6. Lorenc ZP, Bruce S, Werschler WP. Safety and efficacy of a continuous-flow, injection-assisted device in delivery of dermal fillers. Aesthetic Surg J. 2013;33(5):705–12
7. Kablik J, Monheit GD, Yu L, Chang G, Gershkovich J. Comparative physical properties of hyaluronic acid dermal fillers. Dermatologic Surg. 2009;35(Suppl 1):302–12.
8. Le Penske W, Leslie DC, Latini JM, Lerner LB. Injectable penile enhancement procedures: a review of agents, risks, and complications. Urology. 2024;189:126–34.
9. Alter GJ. Editorial comment on "penile girth enhancement with PMMA-based soft tissue fillers". Oxford University Press; 2016. p. 1423.

Clinical Case Series in Hyaluronic Acid-Based Penile Girth Enhancement: Anatomical Considerations, Complications, and Corrective Strategies

10

Contents

Supplementary Information The online version contains supplementary material available at https://doi.org/10.1007/978-981-95-5385-3_10.

D. G. Moon, *Penile Augmentation with Injectable Hyaluronic Acid*,
https://doi.org/10.1007/978-981-95-5385-3_10

10.1 Case 1: Physiologic Time-Dependent Distal Ventral Migration of HA Filler

A 54-year-old male underwent penile girth enhancement (PGE) using hyaluronic acid (HA) filler to address aesthetic concerns regarding penile thickness (Fig. 10.1a). The procedure involved the injection of 10 mL HA filler via a 22G cannula in a single session. The immediate postoperative appearance showed uniform filler distribution and no evidence of complications (Fig. 10.1b). However, at the 4-week follow-up, early signs of distal-ventral migration became evident. Despite prior circumcision, subtle accumulation of filler in the distal shaft and remnant foreskin was noted, leading to mild asymmetry (Fig. 10.1b). By 12 weeks postinjection, progressive filler shifting resulted in further contour changes, with visible redistribution of material toward the distal penis (Fig. 10.1c). The patient expressed interest in additional filler to the right side to address perceived asymmetry. However, clinical assessment suggested that any additional injection at this stage might exacerbate distal pooling rather than correcting the deformity. At the 24-week follow-up, further redistribution of filler had occurred, but in the erect state, no deformities were observed (Fig. 10.1d). A conservative management strategy was adopted, focusing on patient counseling and observation. Given the time-dependent biodegradation of HA filler, retouch procedures were deferred to allow natural resorption and reassessment of contour stability before planning additional intervention.

This case underscores the importance of selecting HA fillers with appropriate rheological properties, including viscosity, cohesiveness, and gel hardness, to minimize physiologic migration. Fillers with a higher degree of cross-linking offer increased structural integrity, helping maintain their position within penile tissues. Additionally, extrusion force should be considered to facilitate smooth and even distribution during injection, ensuring optimal aesthetic outcomes and reducing the likelihood of distal pooling.

Another crucial consideration is the role of circumcision in preventing distal migration. In patients with redundant prepuce, the subpreputial space may serve as a potential reservoir for filler migration, leading to asymmetric deformities.

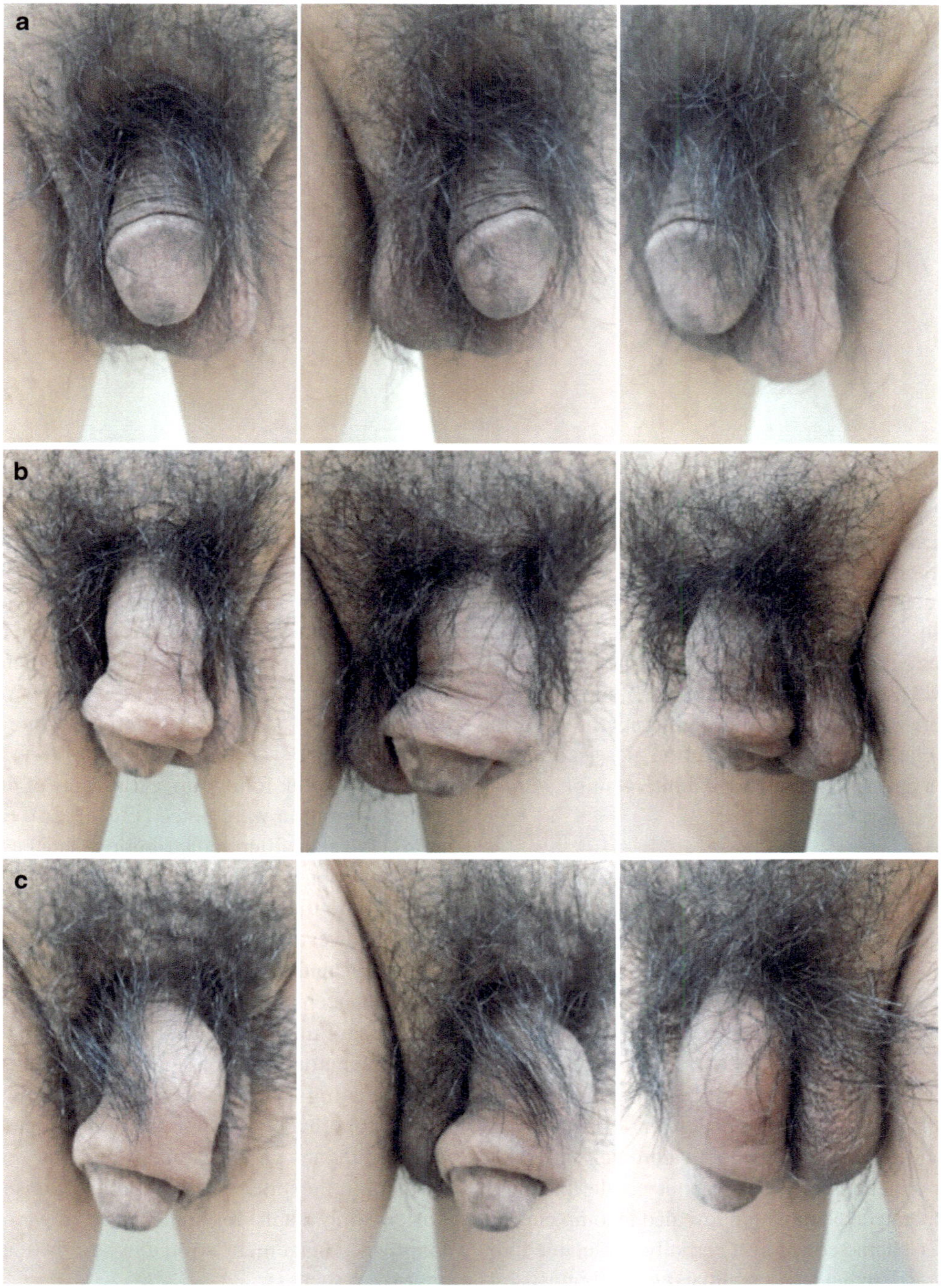

Fig. 10.1 (**a**) Preoperative appearance of the penis before PGE with HA filler in a 54-year-old male (**b**) Immediate postoperative appearance and early signs of distal-ventral migration at 4 weeks postinjection, with subtle accumulation of filler in the distal shaft and remnant foreskin (**c**) At 12 weeks postinjection, progressive shifting of HA filler and contour changes are evident (**d**) At 24 weeks postinjection, further redistribution of filler is visible in the flaccid state, while the erect penis shows no apparent deformity. In this kind of deformity, the patient may ask additional injection in right side, but additional retouched volume mostly go distally. In erect penis, no deformity and better to observe. more time-dependent biodegradation to select retouch time

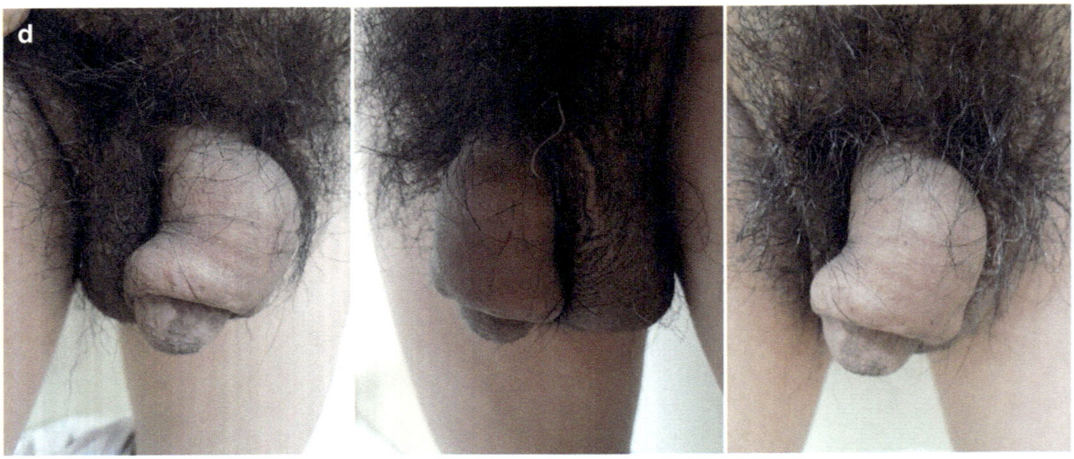

Fig. 10.1 (continued)

Indications for circumcision include phimosis—whether complete, incomplete, or retractable—that could trap filler material distally. In this case, despite thorough counseling and recommendation for circumcision, the patient declined the procedure. This decision underscores the importance of patient-centered care and highlights the need for clinicians to plan follow-up strategies accordingly when patients refuse surgical intervention.

10.2 Case 2: Managing Long-Term Distal Migration, Delayed Circumcision, and HA Remnant Removal in a 55-Year-Old Male

10.2.1 Part 1: Initial PGE and Early Distal Migration

A 55-year-old male underwent penile girth enhancement (PGE) with hyaluronic acid (HA) filler to address concerns about penile thickness. Preoperative examination revealed incomplete phimosis, characterized by a partially retractable foreskin and redundant preputial tissue (Fig. 10.2a). Despite thorough counseling on the potential benefits of preinjection circumcision to prevent filler migration, the patient declined the procedure.

The PGE was performed using a total of 20 mL HA filler administered via a 22G cannula in a single session. The immediate postoperative appearance demonstrated uniform filler distribution with no early complications (Fig. 10.2b).

Figure 10.2 Preoperative appearance showing hemiphimosis with redundant prepuce in a 55-year-old male. Immediate postoperative appearance after 20 mL HA filler injection demonstrating uniform penile girth enhancement. At 24 weeks postinjection, progressive filler redistribution and "Tacobell-like" deformity noted in the flaccid state

At the 4-week follow-up, early signs of distal-ventral migration were noted (Fig. 10.2c). By 12 and 24 weeks, filler redistribution had become more pronounced, leading to a "Tacobell-like" deformity in the flaccid state (Fig. 10.2d, e). The patient, however, expressed no concern regarding this change and remained satisfied with his penile girth enhancement.

This case underscores the dual importance of foreskin anatomy and patient communication in PGE planning. While circumcision is often necessary to prevent distal migration in patients with redundant prepuce, many patients remain resistant despite thorough counseling. Anticipating such resistance and developing adaptive management strategies are critical for long-term success.

10.2.2 Part 2: Minimal Circumcision and Staged Retouching

Two years after the initial procedure, the patient consented to a minimal circumcision to remove redundant prepuce and reduce distal

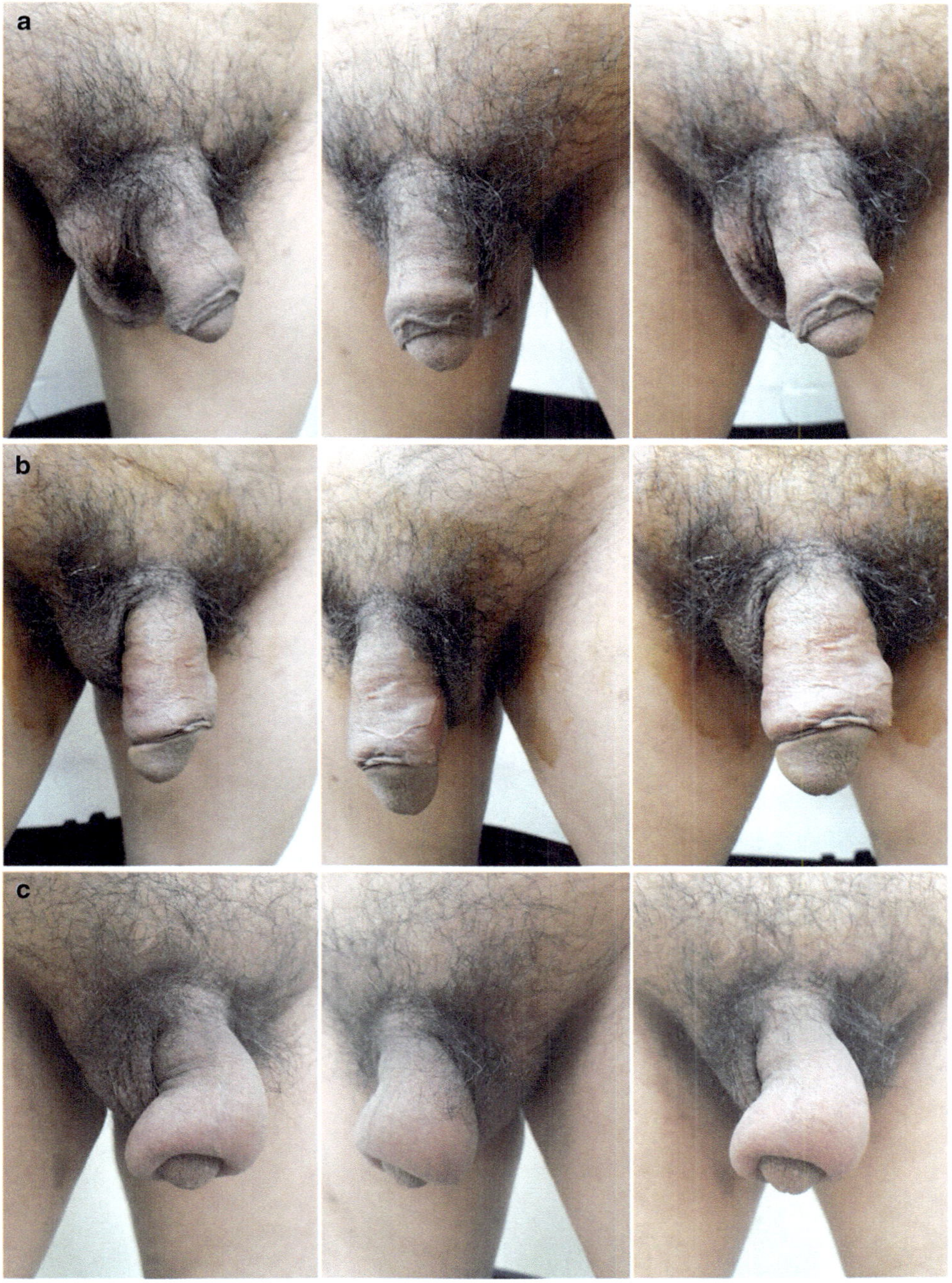

Fig. 10.2 (**a**) Preoperative uncircumcised foreskin (**b**) Immediate postoperative appearance demonstrated uniform filler distribution (**c**) 4 weeks after injection, distal ventral migration of filler made asymmetric appearance (**d**) Aggravated distal ventral migration and asymmetry at 12 weeks after injection (**e**) At 24 weeks postinjection, progressive filler redistribution and "Tacobell-like" deformity noted in the flaccid state R1-27, 23 (**f**) Two years after the initial procedure, the patient consented to a minimal circumcision to remove redundant prepuce and reduced distal pooling of HA filler (**g**) First retouch made distal ventral enlargement despite dorsal injection (**h**) Patient asked for more injection and still good after second retouch (**i**) Overcorrection for dorsal enhancement came to distal ventral and made Tacobell again (**a**) Post-minimal circumcision and (**g**) first retouch improved symmetry but (**i**) third retouch of large volume made distal migration shaped Bell

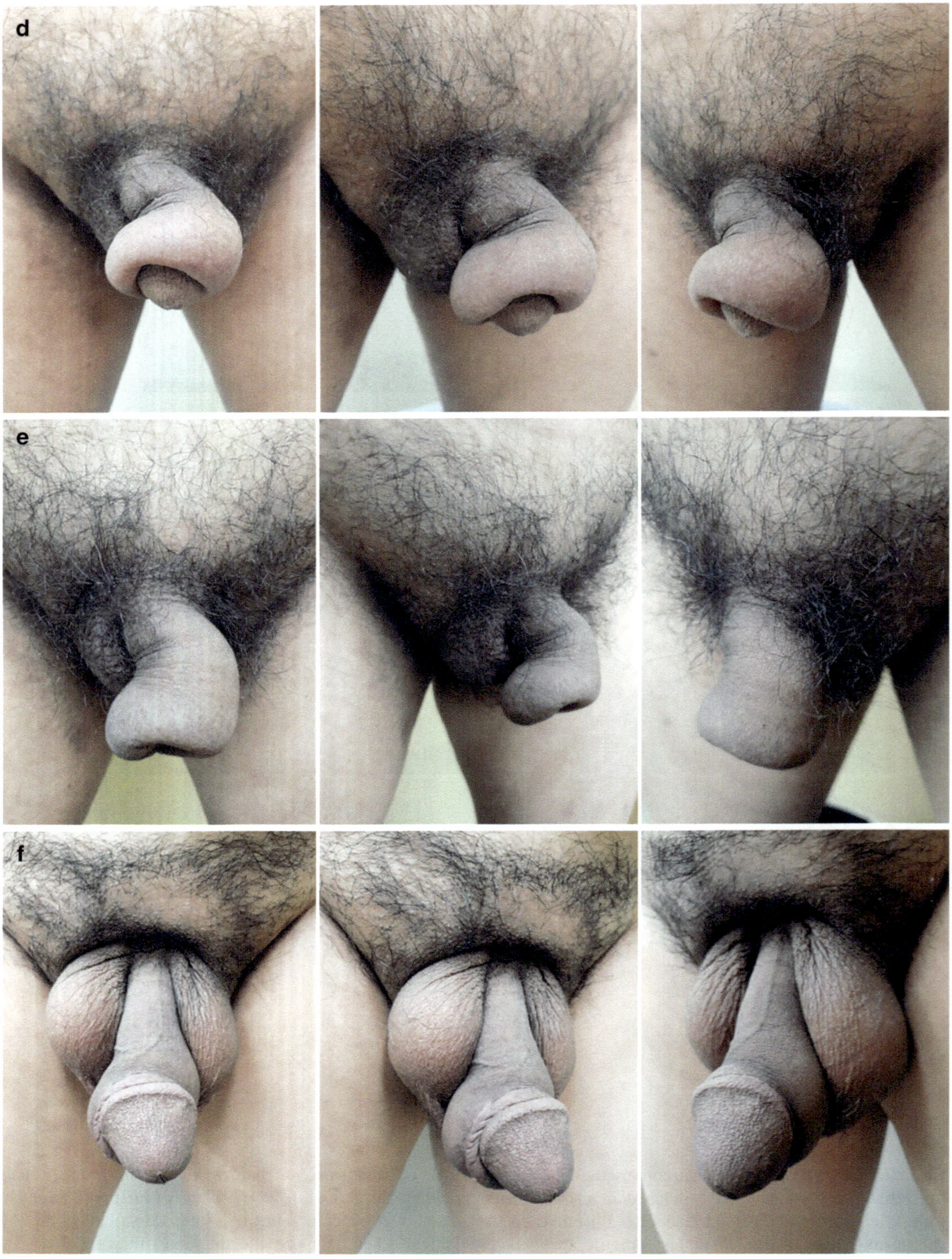

Fig. 10.2 (continued)

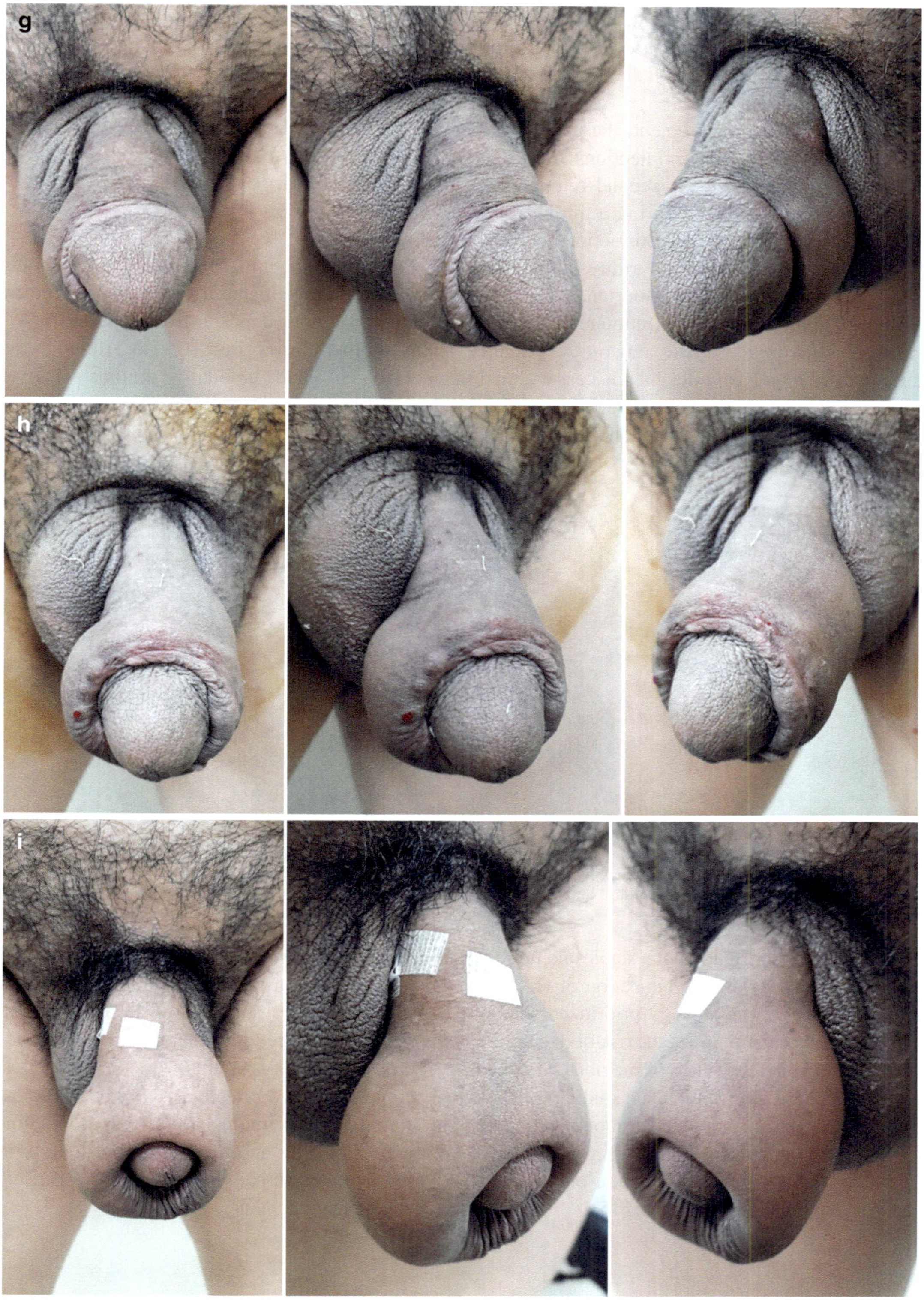

Fig. 10.2 (continued)

pooling of HA filler. Immediately after circumcision, a first retouch procedure was performed, restoring a more symmetrical penile contour (Fig. 10.2f).

Despite initial improvement, the patient later requested additional filler injections to further enhance proximal girth. A second retouch was performed cautiously, but during a third retouch session (April 9, 2020), overcorrection occurred, resulting in a bell-shaped deformity in the distal shaft. This emphasized the importance of careful volume planning and communication with patients regarding realistic outcomes. Patients often desire larger volumes than necessary, envisioning exaggerated results akin to the "Tacobell" shape. However, overcorrection increases the risk of migration and asymmetry. Managing these expectations is crucial for achieving both aesthetic and functional satisfaction.

10.2.3 Part 3: Late-Stage Correction with Hyaluronidase and Reinjection as Case 14 (2024)

By 2024, the patient presented with longstanding asymmetry and palpable irregularities caused by residual HA filler deposits from repeated injections at other clinics (Fig. 10.15a). Although the injected HA had gradually diminished over 4 years, prominent asymmetrical contours remained, resulting in both aesthetic dissatisfaction and tactile discomfort.

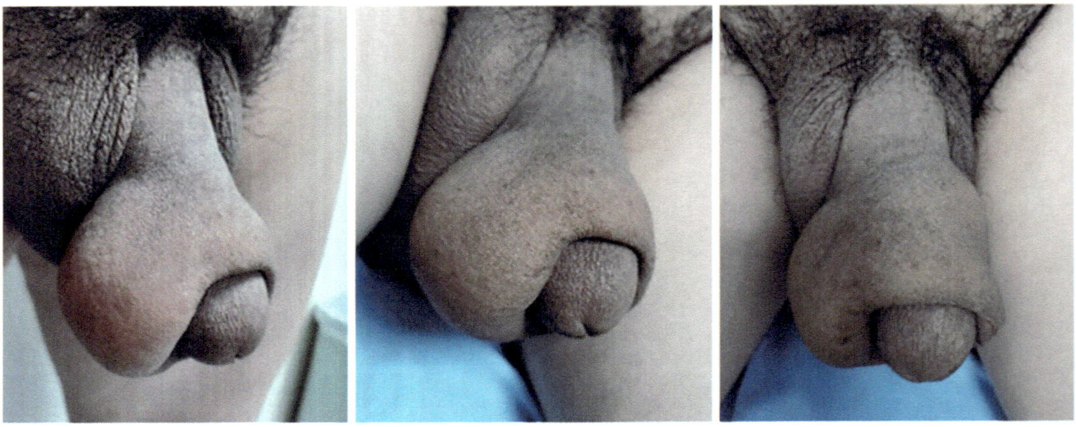

Late-stage correction with hyaluronidase and reinjection will be presented as Case 14

Following confirmation of a stable and uniform base, a carefully planned reinjection of HA filler was undertaken. The strategy prioritized smaller, staged volumes to minimize the risk of overcorrection and prevent recurrence of previous complications. This final intervention successfully restored penile girth and achieved a harmonious, natural appearance. Both the patient and clinician reported high satisfaction with the aesthetic outcome and improved tactile quality (Fig. 10.15).

Summary of Key Principles

1. Assess foreskin anatomy carefully: Redundant prepuce increases the risk of distal migration; preemptive circumcision should be considered in high-risk patients.
2. Communicate effectively with patients: Resistance to circumcision is common; clinicians must counsel patients on long-term implications and align expectations regarding staged management.

3. Avoid overcorrection: Large single-volume injections and repeated retouches increase the likelihood of asymmetry and migration.
4. Use hyaluronidase judiciously: Longstanding HA filler remnants can often be resolved effectively with a single high-dose session.
5. Reinject cautiously after correction: Staged reinjection allows for better control of contour and reduces risk of recurrence.

2. Necessity of Circumcision

Circumcision may be necessary to prevent distal migration with redundant prepuce shown in Case 1 & 2 and senile atrophy and retracted preputial ring in Case 3.

10.3 Case 3: Filler Displacement in a 67-Year-Old Male with Senile Atrophy and Retracted Preputial Ring

A 67-year-old male presented for PGE using HA filler. Preoperative assessment revealed senile atrophy of penile skin and a retracted preputial ring. Despite careful injection technique, the patient developed early filler displacement into the distal shaft and preputial area, likely exacerbated by the lack of tissue elasticity and the reservoir effect created by the retracted ring (Fig. 8.5).

This case underscores the importance of considering age-related anatomical changes when planning PGE. In elderly patients, careful volume selection, slower injection, and possibly pre-injection circumcision may reduce the risk of displacement.

In older patients, senile atrophy of penile skin combined with a retracted preputial ring may further increase the risk of HA filler displacement. In a 67-year-old male (Fig. 10.3a), preexisting tissue laxity and retracted preputial ring created a reservoir effect that contributed to distal migration of filler material. These anatomical changes highlight the need for preoperative assessment and tailored injection strategies in elderly patients.

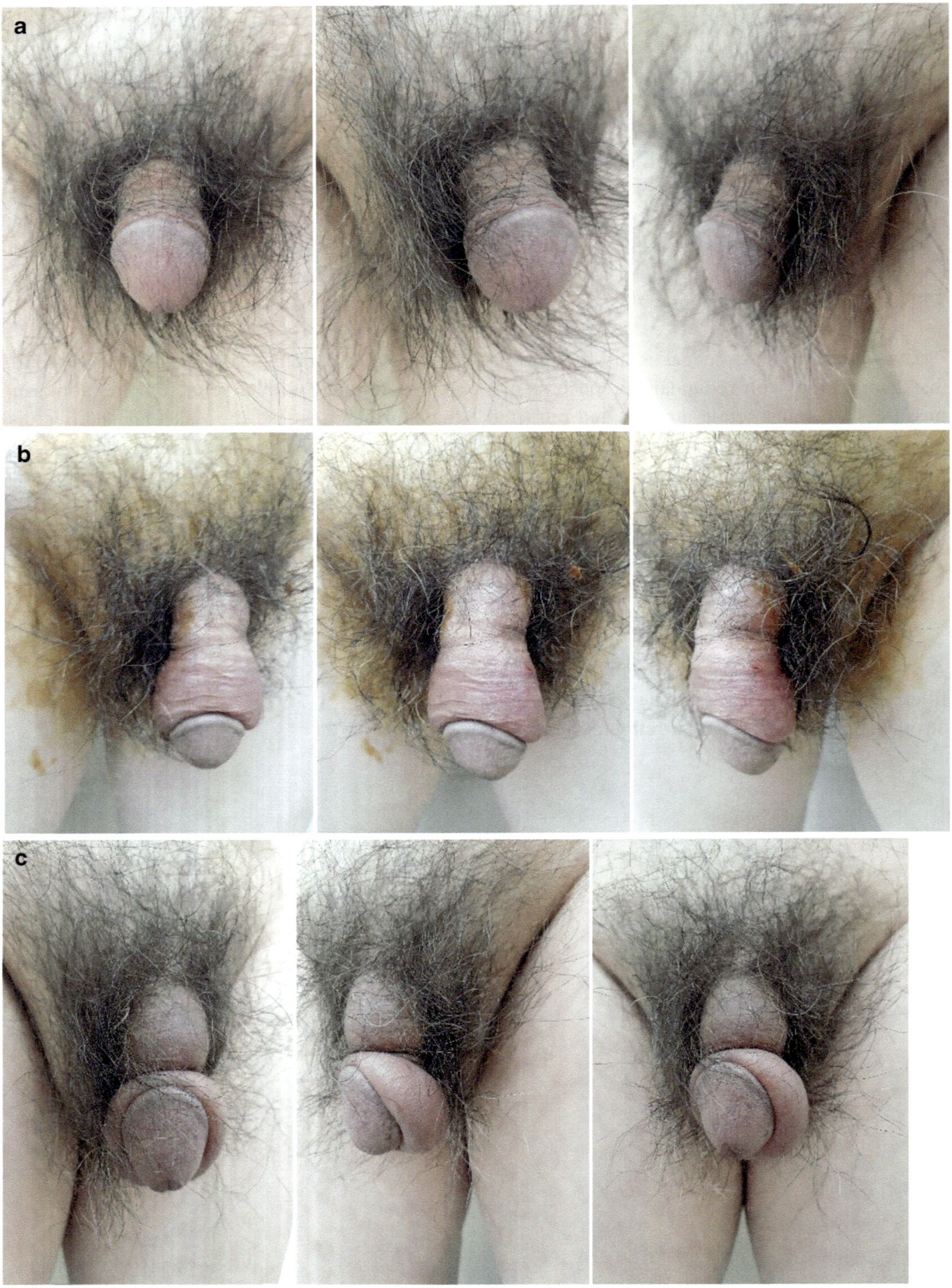

Fig. 10.3 (**a**) Senile atrophy of penile skin and retracted preputial ring were seen (**b**) Well-injected HA gel with even enhancement of girth (**c**) 4 weeks later, separated distal migration by retracted prepuce ring in old person (**d**) 24 weeks later, more separation and prominent distal migration (**e**) 48 weeks later, decreased volume of distal ventral rim

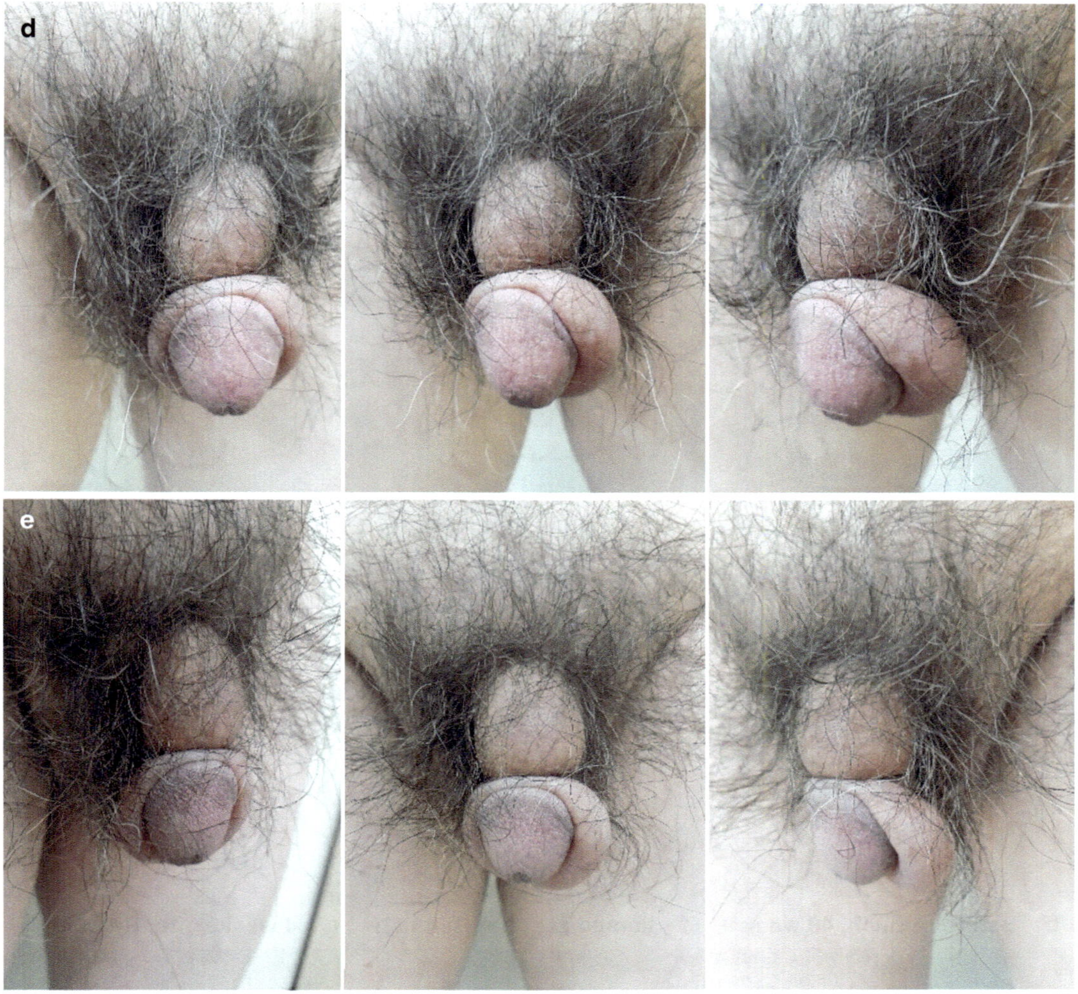

Fig. 10.3 (continued)

10.4 Case 4: Filler Distribution Challenges in a Patient with Previous Circumcision Scar and Adhesions

A 49-year-old male presented for penile girth enhancement (PGE) using hyaluronic acid (HA) filler. Preoperative evaluation revealed a prominent circumferential scar from a previous circumcision and underlying fibrous adhesions. These findings raised concern for potential uneven filler distribution and contour irregularities postinjection.

PGE was performed with a total of 15 mL HA filler using a 22G cannula. Immediate postoperative results showed uniform girth enhancement (Fig. 10.4a, b). However, during follow-ups at 4, 12, and 24 weeks, a progressive distal depression developed along the circumcision line, corresponding to the previous scar tissue and underlying adhesions (Fig. 10.4c, d). At 48 weeks, the depression persisted, although less prominent due to partial filler redistribution (Fig. 10.4e) but final resolution after filler retouch (Fig. 10.4f, g).

This case illustrates how preexisting circumcision scars and fibrous adhesions can act as a mechanical barrier to even filler spread, resulting in contour irregularities. Surgical revision of scar tissue may be considered in refractory cases to

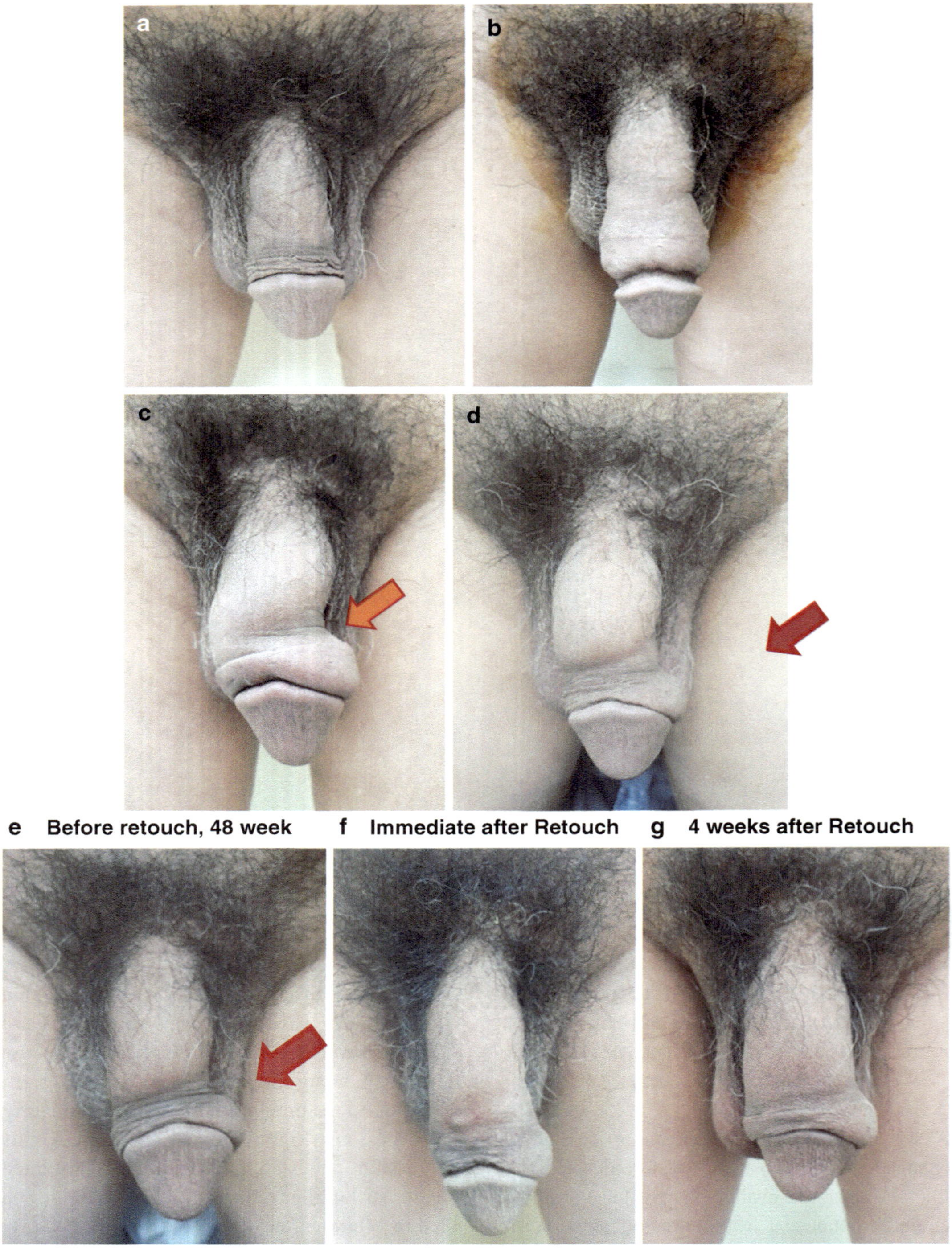

Fig. 10.4 (**a**) Preoperative appearance showing previous circumcision scar. (**b**) Immediate postoperative appearance after 15 mL HA filler injection. At 4 weeks postinjection, early signs of distal depression at the circumcision line, (**c**). At 24 weeks, progressive contour irregularity with filler pooling proximally, (**d**). At 48 weeks, partial resolution of the depression due to partial filler redistribution (**e**), but final resolution after filler retouch (**f**, **g**)

allow better filler distribution during future interventions.

- Previous circumcision scar or underlying adhesions → Can affect filler distribution and require surgical revision if necessary.

3. Injection Technique and Postinjection Management: Strategies for Symmetry and Stability

Achieving a symmetric and aesthetically pleasing penile contour requires careful attention to injection technique, volume planning, and postinjection care. These elements are crucial to minimize common complications such as filler migration, asymmetry, and contour irregularities.

1. Injection Location: Avoid Distal Ventral Placement

The distal ventral region of the penis is particularly susceptible to filler migration because of gravitational forces, dynamic penile movements, and relatively loose connective tissue in this area. Injection of HA filler into this zone significantly increases the risk of distal pooling over time, often resulting in asymmetry, contour deformities, and patient dissatisfaction.

To mitigate these risks, filler should be strategically placed in the proximal and midshaft regions, where tissue support is stronger and more resistant to displacement. Optimal placement within the subdartos plane—between Buck's fascia and dartos fascia—enhances filler stability while minimizing complications such as superficial lumpiness or deep vascular compromise.

10.5 Case 5: Distal Ventral Migration After Large-Volume Initial Injection

A 41-year-old male underwent penile augmentation with a single session of 20 cc HA filler (Fig. 10.5a). At his 4-week postoperative visit, he presented with noticeable asymmetry and a prominent distal ventral bulge caused by early migration of the filler (Fig. 10.5b). Observation was chosen rather than immediate intervention. However, by the 12-week follow-up, further distal ventral migration had occurred, aggravating the asymmetry and contour deformity (Fig. 10.5c). This case illustrates how initial large-volume injections and distal ventral placement can predispose to progressive migration over time.

Key Recommendations

Focus injections on the proximal and midshaft regions, where robust connective tissue offers a more stable anatomical foundation for filler integration.

Avoid depositing filler near the distal ventral aspect to minimize the risk of migration into the subpreputial space or distal shaft, which can lead to progressive asymmetry and contour deformities.

2. Injection Volume and Retouch Strategy: Favoring Staged Sessions for Long-Term Symmetry

Excessive initial injection volumes are strongly associated with filler migration, asymmetry, and contour irregularities. Large single-session doses,

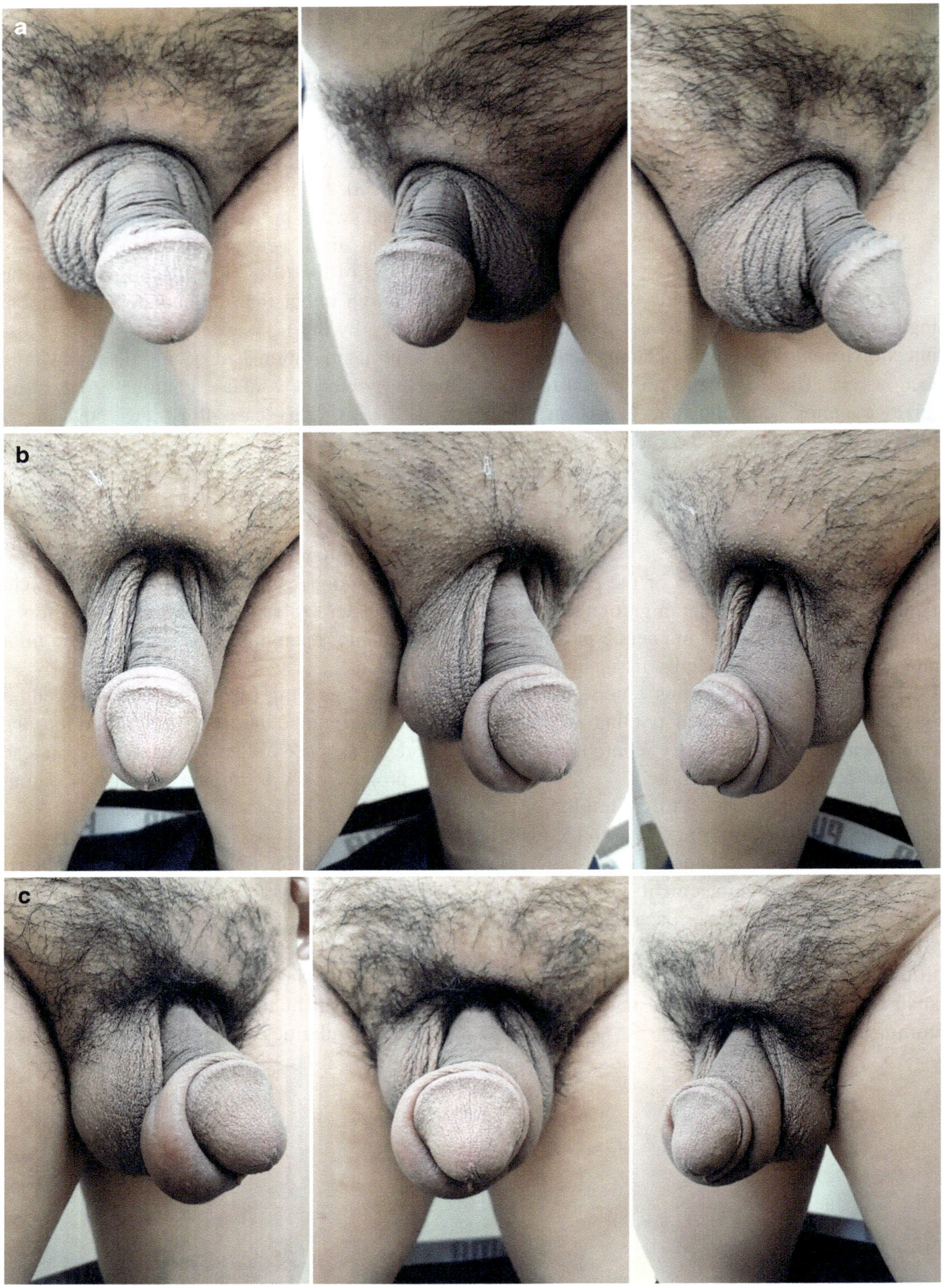

Fig. 10.5 (**a**) Preoperative penis (**b**) 4 weeks after injection, early distal ventral migration of injected filler made asymmetry and a prominent distal ventral bulge (**c**) 12 weeks after injection, further distal ventral migration (**d**) 24 weeks after injection, aggravated distal ventral migration

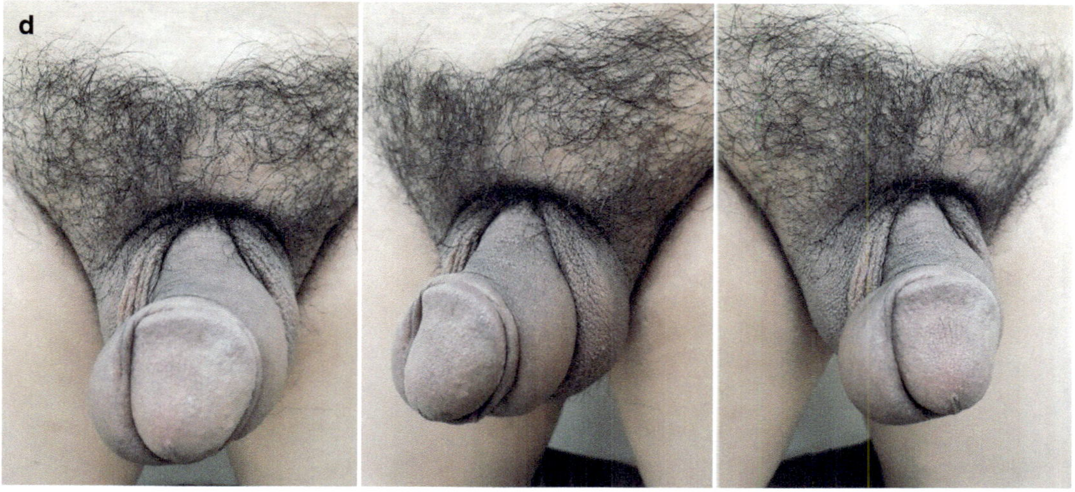

Fig. 10.5 (continued)

particularly ≥20 cc, may overwhelm the subcutaneous tissue's capacity to integrate the material, leading to displacement over time. A staged approach with smaller volumes per session not only allows for better filler distribution but also provides opportunities to address minor irregularities during subsequent visits.

10.6 Case 6: Delayed Aggravation of Distal Migration After Large-Volume Injection

A 42-year-old male received 20 cc of HA filler during a single session. At the 4-week postoperative follow-up, the aesthetic result appeared satisfactory, with no significant asymmetry or migration (Fig. 10.6a, b). However, progressive distal migration was noted at 12 weeks, and by 24 weeks, the patient exhibited aggravated distal ventral bulging and contour asymmetry (Fig. 10.6c, d). This delayed presentation highlights the importance of avoiding large-volume injections and underscores the value of planned, staged augmentation sessions.

Key Recommendations
- *Start conservatively*: Limit initial injection volumes to 10–15 mL and plan 2–3 staged sessions to achieve the desired penile girth while minimizing migration risk.
- *Schedule retouch sessions*: Arrange follow-up retouching at 3–6-month intervals to allow tissue adaptation and address minor contour irregularities effectively.
- *Set expectations early*: During pre-procedure counseling, inform patients that staged augmentation and retouching are integral parts of the treatment plan to ensure optimal aesthetic and functional outcomes.

3. Postinjection Management: Stabilize and Monitor

The first 1–2 weeks following HA filler injection are critical for ensuring optimal integration and preventing complications such as migration, asymmetry, and nodularity. During this period, postinjection care plays a pivotal role in stabilizing the filler material within the subcutaneous tissues.

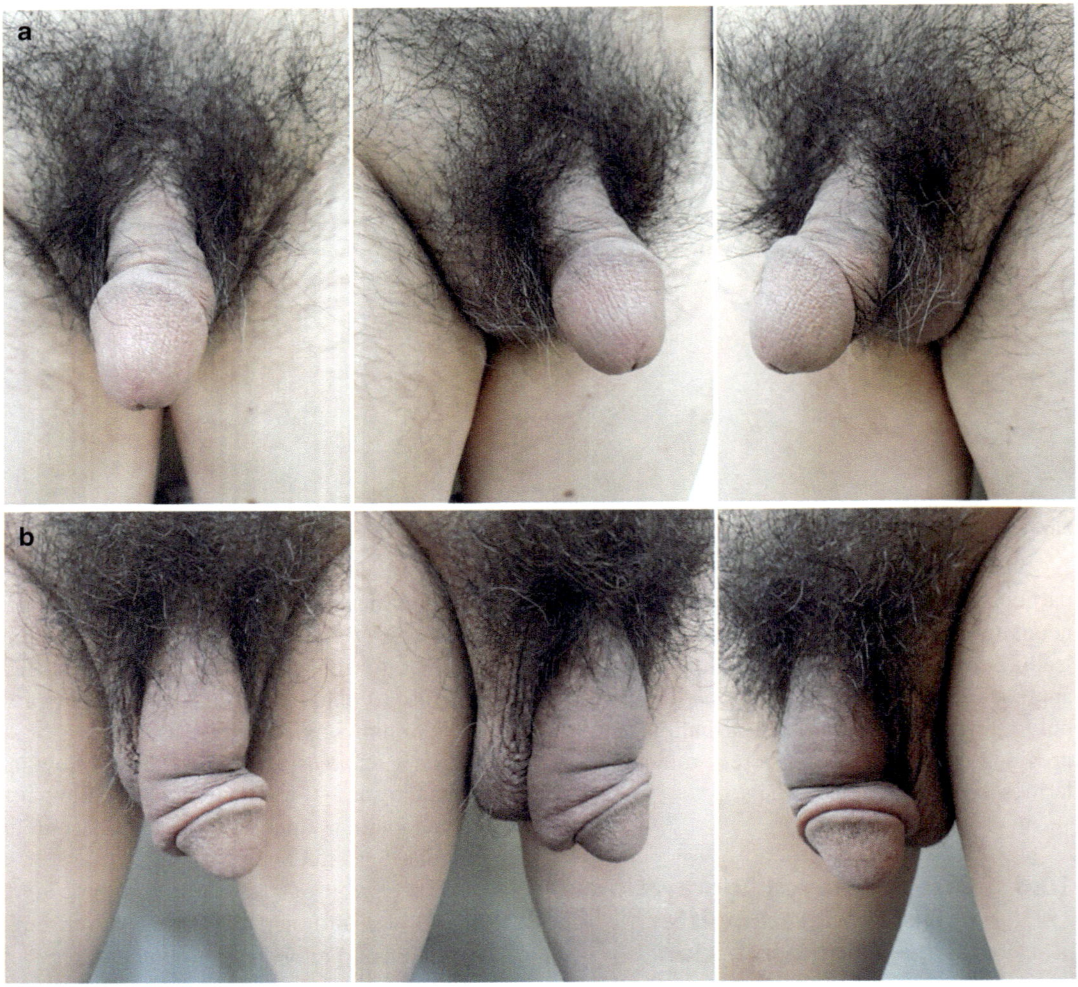

Fig. 10.6 (**a**) Preoperative (**b**) 4 weeks after PGE with HA (**c**) 12 weeks after PGE with HA (**d**) 24 weeks after PGE with HA

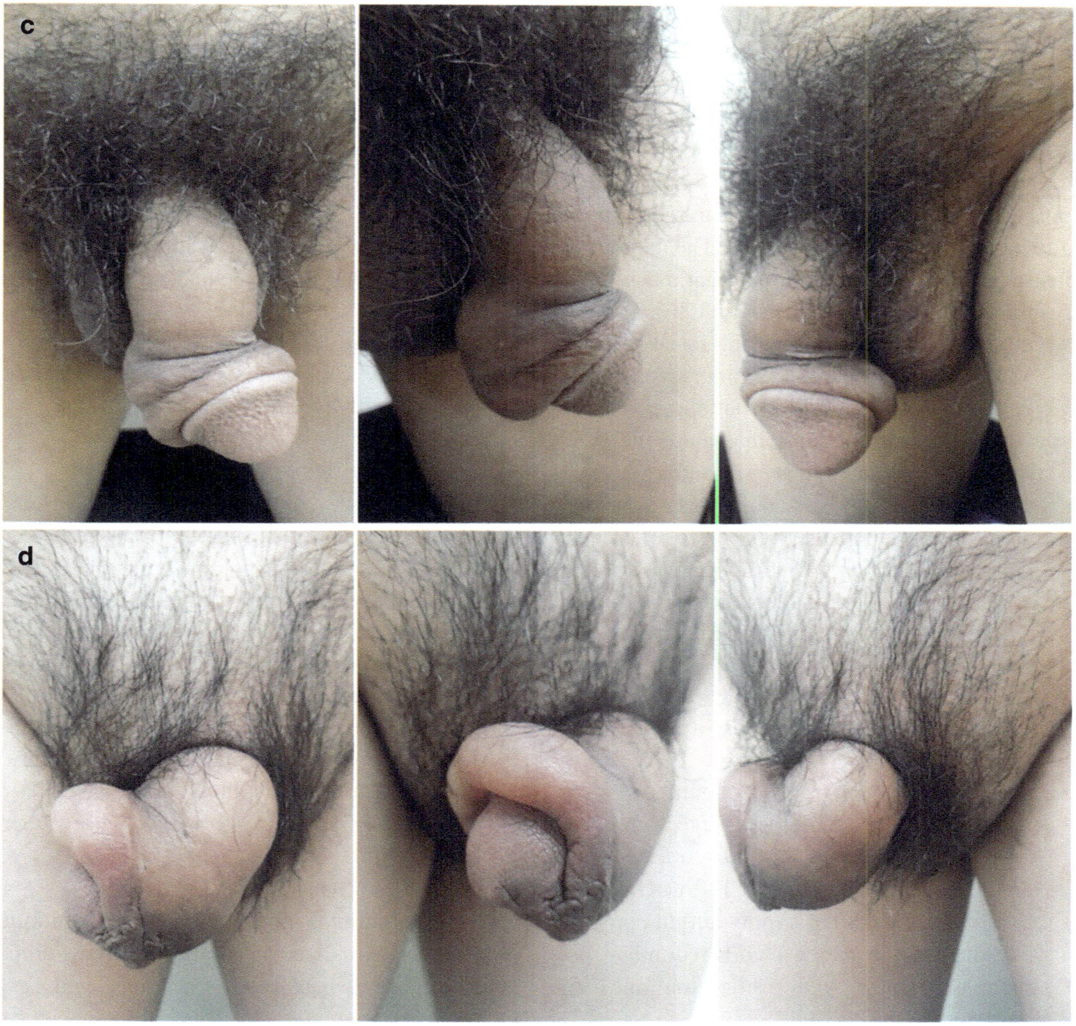

Fig. 10.6 (continued)

- *Manual massage or compressive dressing*: Gentle manual massage, performed under physician guidance, can help distribute the filler evenly and minimize localized accumulation. Alternatively, applying a compressive dressing may assist in maintaining a uniform contour and preventing early migration.
- *Patient instructions*: Patients should be advised to avoid vigorous physical activity, sexual intercourse, and excessive manipulation of the penis during the initial healing phase.
- *Monitoring and early intervention*: Scheduled follow-up visits within the first 2 weeks allow for early identification and correction of minor irregularities through gentle molding or, if necessary, small-volume touch-ups.

Effective postinjection management not only improves aesthetic outcomes but also enhances long-term stability of the augmented contour.

10.7 Case 7: Postinjection Care and Long-Term Stability in a 54-Year-Old Male

A 54-year-old male underwent penile augmentation with 15 cc of HA filler (Fig. 10.7a). Immediate post-procedure evaluation demonstrated a smooth and uniform contour (Fig. 10.7b). The patient was instructed to perform gentle manual massage for 5 min twice daily during the first week and to wear a light compressive dressing for 3–5 days.

At the 4-week follow-up, minor irregularities were noted at the midshaft, but these resolved spontaneously with continued massage (Fig. 10.7c). Subsequent assessments at 12 and 24 weeks showed excellent contour stability and no evidence of migration or asymmetry (Fig. 10.7d, e).

This case highlights the importance of structured postinjection management in promoting even filler distribution and maintaining long-term aesthetic outcomes.

Key Recommendations for Postinjection Management

- *Gentle manual massage*: Encourage patients to perform light, guided massage to promote even filler distribution and correct minor asymmetries during the first 1–2 weeks.
- *Compressive dressing*: Apply a light compressive dressing in patients with redundant prepuce to inhibit filler migration into the subpreputial space.
- *Activity restrictions*: Advise patients to avoid vigorous sexual activity, intense physical exertion, or mechanical pressure on the penis during the initial healing phase to facilitate optimal filler integration.

Clinical Pearls for Achieving Symmetry

"Gradual build-up and meticulous technique are key to achieving symmetry and avoiding the 'Tacobell-like' deformity."

3. Injection Technique and Injector Selection

The choice of injection technique and injector selection plays a crucial role in achieving optimal filler distribution, minimizing complications, and ensuring patient satisfaction. Equally important is the strategy for retouching, which should be approached with careful planning.

Retouching Strategy

- *Staged augmentation*: Multiple small-volume sessions (typically 2–3) are strongly preferred over a single large-volume injection. This approach allows for progressive enhancement, better tissue adaptation, and reduced risk of migration or asymmetry.
- *Patient counseling*: Patients should be informed during pre-procedure consultations that retouch sessions are an integral part of the treatment plan. This sets realistic expectations and fosters long-term satisfaction.

By combining a precise injection technique with an individualized retouching strategy, clinicians can achieve superior symmetry and aesthetic outcomes.

3. Long-Term Considerations
   - Complementary retouch at 2 years to maintain volume and correct minor irregularities.

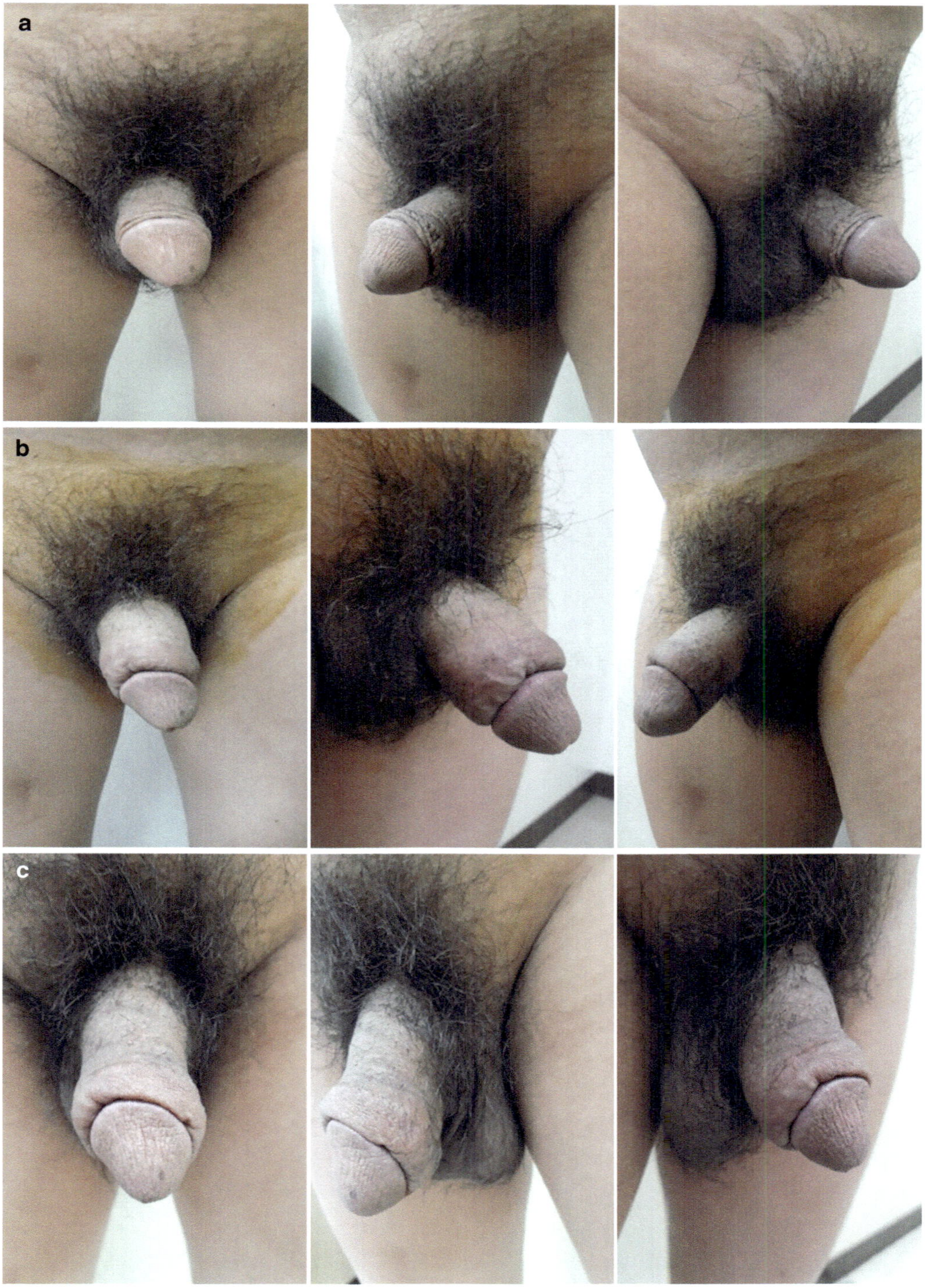

Fig. 10.7 (**a**) Before operation (**b**) Immediate after PGE with HA (**c**) 4 weeks after PGE with HA (**d**) 12 weeks after PGE with HA (**e**) 24 weeks after PGE with HA (**f**) Minor volume reduction and contour softening at the 54-week visit (**g**) Immediate after first retouch at December 24, 2018 (**h**) 4 weeks after first retouch, 2019-01-29 (**i**) 24 weeks after first retouch, 2019-06-03 (**j**) 48 weeks after first retouch. 2019-11-15 (**k**) 54 weeks after first retouch, 2020-01-13 (**l**) second retouch at January 13, 2020

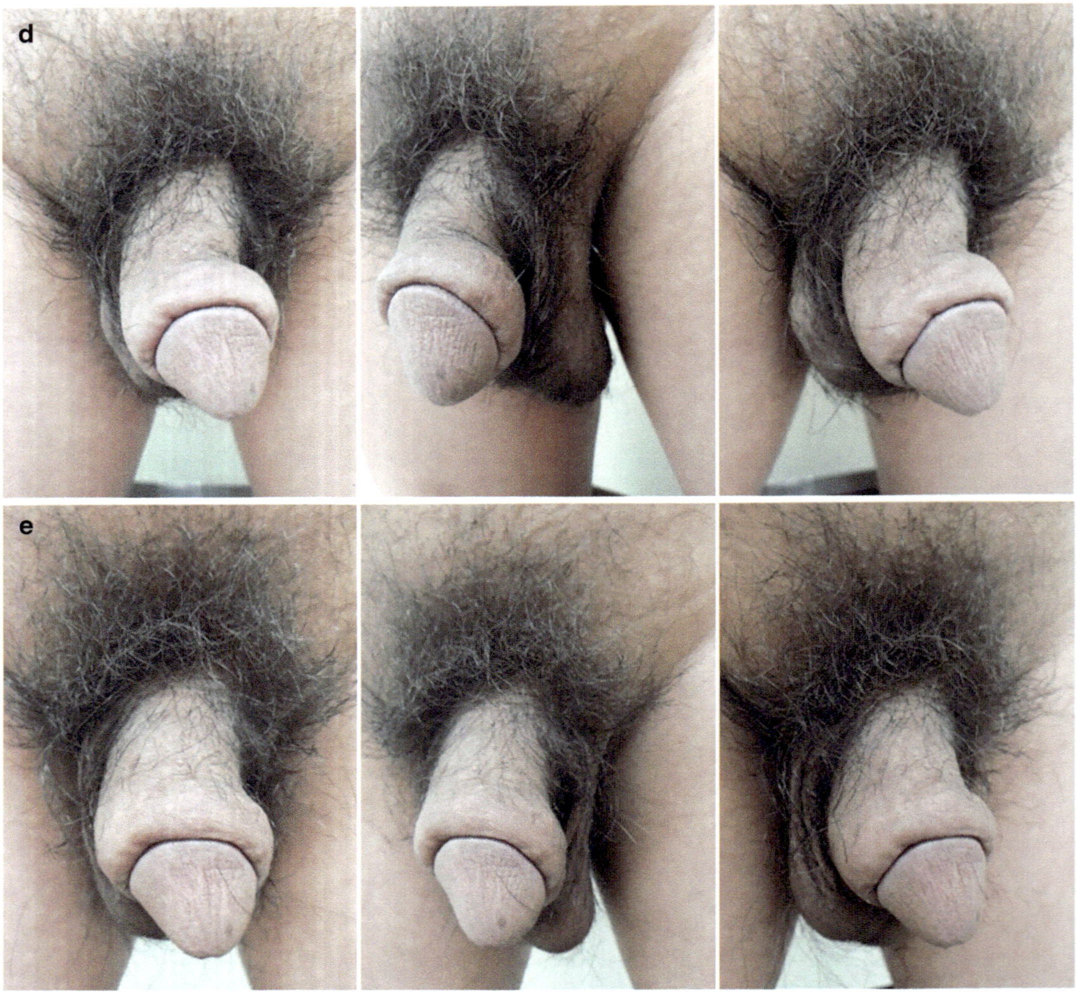

Fig. 10.7 (continued)

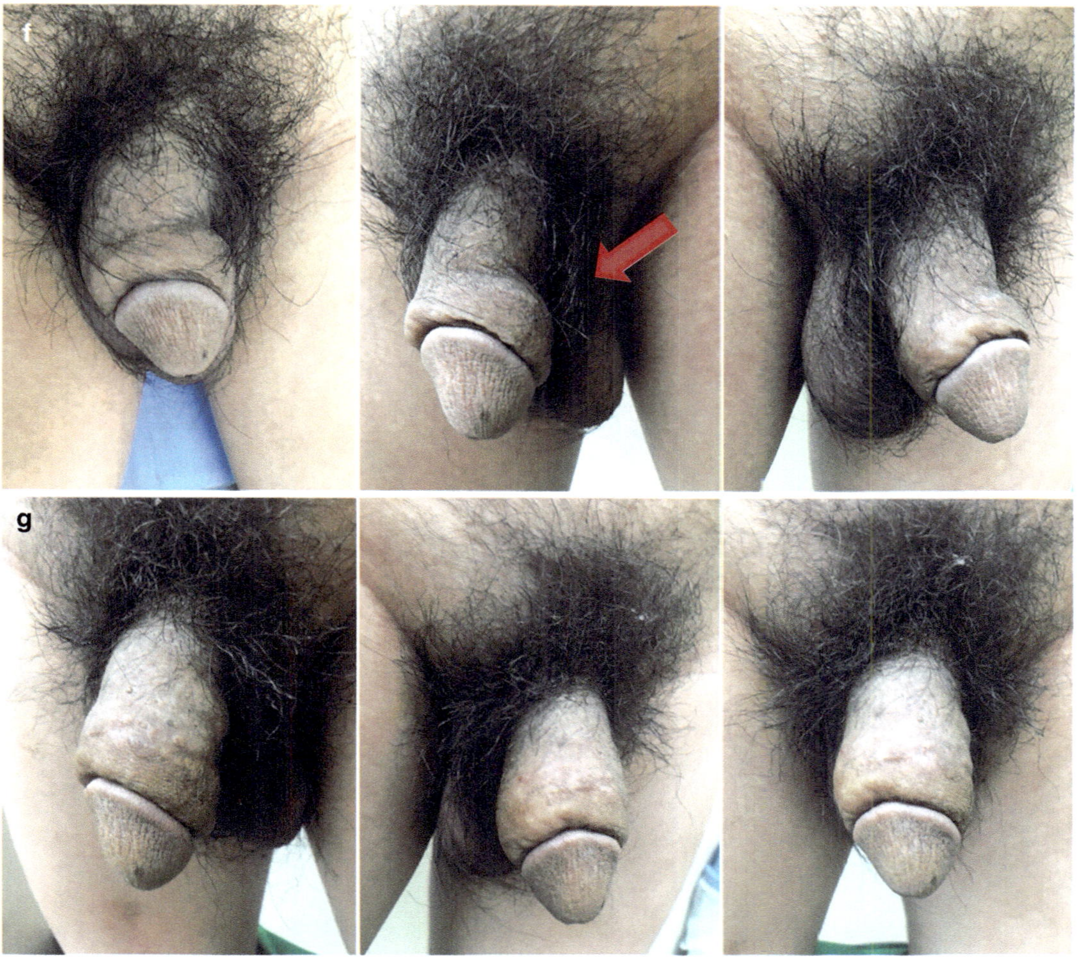

Fig. 10.7 (continued)

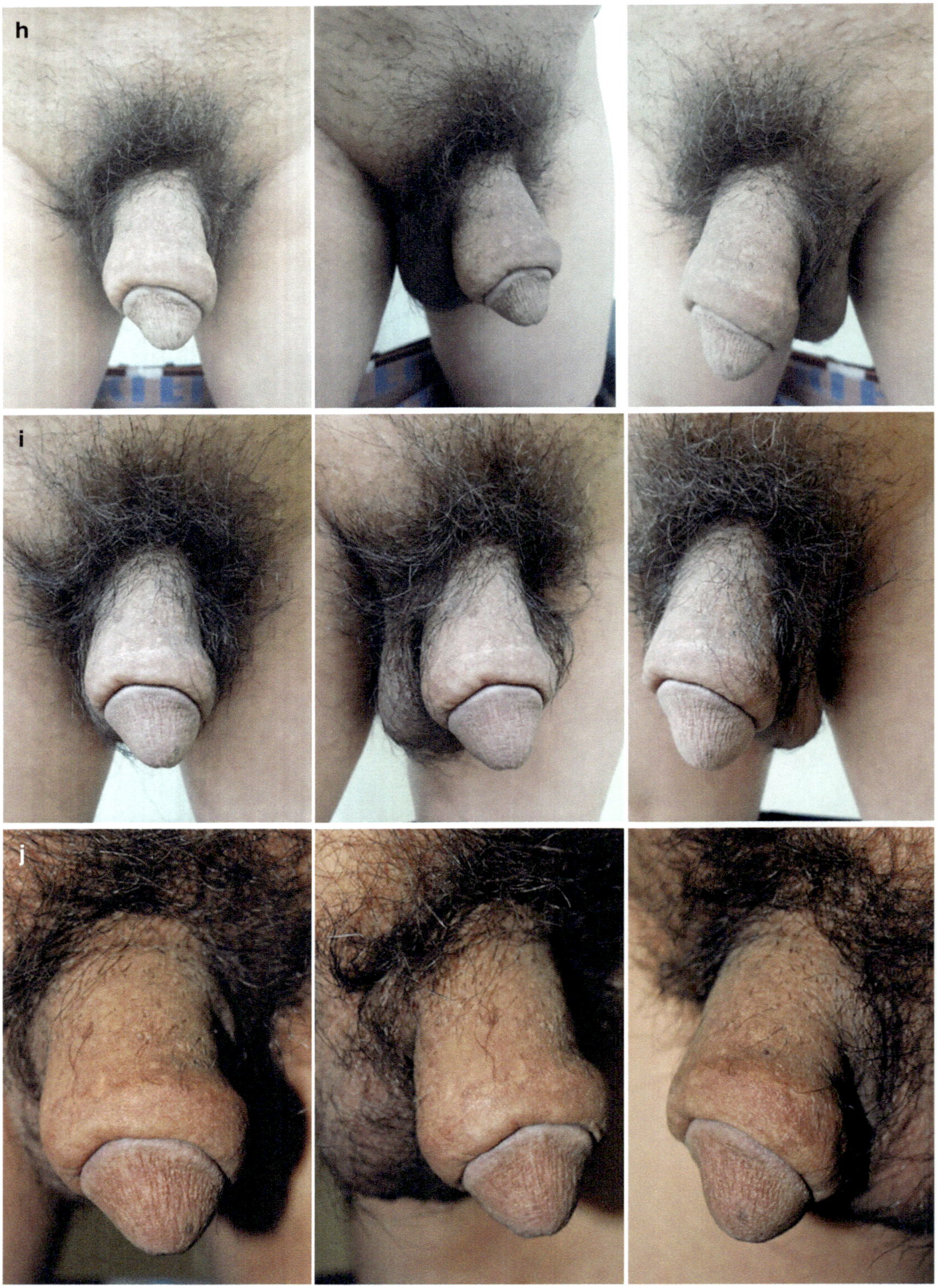

Fig. 10.7 (continued)

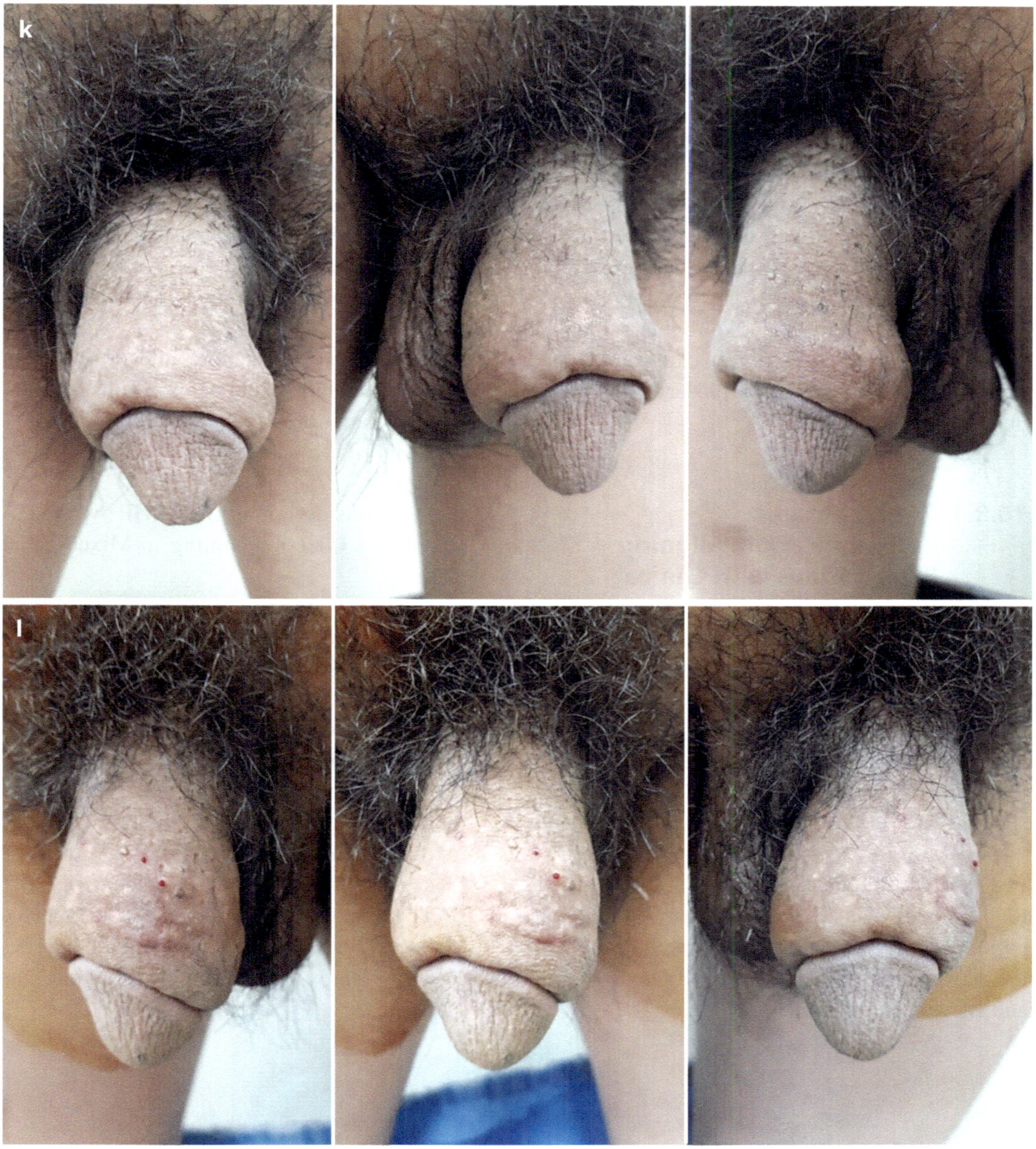

Fig. 10.7 (continued)

10.8 Case 7.1: Postinjection Care and Long-Term Retouching in a 54-Year-Old Male

A 54-year-old male underwent penile augmentation with 15 cc of HA filler at December 18, 2017 (Fig. 10.7a). Immediate post-procedure assessment revealed a smooth and uniform contour (Fig. 10.7b). The patient was instructed to perform gentle manual massage twice daily for 1 week and to wear a light compressive dressing for 3–5 days.

At the 4-week follow-up, minor midshaft irregularities were noted, which resolved with continued massage (Fig. 10.7c). Subsequent assessments at 12 and 24 weeks showed excellent contour stability without evidence of migration or asymmetry (Fig. 10.7d, e).

The patient was followed up to 48 weeks and demonstrated sustained satisfactory volume and symmetry. However, minor volume reduction and contour softening became evident at the 54-week visit at December 24, 2018 (Fig. 10.7f). A second retouch session was performed at this time, restoring the desired girth and correcting subtle irregularities (Fig. 10.7g, h, i, j, k, l).

This extended follow-up highlights the importance of structured postinjection care and planned maintenance retouching to preserve long-term outcomes.

10.8.1 Proper Patient Communication: Aligning Expectations with Clinical Reality

Patients undergoing penile augmentation often desire larger volumes than are medically advisable. However, overcorrection with excessive filler increases the risk of migration, asymmetry, and long-term contour deformities. Final refinements should therefore be carefully planned and openly discussed during pre-procedure consultations.

Clear communication and realistic goal setting are critical to ensuring patient satisfaction, particularly in balancing patient aspirations with the physician's professional assessment of safe and sustainable outcomes.

10.9 Case 8: Photo Presentation of PGE with HA and HA Reinjection at 1-Year Follow-Up in a 39-Year-Old Male (Fig. 10.8)

Summary of Key Principles

- Choose the right HA filler—balance between longevity and safety.
- Consider circumcision in patients with redundant prepuce.
- Avoid large single-volume injections—gradual enhancements yield better results.
- Educate patients on realistic outcomes and the necessity of retouch sessions.

4. Other Considerations for PGE with HA Filler: HA Injection Timing in Mixed-Filler Cases
    - Generally, mixed injection of different fillers is not recommended due to difficulty to find causative filler in case of complication. But mixed injection frequently occurs to increase hardness, compensate deformity, and increase longevity of injected filler.
    - In mixed injection, HA should always be injected after non-HA fillers or after the degradation of the non-HA filler.
    - This sequencing prevents unexpected interactions between different filler types and ensures optimal integration into the tissue.

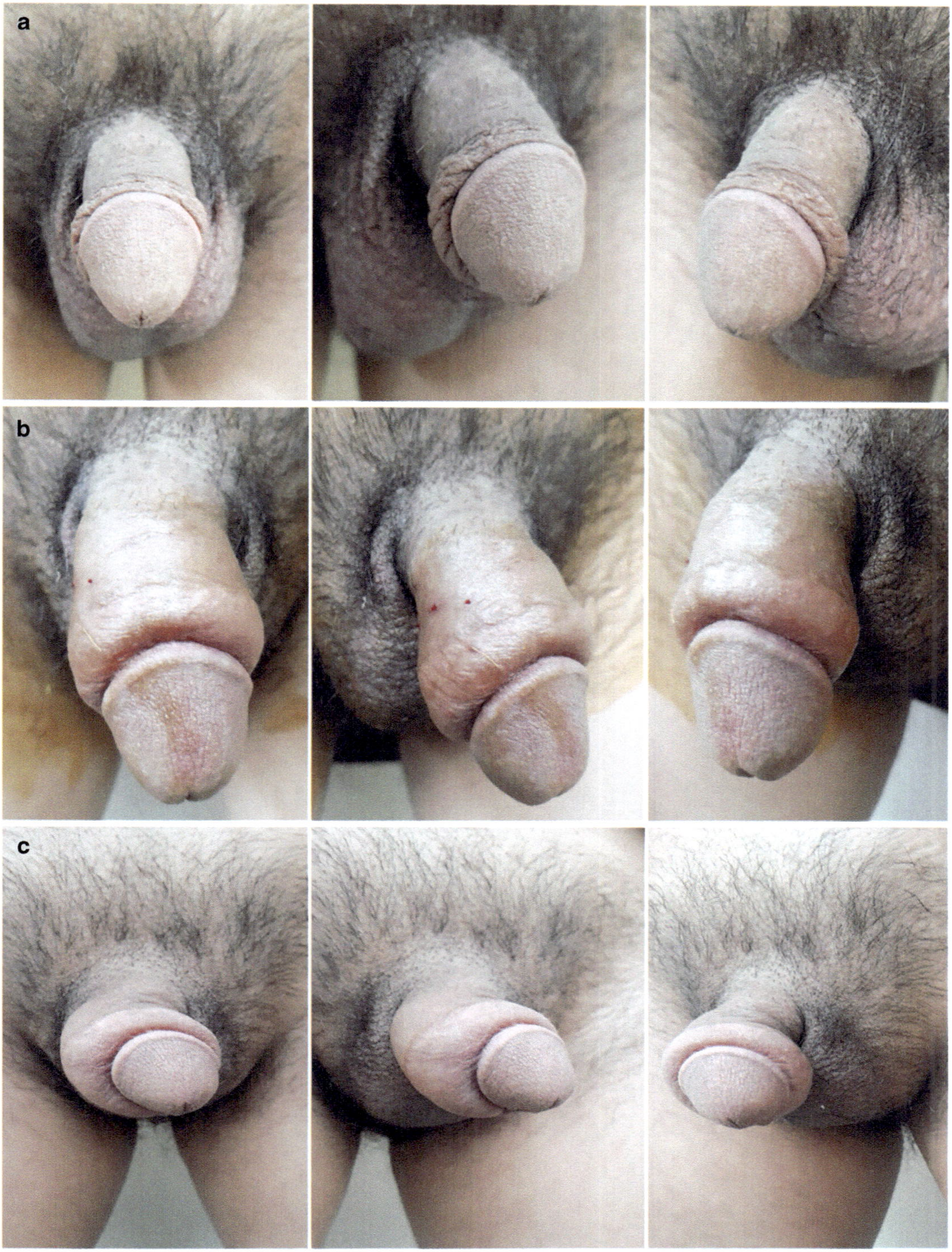

Fig. 10.8 (**a**) Preoperative picture of the penis at 2018-02-07 (**b**) Immediate postoperative picture shows symmetric weel enlarged penile girth (**c**) 4 weeks after PGE with HA shows a little asymmetry due to distal migration (**d**) Prominent distal migration with a little asymmetry at 12 weeks after PGE (**e**) Stabilized morphology of enhance penile girth at 24 weeks after PGE (**f**) Prominent distal rim but much decreased proximal penile body at 48 weeks (**g**) first retouch enhanced volume of penile girth at 48 weeks after initial PGE (**h**) 4 weeks after first retouch shows well-enhanced volume at 2019-03-04 (**i**) 24 weeks after first retouch shows natural appearance of enhanced penis at 2019-07-08

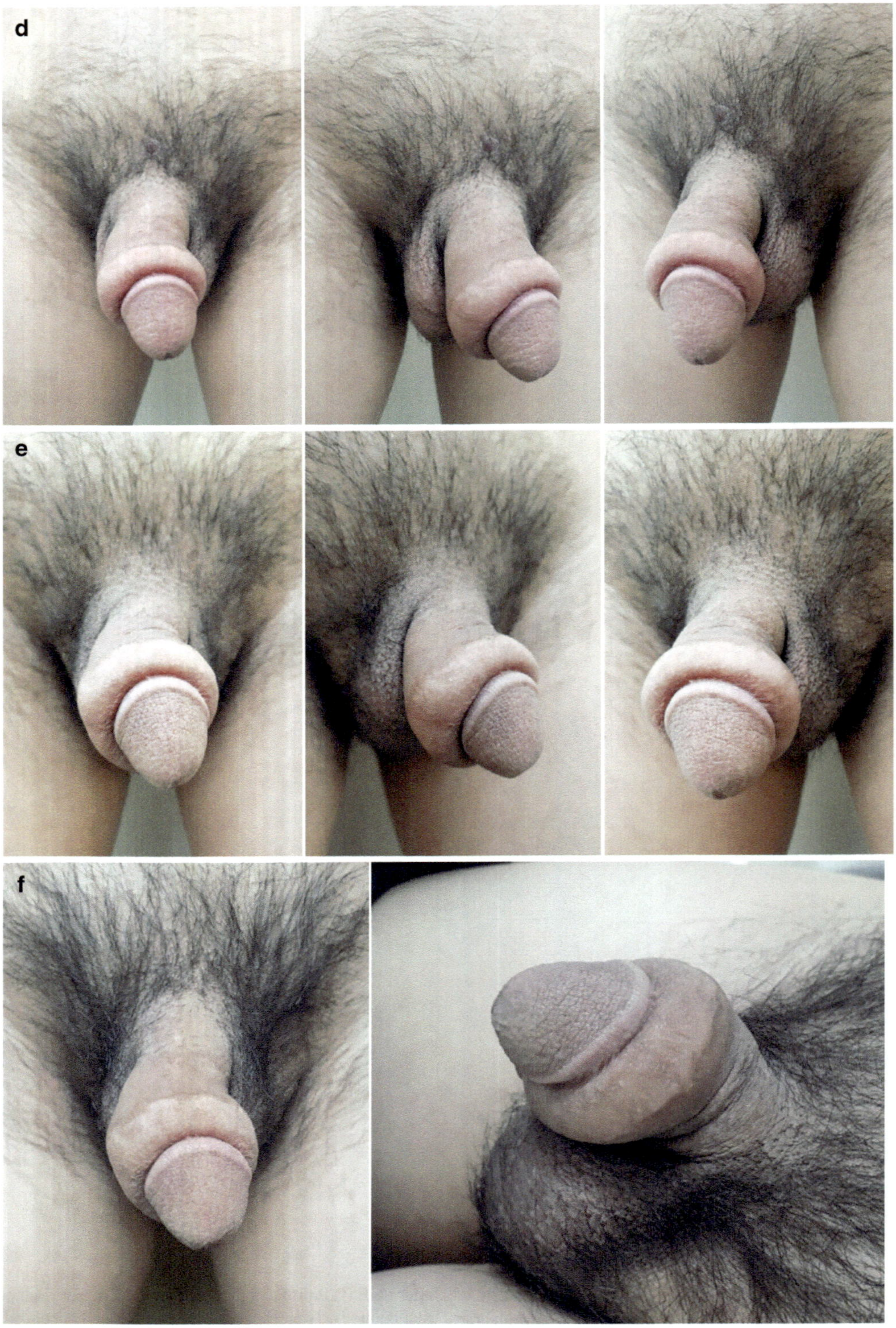

Fig. 10.8 (continued)

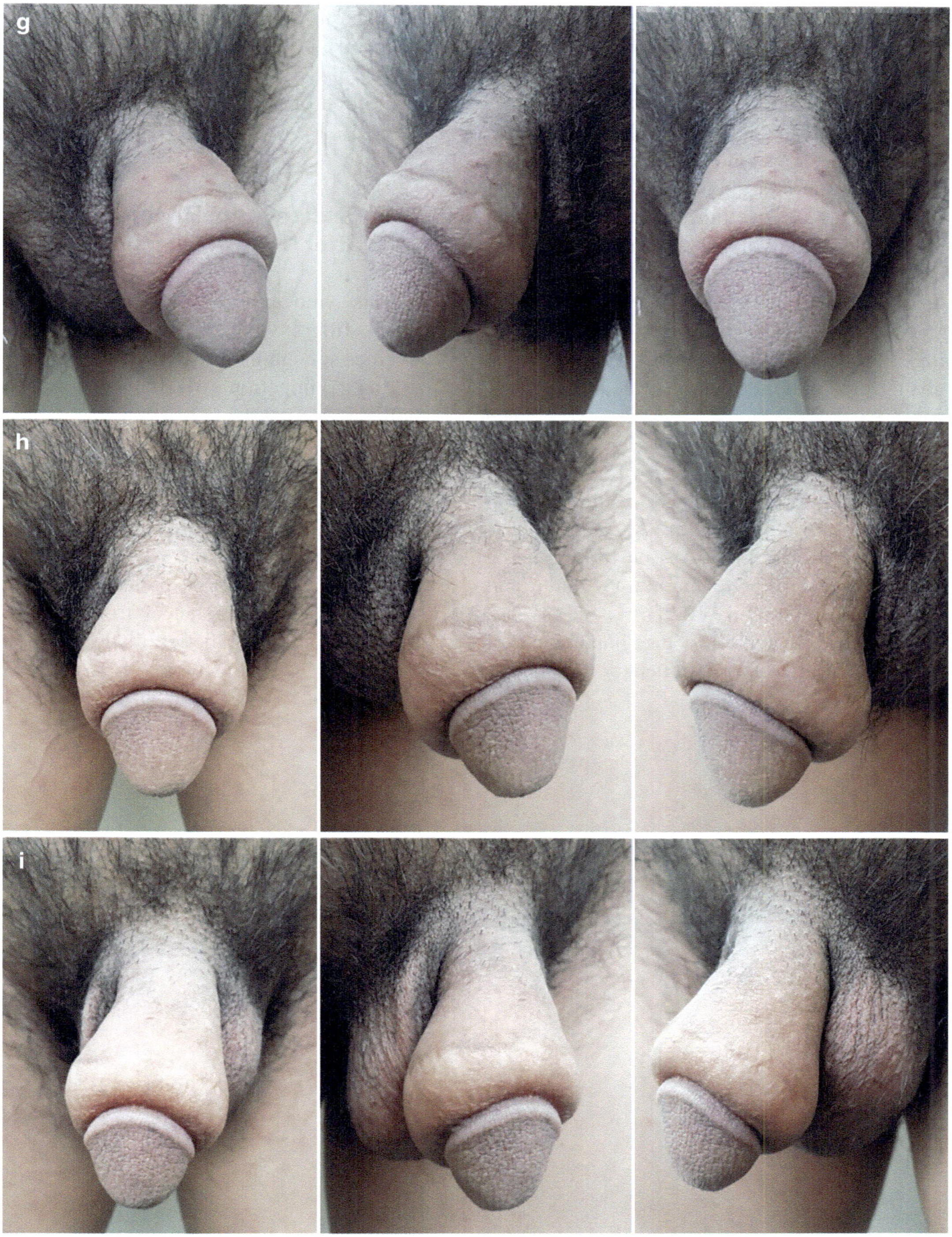

Fig. 10.8 (continued)

10.10 Case 9: HA Injection Following Non-HA Filler for Long-Term Augmentation

A 42-year-old male presented for penile augmentation after previously receiving a non-HA filler injection and glans augmentation by fat transfer at local clinic. Initial evaluation revealed residual volume and acceptable rigidity, but with contour irregularities and uneven distribution (Fig. 10.9a).

At 4 weeks postoperatively, following HA injection to correct deformities and enhance girth, the patient demonstrated improved penile symmetry and a more natural appearance until 24 weeks after operation (Fig. 10.9b–d). Long-term follow-up at 48 weeks showed sustained results without complications (Fig. 10.9e). At that time, a planned retouch session was performed using additional HA filler to maintain volume and refine the contour (Fig. 10.9f).

This case underscores the importance of injecting HA after non-HA fillers or their degradation, ensuring safe integration and predictable results in mixed-filler scenarios.

5. Reinjection of HA in Patients with Previous PLA (e.g., Powerfill®)

10.10.1 Challenges of HA Injection After Non-HA Fillers

- Patients who previously received PLA-based fillers (e.g., Powerfill®) often develop subcutaneous fibrous adhesions, making reinjection of HA technically challenging.
- Due to these adhesions, standard 18G cannula techniques may not be ideal.

Recommended Injection Approach

- Instead of an 18G cannula, a 27G needle with multiple small injections is preferred.
- This minimizes resistance from fibrous adhesions, allowing better distribution of HA.

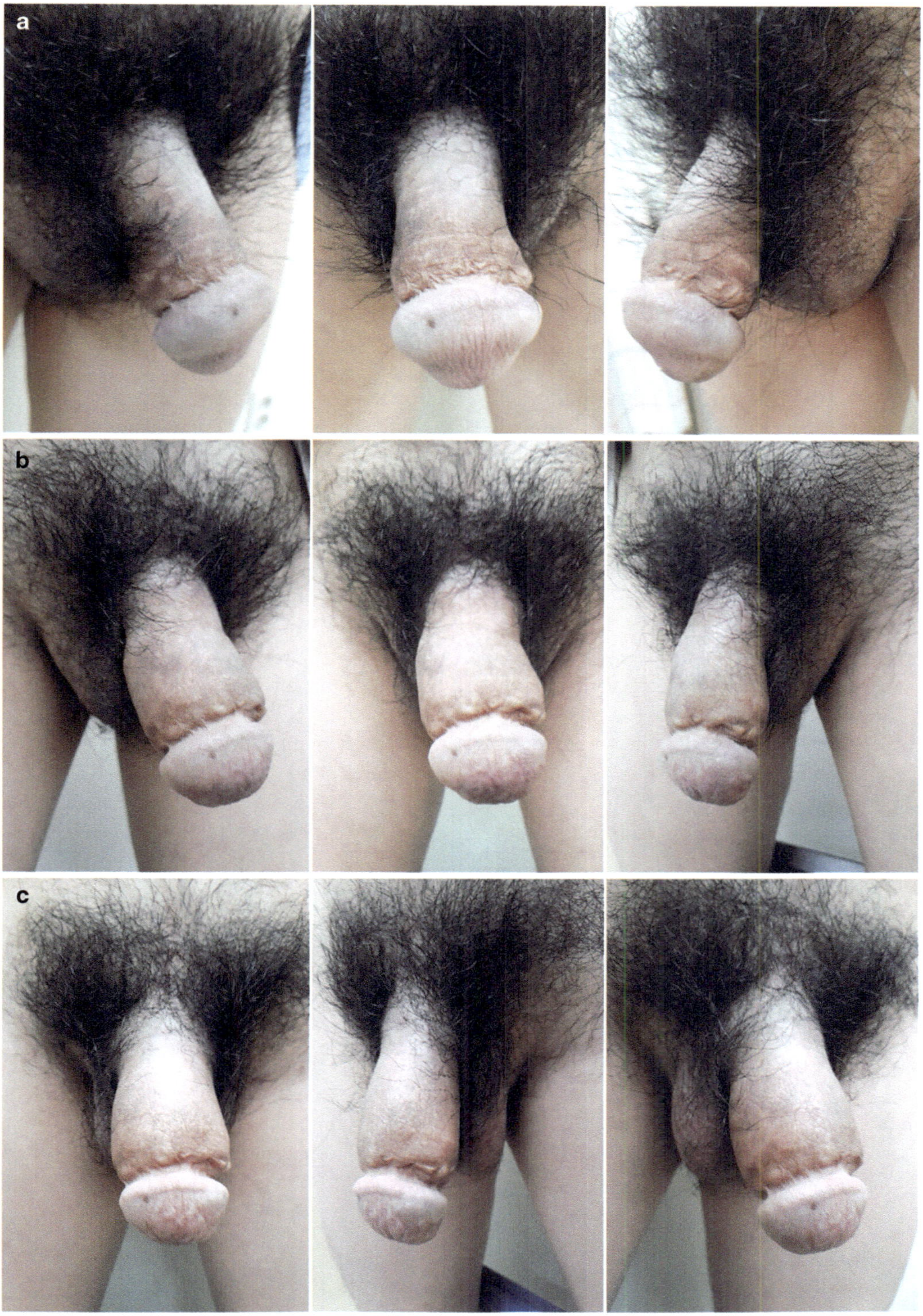

Fig. 10.9 (**a**) Preoperative picture (**b**) At 4 weeks after HA injection for PGE and GPA, improved penile symmetry and a more natural appearance of penile body and glans penis (**c**) 12 weeks (**d**) 24 weeks (**e**) 48 weeks (**f**) Immediate after first retouch for PGE with HA (**g**) injection technique and video clip

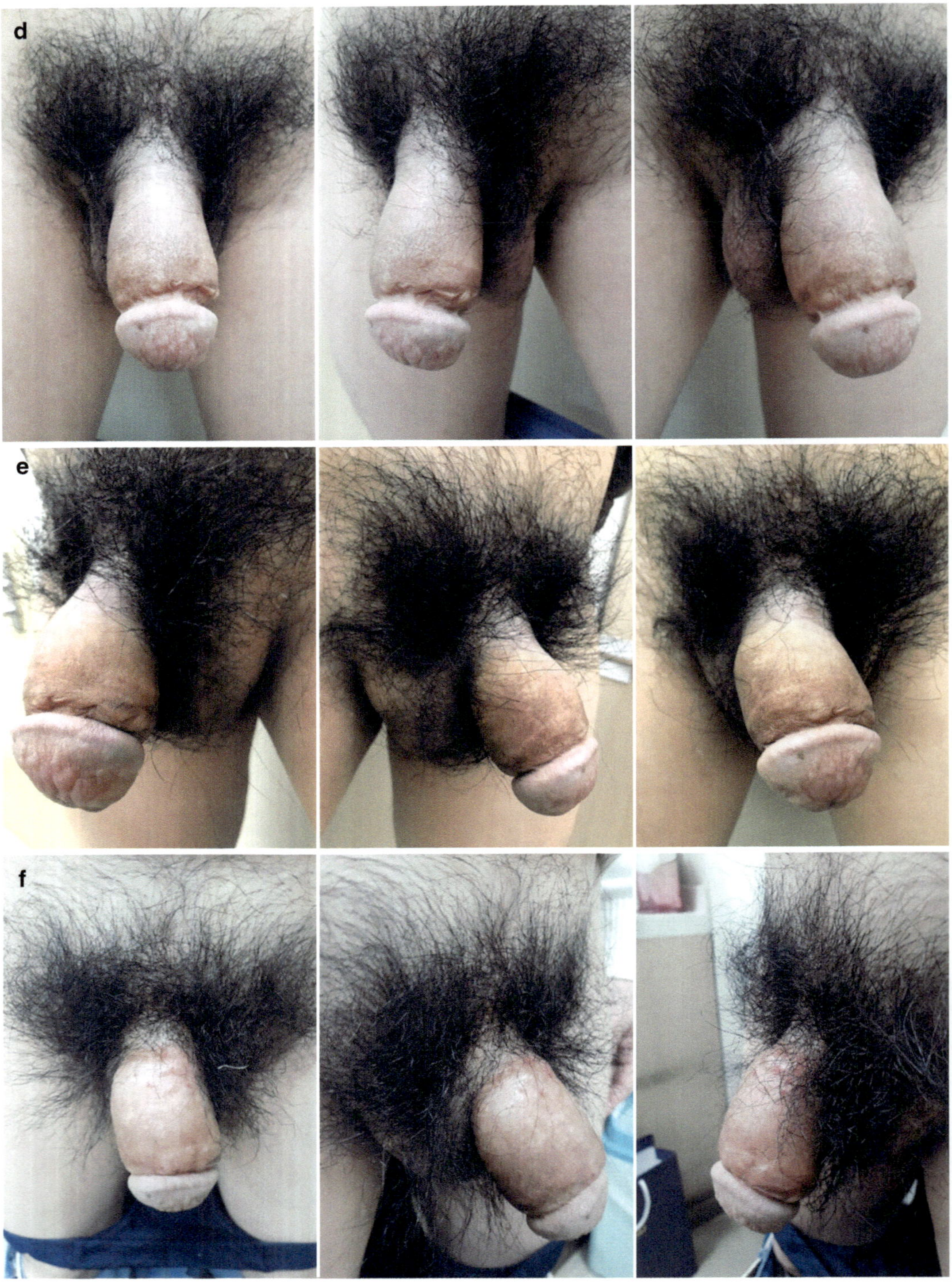

Fig. 10.9 (continued)

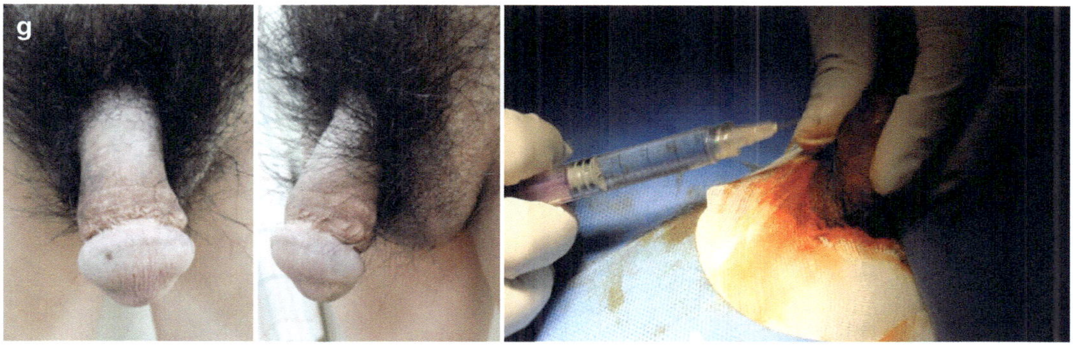

Fig. 10.9 (continued)

10.11 Case 10: Managing PLA History and HA Reinjection in a 42-Year-Old Male

A 42-year-old male with a history of PLA-based filler (Powerfill®) presented for further penile augmentation and correction of glans asymmetric deformity by GPA with fat. Initial evaluation revealed residual PLA material with contour irregularities and fibrous adhesions (Fig. 10.10a). HA filler was carefully injected after the PLA to enhance volume and improve symmetry, using a modified approach to minimize interaction between the two fillers (Fig. 10.10b). At the 4-week follow-up, results were satisfactory with improved aesthetic outcomes (Fig. 10.10c).

At 48 weeks, the patient returned for maintenance augmentation. Reinjection posed technical challenges due to subcutaneous fibrous adhesions from the previous PLA filler, which increased tissue resistance. To address this, a 27G needle was used for multiple small-volume HA deposits, enabling bypass of fibrotic bands and more uniform distribution (Video 10.1, Fig. 10.10c). Post-reinjection assessment confirmed successful correction with enhanced penile contour and patient satisfaction.

This case demonstrates the importance of proper sequencing (HA after non-HA filler) and modifying techniques (small-gauge needle, fractionated dosing) for reinjection in fibrotic tissue.

10.11.1 Clinical Observations: Reinjection in Powerfill® Patients

Until 6 months of follow-up, the patient reported high satisfaction with both the aesthetic and functional outcomes. The presence of subcutaneous fibrous adhesions from the prior PLA filler appeared to stabilize the newly injected HA, preventing migration or asymmetry. This clinical observation suggests that, although reinjection is technically more challenging, it can result in superior long-term contour stability when performed with appropriate technique.

Key Takeaways: HA Reinjection After PLA (Powerfill®)

- HA should always be injected after non-HA fillers to prevent unpredictable filler behavior.
- Patients with prior PLA injections may present fibrotic adhesions, making HA reinjection technically more difficult.
- Use a 27G needle for multiple small-volume injections to improve ease of administration and ensure even distribution.
- Preexisting fibrotic tissue may act as a stabilizing scaffold, reducing HA migration and supporting contour uniformity.

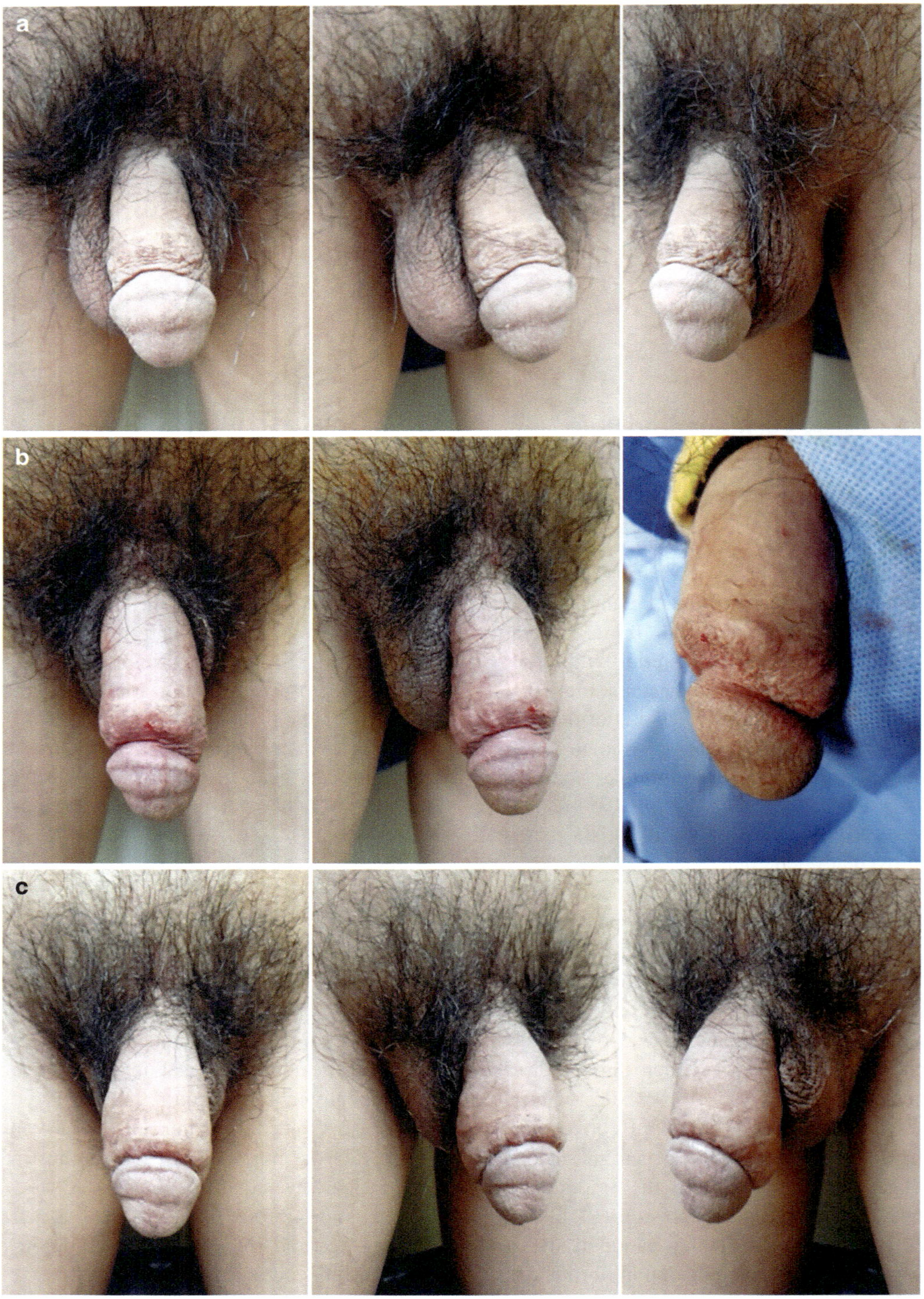

Fig. 10.10 (**a**) Preoperative picture revealed residual PLA material with contour irregularities and glans asymmetry (**b**) Immediate after PGE shows symmetric enlargement of penile girth (**c**) 4 weeks after PGE shows improved volume of penile girth (**d**) 12 weeks after PGE shows natural appearance of penile girth (**e**) 24 weeks after PGE shows natural appearance with maintain volume of girth

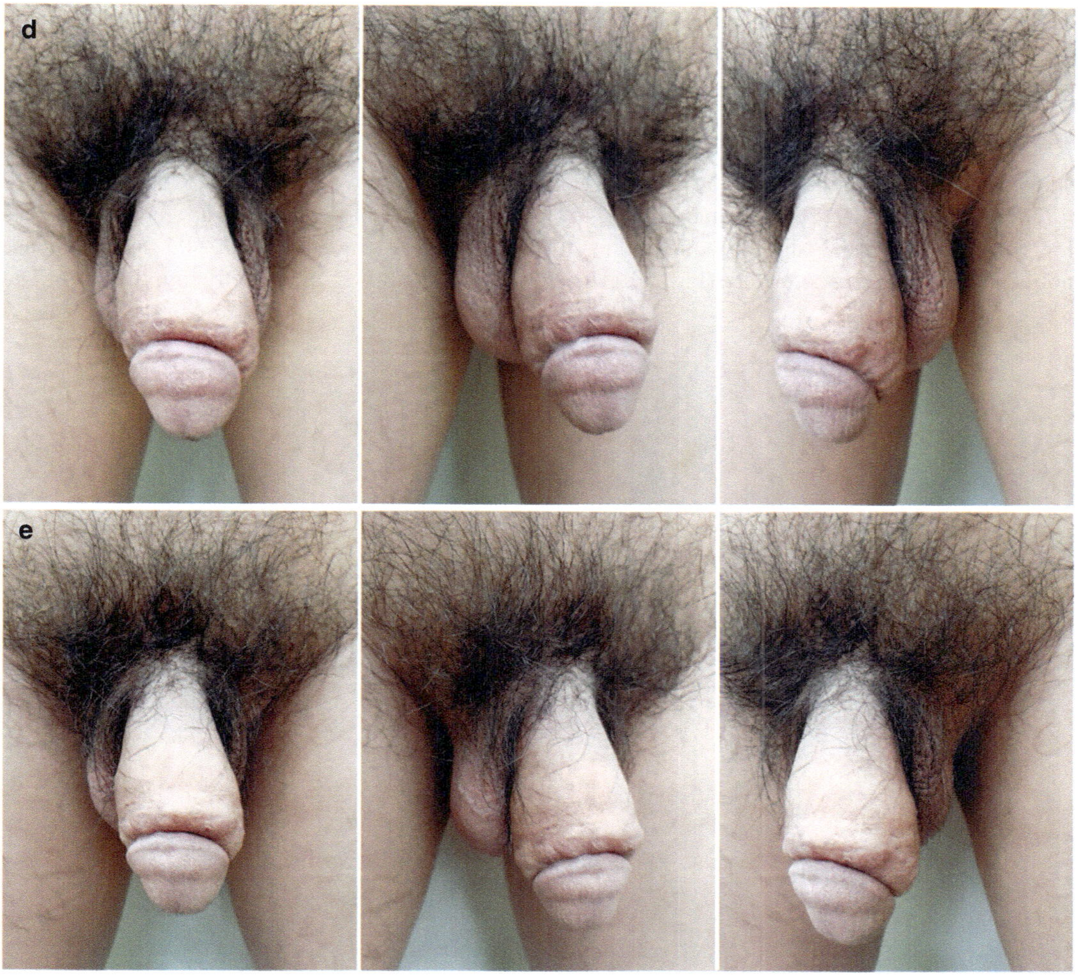

Fig. 10.10 (continued)

4. Remodeling HA Deformity in PGE
   1. Managing Initial Asymmetry and Correction Strategies

      Achieving perfect symmetry in penile girth enhancement (PGE) with HA filler can be challenging, particularly in the early postoperative period. Minor contour irregularities often arise due to uneven filler distribution or variable tissue compliance.

      - Preventive approach: Initial small-volume injections help minimize early asymmetry.

        Starting with small-volume injections during the initial procedure minimizes the risk of overcorrection and facilitates more uniform filler integration. This conservative strategy allows tissue adaptation and creates a stable foundation for subsequent augmentation.
      - Correction methods

        If asymmetry becomes apparent during follow-up, corrective options include:
        – *Retouching with additional HA filler*: Small-volume reinjections can balance uneven areas and restore symmetry.
        – *Hyaluronidase for deformity resolution*: In cases of overcorrection, migrated filler, or persistent nodularity, targeted hyaluronidase administration allows selective HA removal to refine the final contour.

10.12 Case 11: Remodeling HA Asymmetry Over Time in a 41-Year-Old Male

A 41-year-old male enrolled in a PGE clinical study underwent an initial injection of 20 cc HA filler on December 29, 2023. At his 4-week follow-up, he expressed dissatisfaction due to noticeable asymmetric deformity (Fig. 10.11a).

To address the asymmetry, a retouch injection of 10 cc HA was performed 12 weeks after the initial procedure (March 14, 2024) (Fig. 10.11b). While the retouch session improved some irregularities, it resulted in a proximal separated lump observed at 24 weeks (Fig. 10.17d).

At this 6-month follow-up, correction was achieved by injecting 1500 IU hyaluronidase diluted in 1 mL saline directly into the lump. The

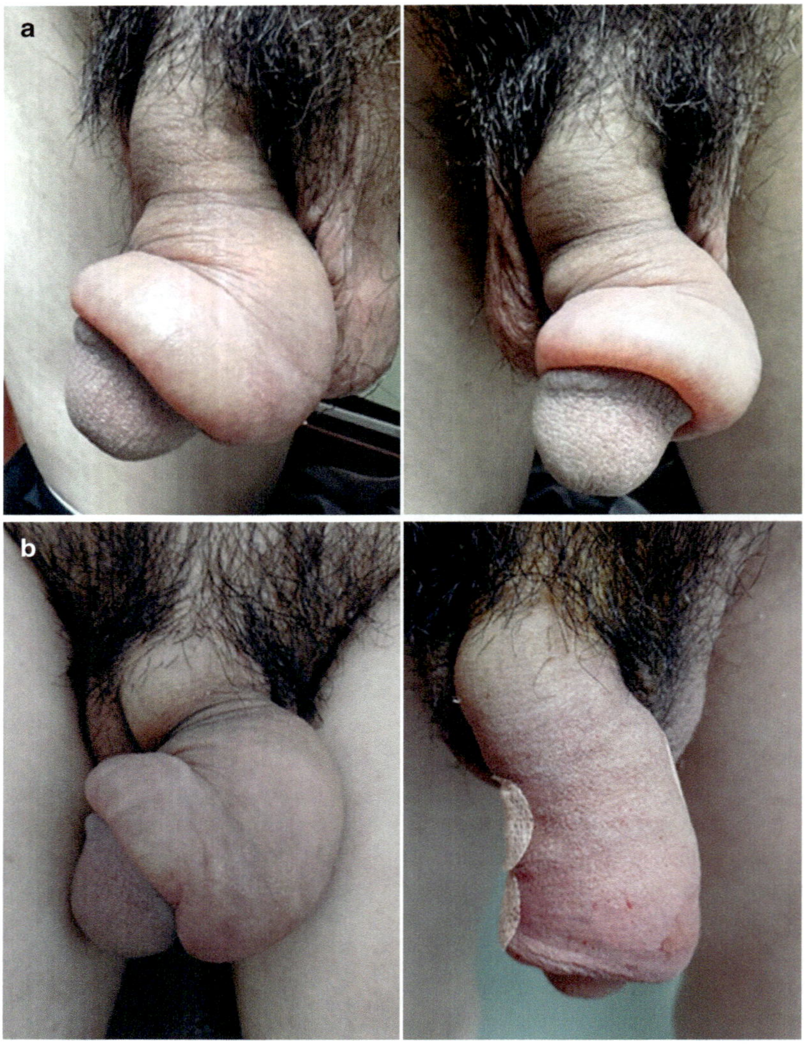

Fig. 10.11 (**a**) Marked distal migration of HA filler and distorted penile body (**b**) Decreased but still distorted penile body at 4 weeks after injection (left), additional 10 cc HA injection corrected deformity (right) (**c**) 24 weeks later, much decreased asymmetry of penile body but two separated proximal and distal lump (**d**) Hyaluronidase injection into proximal lump, video clip (**e**) Complete dissolution of proximal lump within 1 week after hyaluronidase injection

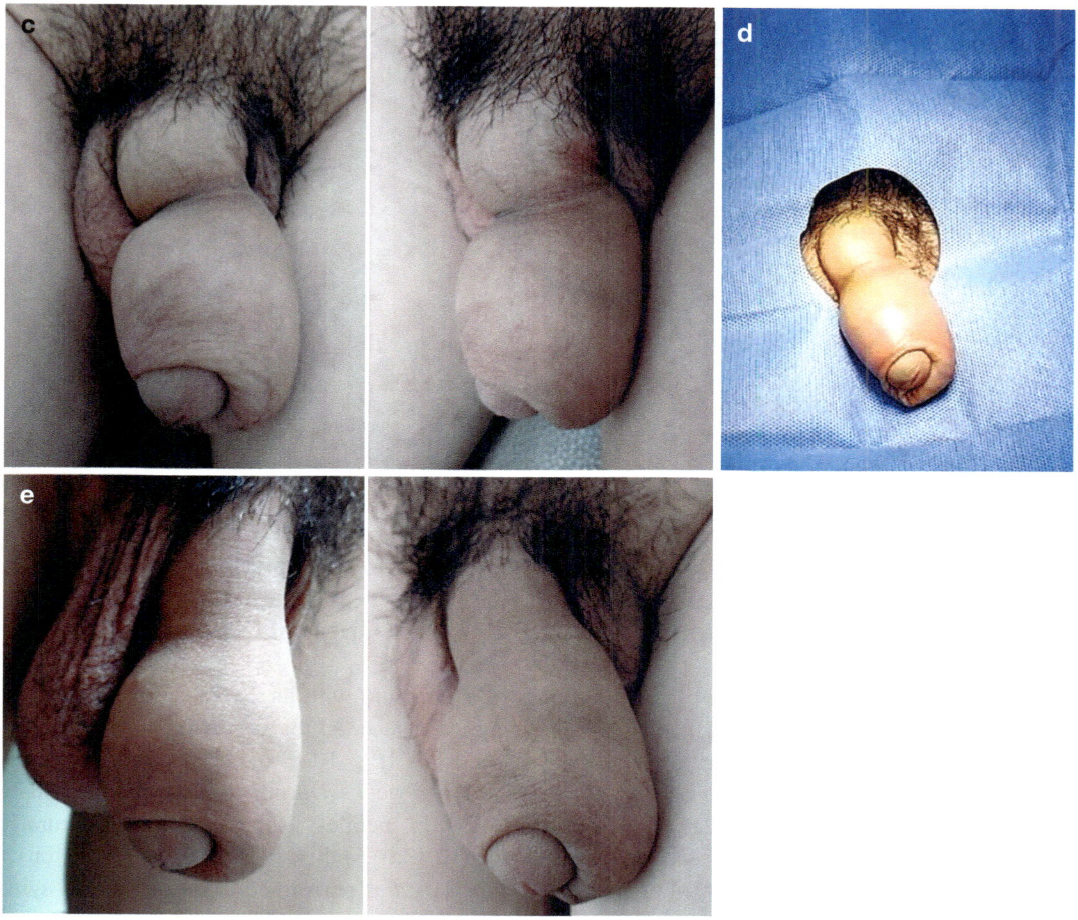

Fig. 10.11 (continued)

intervention completely dissolved the mass within 1 week (Fig. 10.11e). Initially, the patient considered additional hyaluronidase treatment for a left distal lump at 6 months, but he later deferred further intervention, expressing confidence in the procedure and the effectiveness of hyaluronidase.

This case highlights the importance of starting with small-volume injections to reduce early asymmetry and demonstrates how staged retouching combined with hyaluronidase correction can effectively manage complex deformities over time.

2. HA Deformity Correction After Large Initial Volume or Years Postinjection

Although HA fillers are typically expected to biodegrade within 6 months in dermal applications, clinical experience shows that HA can persist for several years when injected into the glans penis or penile shaft. This prolonged retention may be attributed to the unique anatomical characteristics of penile skin, including reduced vascularity and slower tissue turnover compared to facial skin.

Method 1: Puncture and Squeezing Technique

This technique is effective for managing liquefied HA deposits that persist years after the initial injection. By creating multiple punctures with a large-bore needle and applying gentle manual pressure, liquefied filler can be expressed through the puncture sites, reducing localized bulging or nodularity.

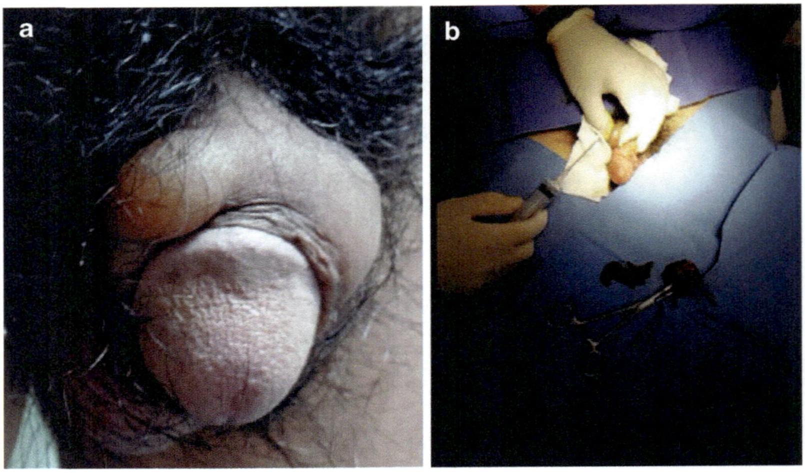

Fig. 10.12 (**a**) Preoperative distal HA lump, (**b**) video clip of puncture and squeezing technique

10.13 Case 12: Correction of a Superficial HA Lump 3.5 Years Postinjection

A patient initially received 22 cc of PLA filler in 2018, followed by an additional 10 cc of HA in 2020. At 3.5 years post-HA injection, he presented with dissatisfaction due to a right distal superficial HA lump (Fig. 10.12a). Correction was performed using the puncture and squeezing technique, resulting in significant improvement of the deformity and patient satisfaction (Fig. 10.12b).

This case illustrates the potential for HA persistence in penile tissues and the utility of simple mechanical techniques for late-stage correction.

Method 1-1: Retouch After Skin Retraction
In cases where significant liquefied HA is expressed using the puncture and squeezing technique, observation is necessary to allow the stretched skin to retract naturally before any further intervention. Attempting immediate retouch may lead to overcorrection or irregularities due to unstable skin tension.

10.14 Case 12 (Continued): Staged Correction and Retouching for Optimal Outcome

After puncture with an 18G needle and manual squeezing successfully expressed most of the liquefied HA (Fig 10.13b), the patient was monitored for 4 weeks. During this time, the previously extended penile skin retracted naturally (Fig. 10.13c). At this stage, a retouch injection of 10 cc HA was performed to restore penile symmetry and volume (Fig. 10.13d). The patient reported high satisfaction with the final result and no recurrence of lumps or irregularities.

This staged approach demonstrates the effectiveness of combining mechanical removal with delayed retouching to achieve optimal aesthetic and functional outcomes.

Method 2: HA Removal Using Hyaluronidase
Hyaluronidase offers a simple and effective solution for removing residual HA filler, even several years after injection. It is particularly useful for addressing asymmetry, nodularity, or overcorrection when mechanical techniques are not feasible.

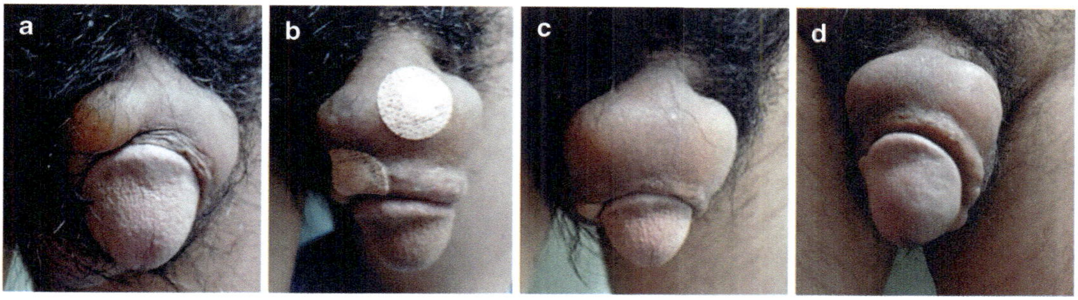

Fig. 10.13 (**a**) Residual bullae of HA, (**b**) a little retracted skin, (**c**, **d**) a retouch of HA restored penile body symmetry and volume

10.15 Case 13: Long-Term HA Remnant Removal in a 54-Year-Old Male

A 54-year-old male presented with dissatisfaction due to left-sided asymmetric residual HA following two Potenfill injections: 20 cc on November 16, 2017 and 10 cc between April and July 2019. At 4–6 years postinjection, he exhibited palpable HA deposits and contour irregularity (Fig. 10.14a, pretreatment).

Correction was achieved by injecting 1500 IU hyaluronidase diluted in 1 mL saline directly into the affected area (Fig. 10.14b, hyaluronidase injection; Video 10.2). The residual HA began softening within 3 days, with complete dissolution observed within 1 week (Fig. 10.14c).

At follow-up, the patient requested restoration of penile girth. Reinjection of HA filler was performed, and results immediately after injection and 48 weeks post-reinjection demonstrated excellent symmetry and volume retention (Fig. 10.14d). The patient reported high satisfaction and no recurrence of asymmetry or irregularities.

This case highlights the effectiveness of hyaluronidase in managing long-standing HA deformities and underscores the importance of staged correction before reinjection for optimal outcomes.

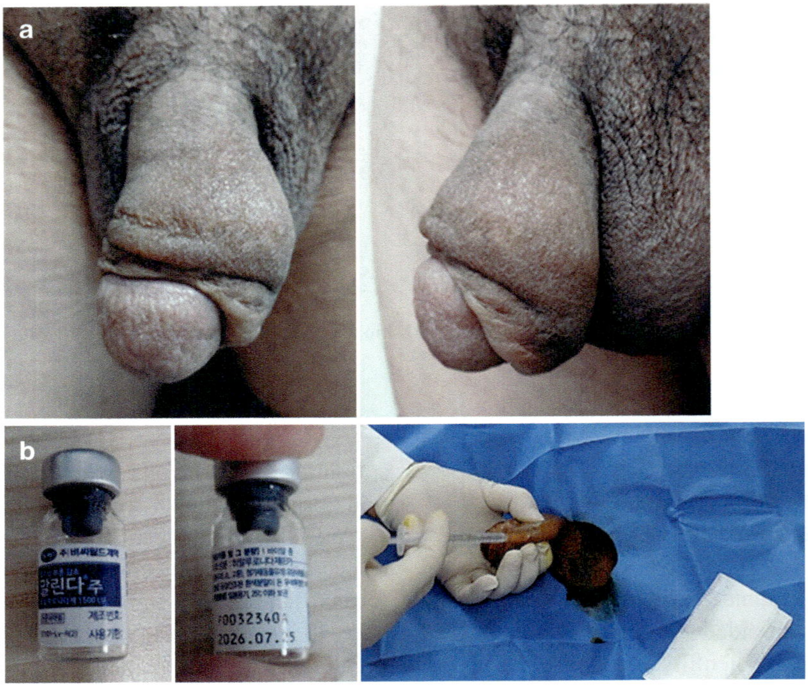

Fig. 10.14 (**a**) Pretreatment photo shows asymmetric remnant of penile body (**b**) Injection of hyaluronidase (**c**) Compared to left picture, almost complete dissolution of HA remnant in middle and right (**d**) Reinjection of HA (Left) and 48 weeks after injection (middle and right) shows symmetrical enhanced penile girth

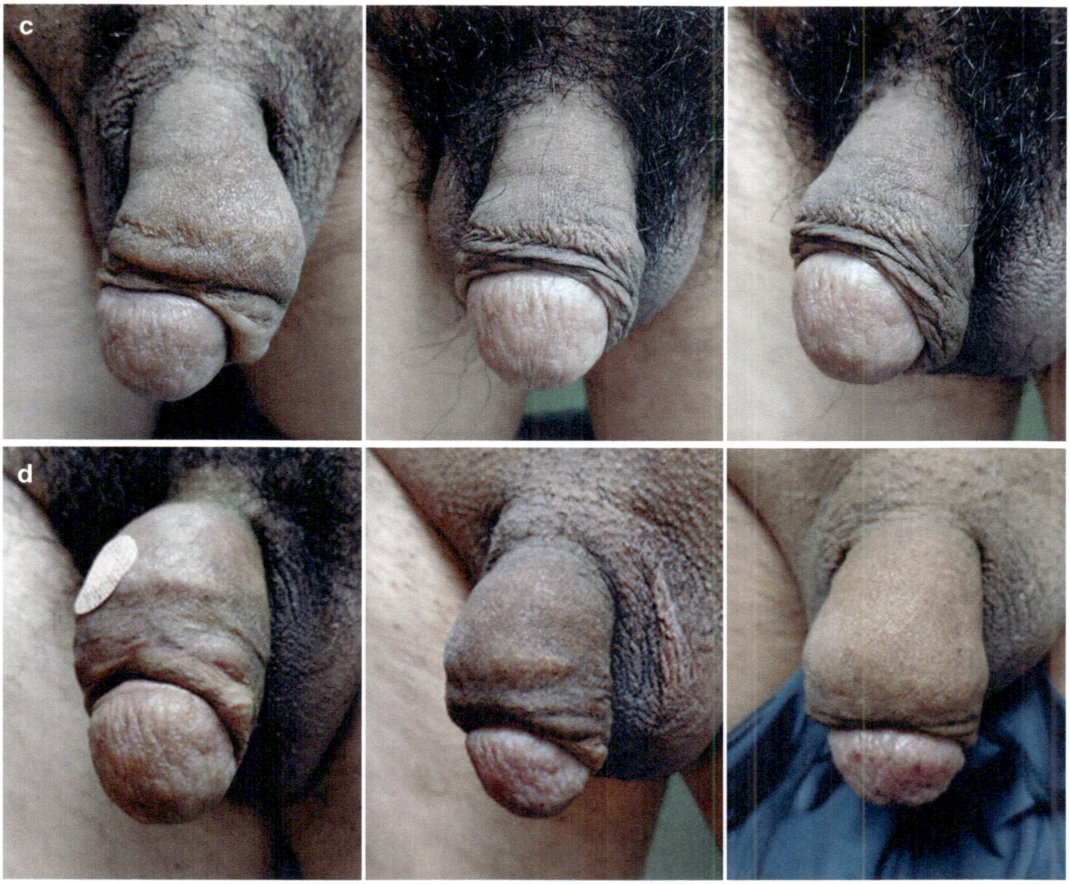

Fig. 10.14 (continued)

10.16 Case 14: Long-Term HA Remnant Removal and Reinjection in a 53-Year-Old Male (Extension of Case 2, Part III)

A 53-year-old male underwent two previous HA filler procedures: 20 cc of Elavie on December 7, 2017, and 10 cc of Potenfill on October 22, 2020. At 4–6 years postinjection, he presented with dissatisfaction due to a left-sided asymmetric HA remnant, leading to contour irregularity and tactile discomfort (Fig. 10.15a, pretreatment).

Correction was performed by injecting 1500 IU of hyaluronidase diluted in 1 mL saline directly into the residual HA deposits (Fig. 10.20b).

At follow-up, the patient requested volume restoration. A staged reinjection of HA filler was performed, and results at 4 and 48 weeks showed excellent symmetry, contour stability, and high patient satisfaction.

This case demonstrates the effectiveness of enzymatic HA removal even years after the initial injection and highlights the value of a staged approach combining hyaluronidase correction with delayed reinjection for optimal long-term results.

10.16.1 The Role of Hyaluronidase in HA-Based PGE

Hyaluronidase is a cornerstone tool for enhancing the safety and versatility of HA-based penile girth enhancement (PGE). In the early phase, it enables

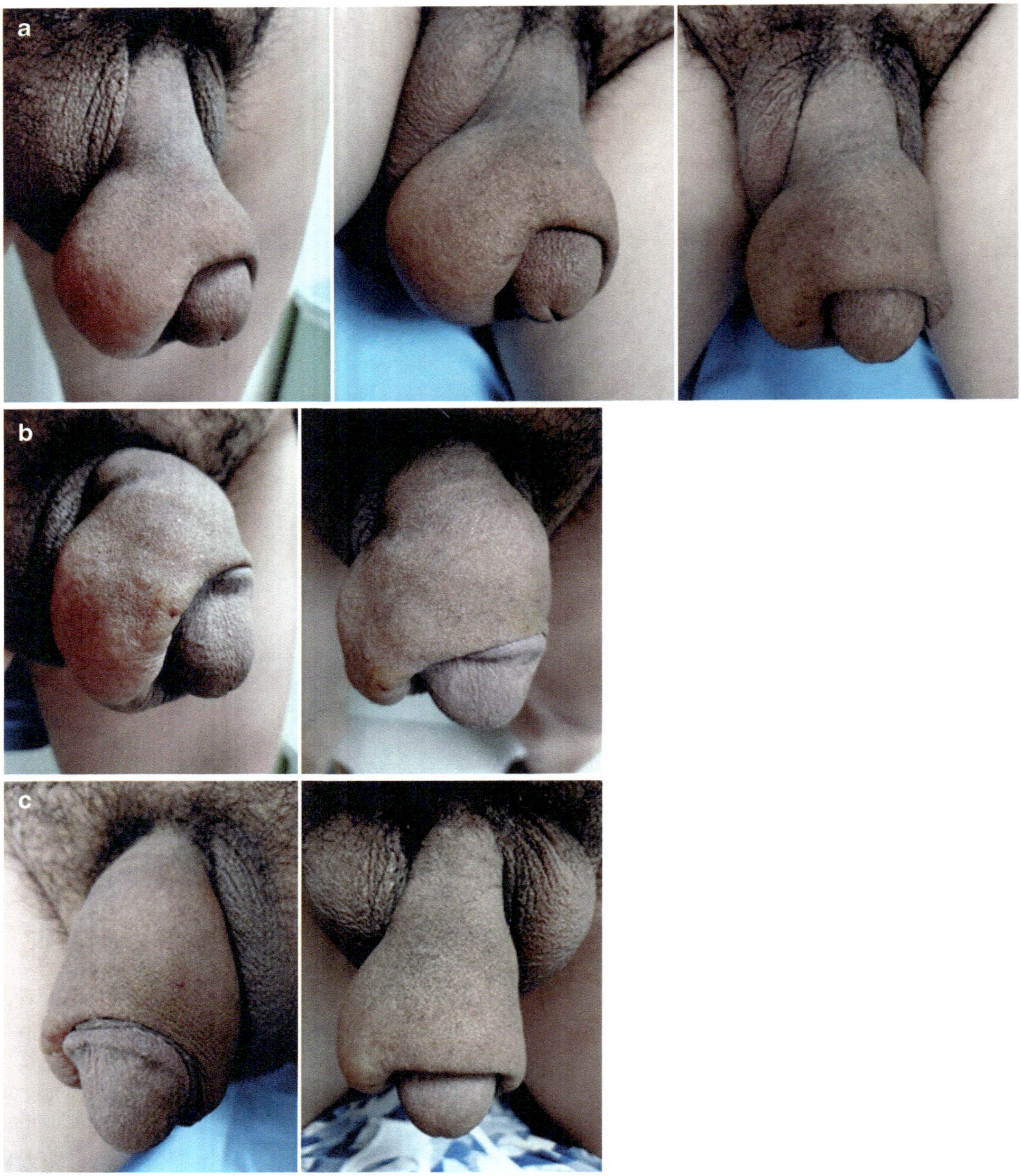

Fig. 10.15 (**a**) 4 years of longstanding asymmetry caused by residual HA filler and repeated HA injection at other clinics (**b**) 18G needle puncture and manual squeezing, (**c**) 4 weeks later, a little decreased but still unsatisfactory at 2024.05.23. 1500 IU hyaluronidase injection was done (**d**) Post-hyaluronidase treatment (1500 IU) in 2024, showing significant resolution of residual HA filler. Softening was observed within 3 days, with complete dissolution achieved within 1 week and no adverse effects (**e**) Reinjection after cleaning with hyaluronidase restored (**f**) penile contour and symmetry at 48 weeks later

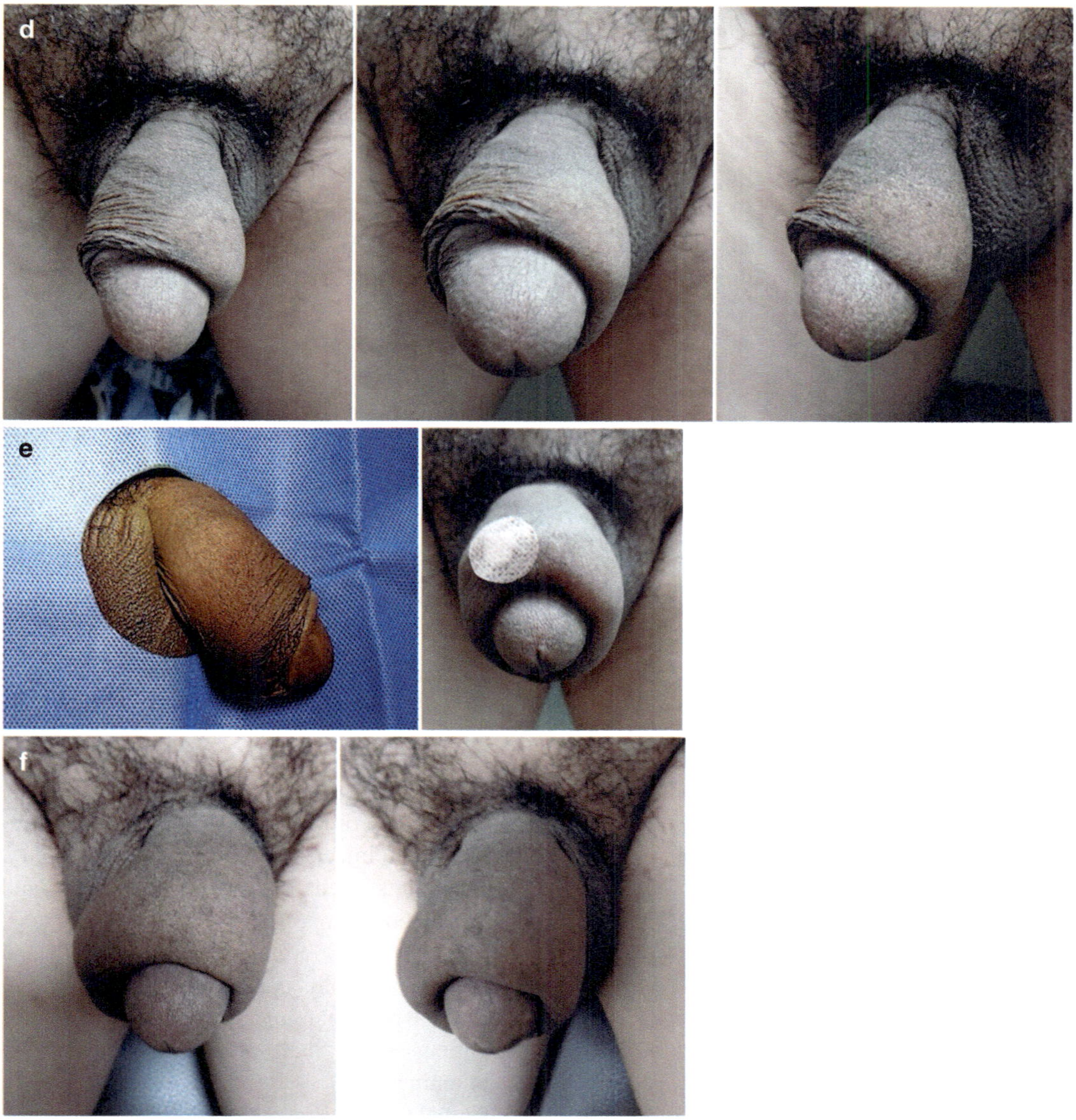

Fig. 10.15 (continued)

rapid correction of contour irregularities, overcorrection, and nodularity. In the late phase, it effectively dissolves residual HA deposits even years after the initial injection, facilitating re-contouring or preparing the tissue for reinjection.

This dual role not only minimizes complications but also increases the confidence of both physicians and patients in HA augmentation. With hyaluronidase as a safety net, concerns about long-term issues such as migration, lump formation, and asymmetry are substantially reduced, making HA the preferred filler for penile augmentation.

Key Takeaways: Hyaluronidase in HA-Based PGE

- Enables early-phase correction of asymmetry and overcorrection
- Effective for late-phase removal of long-standing HA remnants

- Supports reinjection planning by creating a stable tissue foundation
- Enhances the safety and predictability of HA augmentation procedures

Best Practices Box: Key Lessons from Clinical Cases in HA-Based PGE

- Start conservatively: Small-volume initial injections and staged retouching reduce asymmetry and migration risk.
- Anticipate late-phase changes: Regular follow-up detects subtle filler migration and volume shifts.
- Use hyaluronidase confidently: For managing deformities and preparing for reinjection years later.
- Tailor technique to patient history: Prior fillers (e.g., PLA) require modified approaches (smaller needles, fractionated doses).
- Prioritize patient education: Set expectations for maintenance, corrections, and long-term planning.

This chapter illustrates how meticulous technique, patient-specific planning, and long-term management, including the use of hyaluronidase, contribute to successful outcomes in HA-based PGE.

10.17 Conclusion

This 14-case clinical series provides a comprehensive overview of real-world experiences with hyaluronic acid (HA)-based penile girth enhancement (PGE), highlighting the nuanced interplay between anatomy, technique, and long-term outcomes. The cases underscore that patient-specific factors—such as preputial anatomy, age-related changes, and prior filler exposure—must guide injection planning and volume selection. Complications including distal migration, nodularity, and asymmetry were most effectively managed through a combination of conservative observation, hyaluronidase application, and staged reinjections. Importantly, proper postinjection care and proactive patient education proved critical to procedural success and satisfaction. These findings emphasize that successful PGE with HA is not a one-time event but a process requiring precision, patience, and personalized follow-up strategies.

Case Summary: Clinical Insights from 14 HA-Based Penile Girth Enhancement (PGE) Cases

This case series presents diverse clinical experiences with HA-based penile girth enhancement (PGE), offering key insights into procedural strategy, filler behavior, and long-term management:

- Case 1 (54M): Demonstrated *physiologic distal migration* despite uniform initial results. Conservative monitoring led to natural stabilization without retouch. Emphasized importance of gel rheology, circumcision, and patient counseling.
- Case 2 (55M): A staged journey from early filler migration to deformity, delayed circumcision, and multiple retouches over 4 years. Final correction with hyaluronidase and strategic reinjection restored symmetry. Highlights need for long-term planning and patient education.
- Case 3 (67M): Severe *distal migration* caused by senile atrophy and retracted preputial ring. Emphasized anatomical risk factors in elderly patients, and the value of injection site planning.
- Case 4 (49M): Presented filler entrapment and asymmetry due to circumcision scar and adhesions. Retouching improved results. Suggests need for preinjection scar assessment and possible revision.
- Case 5 (41M): Large single-session injection (20 cc) led to *progressive distal ventral migration*. Underscores risk of overcorrection and the need to avoid distal ventral deposits.
- Case 6 (42M): Initially stable at 4 weeks post-20 cc injection, but late-onset migration worsened by 24 weeks. Highlights delayed behavior of high-volume HA and benefit of conservative dosing.

- Cases 7 and 8 (54M): Exemplary postinjection management with structured massage and compressive dressing. Minor irregularities resolved spontaneously; retouch at 1 year yielded stable long-term results. Model for best practices.
- Case 9 (42M): HA injection over prior *non-HA filler* improved symmetry without complications. Long-term follow-up showed safety of proper sequencing (HA after non-HA).
- Case 10 (42M): Reinjection after Powerfill® (PLA) exposure required special technique using a 27G needle. Despite fibrotic adhesions, the result was symmetrical with no migration. Fibrosis may have offered scaffold-like stability.
- Case 11 (41M): Asymmetry after initial 20 cc injection partially improved with retouch but required hyaluronidase for complete correction. Demonstrates combined approach of filler and enzyme.
- Case 12: Late-onset superficial HA deformity *3.5 years* postinjection successfully corrected using puncture and squeezing. Subsequent skin retraction allowed delayed retouch with good aesthetic outcome.
- Case 13 (54M): Presented with persistent HA lump *6 years* post-Potenfill. A single session of 1,500 IU hyaluronidase fully resolved the deformity. Reinjection restored symmetry with long-term stability.
- Case 14 (53M): Recurrent asymmetry after two HA injections was managed by puncture, squeezing, and hyaluronidase, followed by staged reinjection. Reinforced principles of staged correction after enzymatic cleanup.

Integrated Lessons from the Series

- Start conservatively: Limit initial injection volumes and favor staged augmentation.
- Anatomy matters: Redundant prepuce, senile atrophy, and scarring significantly impact outcomes.
- Hyaluronidase is essential: Useful both early and late for managing asymmetries or overcorrection.
- Retouch timing is strategic: Stabilization before reinjection yields more predictable outcomes.
- Patient education is pivotal: Clear communication around risks, expectations, and follow-up improves satisfaction and compliance.

Case No.	Age	Initial HA volume	Main complication	Intervention	Outcome
1	54	10 mL HA	Physiologic distal-ventral migration	Observation only	Stable in erect state, no retouch
2	55	20 mL HA	Severe distal migration over 4 years	Delayed circumcision, hyaluronidase, reinjection	Restored contour, long-term satisfaction
3	67	Not specified	Filler displacement due to senile atrophy, preputial ring	None	Migration persisted, underscores anatomical risk
4	49	15 mL HA	Depression at circumcision scar line	Retouching	Final resolution with retouch
5	41	20 mL HA	Distal ventral bulge by 12??4 weeks	Observation	Persistent deformity, emphasizes injection site caution
6	42	20 mL HA	Delayed migration after 12??4 weeks	Observation	Aggravated bulge, suggests staged injection preferable
7	54	15 mL HA	Minor irregularity at 4 weeks	Massage, compressive dressing	Stable at 24 weeks
8	54	10 mL HA (retouch)	Volume loss at 54 weeks	Retouch with 10 mL HA	Stable, long-term symmetry

Case No.	Age	Initial HA volume	Main complication	Intervention	Outcome
9	42	HA post-PLA	Contour irregularities	HA reinjection after PLA	Good result, long-term stability
10	42	HA post-Powerfill	Fibrous adhesions	27G needle, small deposits	Symmetry maintained, no migration
11	41	20 + 10 mL HA	Proximal lump	Hyaluronidase	Deformity resolved
12	56	10 mL HA	Superficial lump 3.5 years post	Puncture + squeezing, delayed retouch	Restored volume, symmetry
13	54	20 + 10 mL HA	Asymmetric remnant 6 yrs post	Hyaluronidase + reinjection	Excellent contour, stable at 48 weeks
14	53	20 + 10 mL HA	Left-sided lump, long-term	Hyaluronidase + delayed reinjection	Symmetry restored, high satisfaction

Further Readings

1. Zucchi A, Costantini E, Cai T, et al. Hyaluronic acid in andrology: a narrative review. Int J Impot Res. 2021;33(6):637–46. https://doi.org/10.1038/s41443-021-00461-8.
2. Kim JJ, Kwak TI, Jeon BG, Moon DG. Effects of glans penis augmentation using hyaluronic acid gel for premature ejaculation. Int J Impot Res. 2004;16(6):547–51. https://doi.org/10.1038/sj.ijir.3901226.
3. Ahn ST, Kwak TI, Park KS, Kim JJ, Moon DG. Complications of glans penis augmentation. Int J Impot Res. 2019;31(4):245–55. https://doi.org/10.1038/s41443-019-0121-4.
4. Reyes-Vallejo L, Vélez-Montoya R, Rodríguez-De La Rosa M, et al. Delayed-onset nodules after hyaluronic acid injections: management and prevention. Dermatol Surg. 2019;45(11):1403–10. https://doi.org/10.1097/DSS.0000000000001881.
5. Lee WJ, Kim WT, Kim YJ, et al. Long-term persistence of hyaluronic acid filler in penile subcutaneous tissue: a retrospective ultrasonographic study. Urology. 2021;147:249–53. https://doi.org/10.1016/j.urology.2020.07.024.
6. De Boulle K, Heydenrych I. Patient factors influencing dermal filler complications: prevention, assessment, and treatment. Dermatol Surg. 2015;41(Suppl 1):S72–6. https://doi.org/10.1097/DSS.0000000000000284.
7. Beleznay K, Carruthers JD, Humphrey S, Carruthers A. Avoiding and treating blindness from fillers: a review of the world literature. Plast Reconstr Surg. 2021;147(1):24e–32e. https://doi.org/10.1097/PRS.0000000000007506.

Part III

Glans Penis Augmentation

Premature Ejaculation: Integrating Pathophysiology with Current Treatment Modalities

11

Contents

11.1 Introduction

Premature ejaculation (PE) is among the most prevalent male sexual dysfunctions, affecting up to 30% of men worldwide and significantly impairing quality of life for patients and their partners [1]. According to the International Society for Sexual Medicine (ISSM), PE is categorized into lifelong PE (present since the first sexual experiences) and acquired PE (developing after a period of normal ejaculatory control). The diagnostic criteria include ejaculation within about 1 min of vaginal penetration in lifelong PE or a bothersome reduction to less than 3 min in acquired PE, inability to delay ejaculation, and associated distress or interpersonal difficulties [2, 3].

This chapter provides an integrated review of PE pathophysiology and current treatments, establishing the rationale for GPA as a novel intervention.

Advancements in neuroimaging, molecular genetics, and neurophysiology have expanded our understanding of PE's pathophysiology,

D. G. Moon, *Penile Augmentation with Injectable Hyaluronic Acid*,
https://doi.org/10.1007/978-981-95-5385-3_11

revealing a multifactorial etiology that complicates treatment strategies. Conventional therapies such as selective serotonin reuptake inhibitors (SSRIs) and topical anesthetics offer symptomatic relief but suffer from high discontinuation rates and varying efficacy [4, 5]. Recently, attention has turned to novel approaches, including GPA with HA filler, which targets peripheral hypersensitivity in the glans penis. This chapter integrates pathophysiological knowledge with current treatment options to establish a foundation for GPA as a logical, mechanism-based intervention.

11.2 Pathophysiology of Premature Ejaculation

11.2.1 Central Nervous System Contributions

Ejaculation is a coordinated reflex involving cortical, subcortical, and spinal centers. The medial preoptic area (MPOA), paraventricular nucleus (PVN), and subparafascicular thalamus play central roles in integrating sensory input and coordinating motor output via the spinal generator of ejaculation (SGE) located in mid-lumbar segments [6, 7]. Functional MRI studies reveal hypoactivation of inhibitory brain regions such as the medial prefrontal cortex and anterior cingulate cortex in PE patients, suggesting impaired top-down control over the ejaculatory reflex [8] (Fig. 11.1).

11.2.2 Neurotransmitter Systems

Serotonin (5-HT) acts as a key inhibitory neurotransmitter. Deficiency of synaptic 5-HT and polymorphisms in the serotonin transporter gene (5-HTTLPR) have been linked to reduced inhibitory tone and rapid ejaculation [9, 10]. Dopamine (DA), by contrast, facilitates ejaculation through mesolimbic pathways. Excess dopaminergic activity in the nucleus accumbens accelerates ejaculation and contributes to PE [11, 12].

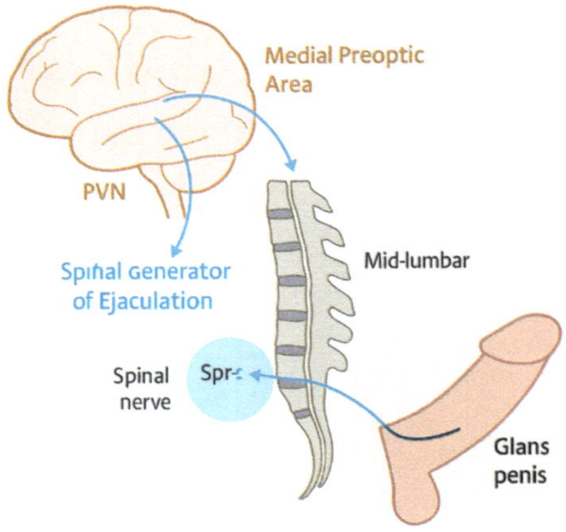

Fig. 11.1 Neural pathways involved in ejaculation control

Oxytocin, a hypothalamic neuropeptide, enhances smooth muscle contractions during emission and expulsion phases, with elevated levels noted in men with PE [13].

Peripheral Sensory Mechanisms.

The dorsal nerve of the penis transmits tactile stimuli to the SGE. Hypersensitivity of the glans penis, evidenced by reduced thresholds in biothesiometry and shortened latencies in dorsal nerve somatosensory evoked potential (DNSEP) studies, is a hallmark of PE [14, 15]. This peripheral hypersensitivity suggests a viable target for local interventions (Fig. 11.2).

11.2.3 Hormonal and Endocrine Factors

Hormonal imbalances also contribute to ejaculatory control. Elevated testosterone levels may shorten IELT by enhancing dopaminergic tone [16]. Hyperthyroidism is associated with accelerated ejaculation, whereas hypothyroidism delays it [17]. Low prolactin levels are linked to increased sexual drive and PE, while elevated cortisol from hypothalamic-pituitary-adrenal (HPA) axis dysregulation may heighten sympathetic activity and reduce ejaculatory control [18, 19] (Fig. 11.3).

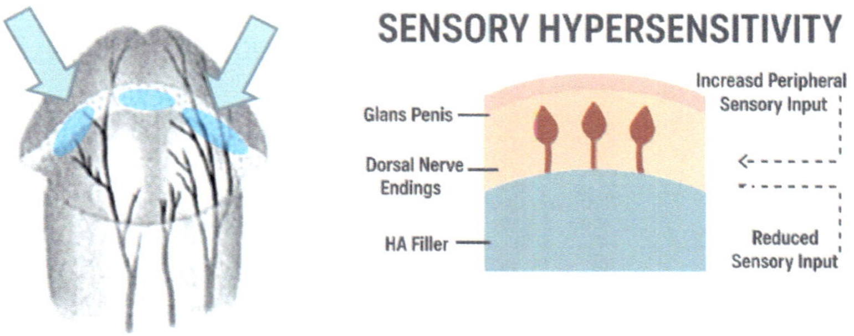

Fig. 11.2 Tentative mechanism of GPA with HA for treatment of PE

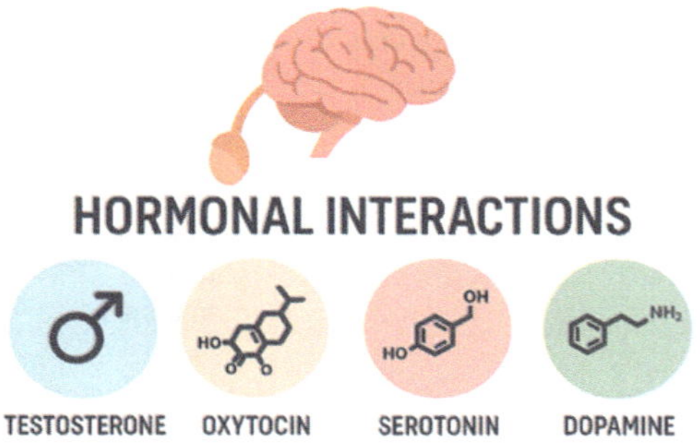

Fig. 11.3 Hormonal interaction of ejaculation

11.2.4 Autonomic Dysregulation

Sympathetic hyperactivity originating from T10–L2 spinal segments plays a role in lifelong PE. Heart rate variability studies demonstrate increased adrenergic tone in PE patients, supporting autonomic dysregulation as a contributor [20].

11.3 Current Treatment Modalities and Their Pathophysiological Targets

11.3.1 Pharmacological Therapies

Selective serotonin reuptake inhibitors (SSRIs) remain the cornerstone of pharmacological treatment for PE. By enhancing serotonergic neurotransmission, SSRIs increase central inhibitory control over the ejaculatory reflex. Dapoxetine, a short-acting SSRI, is currently the only approved drug specifically for PE and has demonstrated efficacy in multiple randomized controlled trials [21]. Daily use of longer-acting SSRIs such as paroxetine, fluoxetine, and sertraline also improves IELT but is often limited by adverse effects including nausea, fatigue, and sexual dysfunction, contributing to high discontinuation rates approaching 90% over 2 years [22, 23]. Notably, paroxetine has been identified as the most effective among SSRIs, with studies reporting an eightfold increase in IELT compared to placebo [24].

Topical anesthetics such as lidocaine-prilocaine sprays and creams provide another option by reducing glans sensitivity, thus delaying ejaculation [25]. Placebo-controlled studies have shown significant improvements in IELT and patient satisfaction, but side effects such as penile numbness and the potential for transference to a partner limit their acceptability [26]. These preparations are most appropriate for patients seeking nonsystemic, on-demand treatments.

Phosphodiesterase type 5 inhibitors (PDE5Is), though primarily indicated for erectile dysfunction, have demonstrated adjunctive benefits in PE patients, particularly in those with comorbid erectile issues. Their proposed mechanism involves nitric oxide-mediated smooth muscle relaxation and potential reduction of penile hypersensitivity [27]. Meta-analyses indicate that combining PDE5Is with SSRIs offers superior outcomes over SSRIs alone, yet PDE5Is remain less effective as monotherapy for PE [28].

Tramadol, an opioid analgesic with serotonergic activity, has also been explored as an on-demand option for PE. Several studies report

Table 11.1 Pharmacological therapies

Treatment	Target mechanism	Efficacy	Limitations
SSRIs (e.g., dapoxetine)	↑ Serotonin transmission	IELT increased up to 8× baseline	Side effects, poor adherence [23, 24]
Topical anesthetics	↓ Glans sensitivity (PNS modulation)	IELT significantly increased	Numbness, partner transference [25]
PDE5 inhibitors	↓ Penile hypersensitivity	Modest IELT benefit in PE + ED	Not first-line for PE alone [26]
Tramadol	Mixed serotonergic/opioid activity	IELT prolongation	Dependency, dizziness, nausea [27]

significant IELT improvements, but concerns regarding dependency and side effects such as dizziness, nausea, and somnolence restrict its long-term use [29, 30] (Table 11.1).

11.4 Behavioral Therapies

Behavioral interventions, including the stop-start and squeeze techniques, aim to train patients to recognize and delay their ejaculatory response [31]. These methods require considerable patient commitment and practice. While they have shown variable success rates, evidence suggests they are most effective when combined with pharmacotherapy. Cognitive behavioral therapy (CBT) addresses psychological contributors to PE, such as performance anxiety and maladaptive sexual beliefs. Recent studies demonstrate that CBT combined with pharmacotherapy produces superior outcomes compared to either modality alone, supporting a multimodal approach [32, 33] (Table 11.2).

Table 11.2 Behavioral therapies

Therapy	Target mechanism	Limitations
Stop-start, squeeze techniques	Retrain sensory-motor control	Labor-intensive, variable efficacy
Cognitive behavioral therapy	Reduce anxiety, improve self-regulation	Slow onset, requires high patient commitment

11.5 Surgical and Minimally Invasive Therapies

Selective dorsal neurectomy (SDN) involves partial resection of the dorsal penile nerve to reduce glans sensitivity. While small random-

Table 11.3 Surgical and minimally invasive therapies

Procedure	Target Mechanism	Evidence	Limitations
Selective dorsal neurectomy	↓ Dorsal nerve sensory input	IELT improved in small RCTs [12–14]	Numbness, potential for sexual dissatisfaction
GPA with HA filler	↓ Glans sensitivity (cushioning effect)	IELT and satisfaction improved [32, 33]	Reabsorption over time; touch-ups required
Neuromodulation (pulsed RF)	Modulate dorsal nerve excitability	Promising pilot data [18, 19]	Requires validation in larger RCTs

ized controlled trials and observational studies report significant IELT increases post-SDN, the procedure carries risks such as penile numbness, altered sensation, and decreased sexual satisfaction [34, 35].

Glans penis augmentation (GPA) using hyaluronic acid filler offers a minimally invasive alternative to SDN. By creating a cushioning effect in the submucosa of the glans penis, GPA attenuates sensory input from the dorsal nerve. Clinical trials demonstrate IELT improvements lasting up to 9 months, high patient and partner satisfaction, and a favorable safety profile [36, 37]. The reversibility of GPA via hyaluronidase further enhances its appeal as a safe and temporary intervention.

Neuromodulation techniques, such as pulsed radiofrequency and cryoablation of the dorsal nerve, are emerging as potential PE treatments. Pilot studies have reported promising outcomes, but larger, multicenter trials are needed to establish efficacy and safety [38, 39] (Table 11.3).

11.5.1 Integrating Pathophysiology with Treatment Selection

The pathophysiological understanding of PE underscores the need for multimodal therapy targeting both central and peripheral mechanisms. GPA with HA filler uniquely addresses peripheral hypersensitivity by modulating sensory input at the glans level, complementing pharmacological and behavioral interventions (Fig. 11.4).

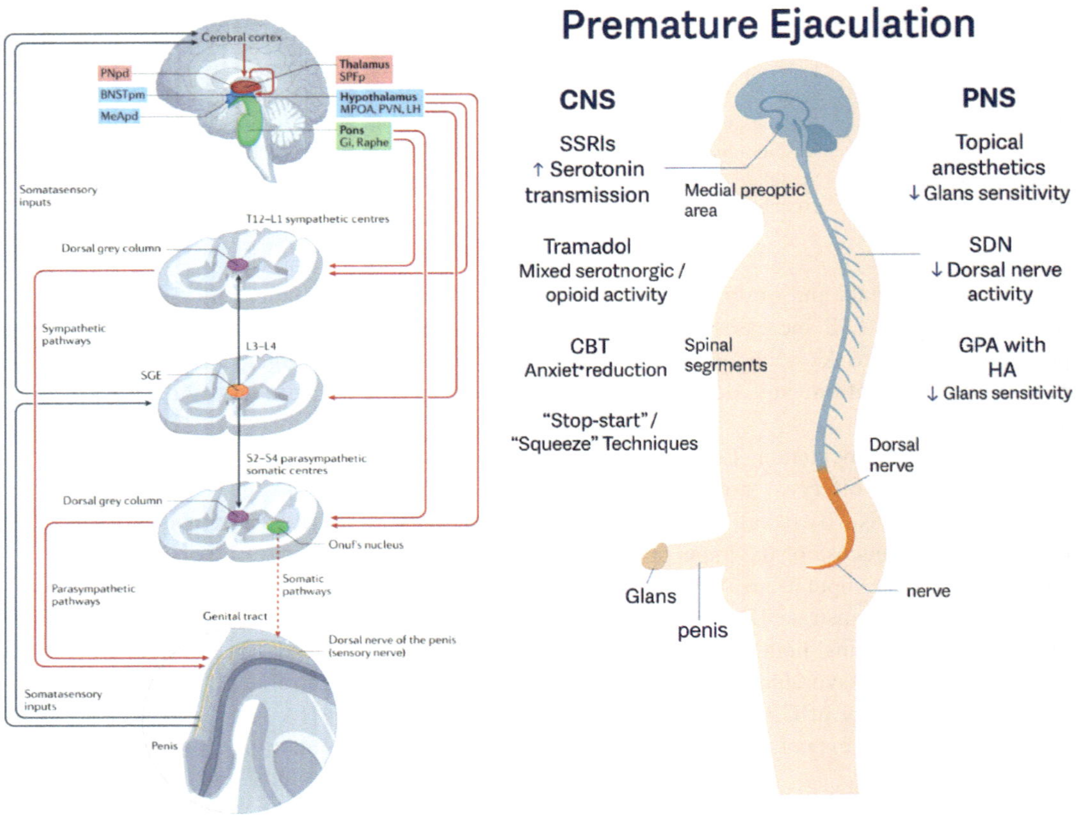

Fig. 11.4 Neuroanatomical mechanisms of ejaculation and PE treatment

11.6 Positioning GPA with HA Filler as a Mechanism-Based Therapy

GPA offers a patient-friendly, reversible approach to PE management by targeting the peripheral sensory component of ejaculatory control. Its minimally invasive nature and favorable safety profile position it as an attractive option for men with lifelong PE, particularly those unresponsive or intolerant to conventional therapies [12, 40].

11.7 Take-Home Messages for Clinicians

- PE involves central, peripheral, hormonal, and autonomic dysregulation.
- Pharmacotherapy remains first-line but is limited by side effects and adherence issues.
- GPA with HA filler is a promising, reversible option targeting peripheral hypersensitivity.
- Multimodal, personalized approaches are key to effective PE management.

11.8 Conclusion

PE management must evolve beyond symptomatic control to address its multifactorial pathophysiology. GPA with HA filler exemplifies this shift by providing a minimally invasive, mechanism-based intervention. As clinical evidence continues to accumulate, GPA may establish itself alongside SSRIs as a cornerstone therapy for lifelong PE, particularly in men with penile hypersensitivity and refractory cases.

References

1. Salonia A, Bettocchi C, Boeri L, Capogrosso P, Carvalho J, Cilesiz NC, et al. European Association of Urology guidelines on sexual and reproductive health—2021 update: male sexual dysfunction. Eur Urol. 2021;80(3):333–57.
2. McMahon CG, Althof SE, Waldinger MD, Porst H, Dean J, Sharlip ID, et al. An evidence-based definition of lifelong premature ejaculation: report of the International Society for Sexual Medicine (ISSM) ad hoc committee for the definition of premature ejaculation. J Sex Med. 2008;5(7):1590–606.
3. Rowland DL, Patrick DL, Rothman M, Gagnon DD. The psychological burden of premature ejaculation. J Urol. 2007;177(3):1065–70.
4. Waldinger MD. The neurobiological approach to premature ejaculation. J Urol. 2002;168(6):2359–67.
5. Giuliano F, Clement P. Neuroanatomy and physiology of ejaculation. Annu Rev Sex Res. 2005;16(1):190–216.
6. Truitt WA, Coolen LM. Identification of a potential ejaculation generator in the spinal cord. Science. 2002;297(5586):1566–9.
7. Coolen LM. Neural control of ejaculation. J Comp Neurol. 2005;493(1):39–45.
8. Yang X, Gao M, Zhang L, Liu L, Liu P, Sun J, et al. Central neural correlates during inhibitory control in lifelong premature ejaculation patients. Front Hum Neurosci. 2018;12:206.
9. Janssen PK, van Schaik R, Olivier B, Waldinger MD. The 5-HT2C receptor gene Cys23Ser polymorphism influences the intravaginal ejaculation latency time in Dutch Caucasian men with lifelong premature ejaculation. Asian J Androl. 2014;16(4):607–10.
10. van Raaij JJ, Serefoglu EC, van Amelsvoort TA, Janssen PK. Possible pathophysiologic roles of neurotransmitter systems in men with lifelong premature ejaculation: a scoping review. Sex Med Rev. 2024;12(4):638–51.
11. Jern P, Santtila P, Witting K, Alanko K, Harlaar N, Johansson A, et al. Premature and delayed ejaculation: genetic and environmental effects in a population-based sample of Finnish twins. J Sex Med. 2007;4(6):1739–49.
12. Coskuner ER, Ozkan B. Premature ejaculation and endocrine disorders: a literature review. World J Mens Health. 2021;40(1):38.
13. Corona G, Mannucci E, Forti G, Maggi M. Hypogonadism, ED, metabolic syndrome and obesity: a pathological link supporting cardiovascular diseases. Int J Androl. 2009;32(6):587–98.
14. Krysiak R, Kowalcze K, Okopień B. Sexual function and depressive symptoms in men with hypoprolactinaemia secondary to overtreatment of prolactin excess: a pilot study. Endocrinol Diabetes Nut. 2022;69(4):279–88.
15. Zorba OU, Cicek Y, Uzun H, Cetinkaya M, Önem K, Rifaioğlu MM. Autonomic nervous system dysfunction in lifelong premature ejaculation: analysis of heart rate variability. Urology. 2012;80(6):1283–6.
16. Park HJ, Park NC, Kim TN, Baek SR, Lee KM, Choe S. Discontinuation of dapoxetine treatment in patients with premature ejaculation: a 2-year prospective observational study. Sex Med. 2017;5(2):e99–e105.
17. Mondaini N, Fusco F, Cai T, Benemei S, Mirone V, Bartoletti R. Dapoxetine treatment in patients with lifelong premature ejaculation: the reasons of a "Waterloo". Urology. 2013;82(3):620–4.
18. Waldinger M, Zwinderman A, Schweitzer D, Olivier B. Relevance of methodological design for the interpretation of efficacy of drug treatment of premature ejaculation: a systematic review and meta-analysis. Int J Impot Res. 2004;16(4):369–81.
19. Dinsmore WW, Hackett G, Goldmeier D, Waldinger M, Dean J, Wright P, et al. Topical eutectic mixture for premature ejaculation (TEMPE): a novel aerosol-delivery form of lidocaine-prilocaine for treating premature ejaculation. BJU Int. 2007;99(2):369–75.
20. Xia J-D, Han Y-F, Zhou L-H, Chen Y, Dai Y-T. Efficacy and safety of local anaesthetics for premature ejaculation: a systematic review and meta-analysis. Asian J Androl. 2013;15(4):497.
21. Sridharan K, Sivaramakrishnan G, Sequeira RP, Al-Khaja KA. Pharmacological interventions for premature ejaculation: a mixed-treatment comparison network meta-analysis of randomized clinical trials. Int J Impot Res. 2018;30(5):215–23.
22. Martyn-St James M, Cooper K, Ren S, Kaltenthaler E, Dickinson K, Cantrell A, et al. Phosphodiesterase type 5 inhibitors for premature ejaculation: a systematic review and meta-analysis. Eur Urol Focus. 2017;3(1):119–29.
23. Sharma AP, Sharma G, Tyagi S, Devana SK, Mavuduru RS, Bora GS, et al. Safety and efficacy of "on-demand" tramadol in patients with premature ejaculation: an updated meta-analysis. Int Braz J Urol. 2021;47(5):921–34.
24. Cormio L, Massenio P, La Rocca R, Verze P, Mirone V, Carrieri G. The combination of dapoxetine and behavioral treatment provides better results than dapoxetine alone in the management of patients with lifelong premature ejaculation. J Sex Med. 2015;12(7):1609–15.

25. Basal S, Goktas S, Ergin A, Yildirim I, Atim A, Tahmaz L, et al. A novel treatment modality in patients with premature ejaculation resistant to conventional methods: the neuromodulation of dorsal penile nerves by pulsed radiofrequency. J Androl. 2010;31(2):126–30.
26. Prologo JD, Snyder LL, Cherullo E, Passalacqua M, Pirasteh A, Corn D. Percutaneous CT-guided cryoablation of the dorsal penile nerve for treatment of symptomatic premature ejaculation. J Vasc Interv Radiol. 2013;24(2):214–9.
27. Zhang GX, Yu LP, Bai WJ, Wang XF. Selective resection of dorsal nerves of penis for premature ejaculation. Int J Androl. 2012;35(6):873–9.
28. Tang Q-L, Song T, Han Y-F, Yang B-B, Chen J-H, Xu Z-P, et al. The application of intraoperative neurophysiological monitoring in selective dorsal neurotomy for primary premature ejaculation: a prospective single-center study. Asian J Androl. 2023;25(1):137–42.
29. Ambusaidi H, Alshuaibi M, Zugail AS, Beley S. The role of surgical therapy in the management of premature ejaculation: a narrative review. Transl Androl Urol. 2023;12(10):1589.
30. Ahn ST, Shim JS, Bae WJ, Kim SW, Kim JJ, Moon DG. Efficacy and safety of penile girth enhancement using hyaluronic acid filler and the clinical impact on ejaculation: a multi-center, patient/evaluator-blinded, randomized active-controlled trial. World J Mens Health. 2021;40(2):299.
31. Alahwany A, Ragab MW, Zaghloul A, Abdallah H, Mostafa T. Hyaluronic acid injection in glans penis for treatment of premature ejaculation: a randomized controlled cross-over study. Int J Impot Res. 2019;31(5):348–55.
32. Herrmann JL, Hoffmann RK, Ward CE, Schulman JM, Grekin RC. Biochemistry, physiology, and tissue interactions of contemporary biodegradable injectable dermal fillers. Dermatologic Surg. 2018;44:S19–31.
33. Gul M, Bocu K, Serefoglu EC. Current and emerging treatment options for premature ejaculation. Nat Rev Urol. 2022;19(11):659–80.
34. Maggi M, Buvat J, Corona G, Guay A, Torres LO. Hormonal causes of male sexual dysfunctions and their management (hyperprolactinemia, thyroid disorders, GH disorders, and DHEA). J Sex Med. 2013;10(3):661–77.
35. Soni KK, Jeong H-S, Jang S. Neurons for ejaculation and factors affecting ejaculation. Biology. 2022;11(5):686.
36. Geng B, Gao M, Wu J, Liu C, Piao R, Yang G, et al. Functional connectivity of nucleus accumbens is associated with lifelong premature ejaculation in male adults: a resting-state fMRI study. Clin Neuroradiol. 2022;32:1–9.
37. Zhang T, Tang D, Cai H, Zhang B, Yang Y, Zhang C, et al. Selective functional hyperconnectivity in the middle temporal gyrus subregions in lifelong premature ejaculation. J Sex Med. 2020;17(8):1457–66.
38. Perretti A, Catalano A, Mirone V, Imbimbo C, Balbi P, Palmieri A, et al. Neurophysiologic evaluation of central-peripheral sensory and motor pudendal pathways in primary premature ejaculation. Urology. 2003;61(3):623–8.
39. Sun Z, Liao Z, Zheng Q, Chen J, Lv B, Bao C, et al. A study of differences in penile dorsal nerve somatosensory evoked potential testing among healthy controls and patients with primary and secondary premature ejaculation. J Sex Med. 2021;18(4):732–6.
40. Krassioukov A, Elliott S. Neural control and physiology of sexual function: effect of spinal cord injury. Top Spinal Cord Inj Rehabil. 2017;23(1):1–10.

Development and Clinical Applications of Glans Penis Augmentation with Injectable Hyaluronic Acid Gel

12

Contents

12.1 Introduction

Penile augmentation is an area of growing interest globally, driven by societal shifts, media influence, and patient demand for aesthetic and functional enhancement. Surgical interventions, including dermofat grafts, silicone implants, and ligamentolysis, have historically been used but carry risks such as scarring, deformity, and patient dissatisfaction [1, 2]. Patients often report disproportionate penile morphology following girth enhancement procedures, highlighting a clear clinical need for glans augmentation. Although augmentation phalloplasty is not an established procedure, the demand for penile augmentation continues to increase as the media promotes a standard for normalcy among males and advertisements create interest in corrective surgery. The current main augmentation phalloplasty techniques are girth enhancement and penile lengthening procedures. There is no argument against glans penis augmentation (GPA) for hypospadias repair and penile reconstruction for congenital micropenis or secondary micropenis (iatrogenic, infection, or trauma). The current penile girth enhancement (PGE) technique may produce an iatrogenic penile deformity of a thick penile body with a relatively small glans penis. In addition to some patients' complaints of poor glans tumescence during normal erection [3], a small glans and lack of tumescence are evident after penile prosthesis implantation [4, 5].

Before the early 2000s, glans augmentation had not been standardized due to technical chal-

D. G. Moon, *Penile Augmentation with Injectable Hyaluronic Acid*,
https://doi.org/10.1007/978-981-95-5385-3_12

lenges and lack of suitable biomaterials. Hyaluronic acid (HA) gel, with its excellent biocompatibility and widespread use in soft-tissue augmentation, emerged as an ideal candidate [6, 7]. The innovation of GPA using HA gel addressed both aesthetic concerns and functional issues, positioning it as a groundbreaking advance in sexual medicine.

12.2 Preclinical Studies: Establishing Feasibility

12.2.1 Technical Feasibility and Histological Potential Space

Initial animal studies involved submucosal injections of Restylane® (Q-Med, Sweden) into the glans penis of New Zealand White rabbits. Using a 30G needle, the filler was delivered carefully to avoid overdistension of the mucosa. Histological analysis at 3 months post-injection revealed potential spaces within the dermis capable of accommodating HA gel without inflammatory changes.

Moon et al. (2003) reported the presence of Alcian blue-stained gel localized in these potential spaces, confirming retention and biocompatibility [8]. Histological sections at 3 months post-injection demonstrate Alcian blue-stained HA gel retained in defined tissue spaces (Fig. 12.1). Post-hyaluronidase treatment confirmed biodegradability and biocompatibility.

12.2.2 Long-Term Retention and Biocompatibility: Beagle Dog Model

In subsequent studies, Perlane® was injected into the glans of 14 Beagle dogs. Gross and histological observations at 3 and 6 months post-injection demonstrated excellent filler retention and no signs of tissue reaction or necrosis [8] (Figs. 12.2 and 12.3)

These studies provided the basis for human trials, demonstrating feasibility, biocompatibility, and long-term volume retention of HA gel in glans tissue.

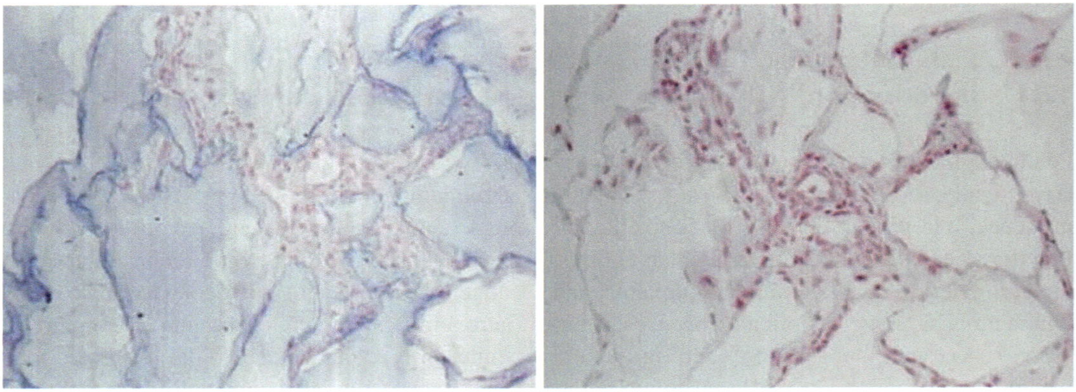

Fig. 12.1 Histological sections at 3 months post-injection of hyaluronic acid gel into the mucosa of the rabbit glans penis
Left: Various cavities within the tissue contain Alcian blue-stained hyaluronic acid gel, indicating successful retention of the filler material (x200 magnification)
Right: After treatment with hyaluronidase, the Alcian blue stain reveals the enzymatic digestion of the hyaluronic acid gel, confirming its biodegradability and biocompatibility (x200 magnification)

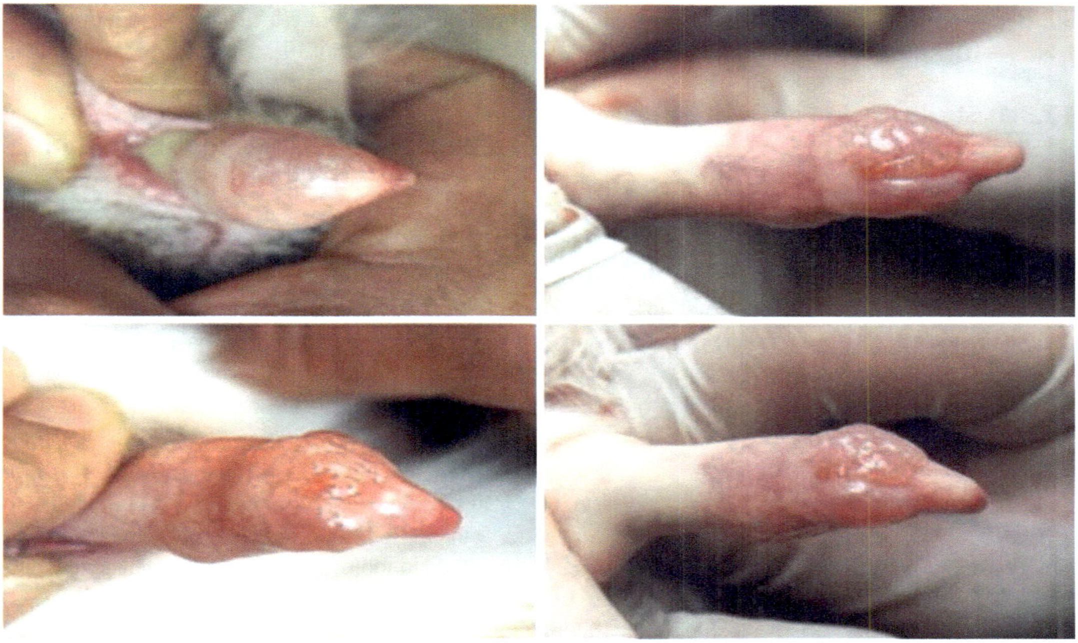

Fig. 12.2 Gross appearance of the canine glans penis after hyaluronic acid gel injection. The photograph demonstrates the visible augmentation and volume enhancement of the glans penis immediately after injection, illustrating the feasibility of subcutaneous filler placement. Implants were well maintained until 6 months

Upper left: glans penis before injection, showing baseline morphology

Upper right: immediately after injection, demonstrating significant volume augmentation

Lower left: three months post-injection, showing well-maintained implant volume and shape

Lower right: six months post-injection, with implants remaining intact and stable without significant volume loss

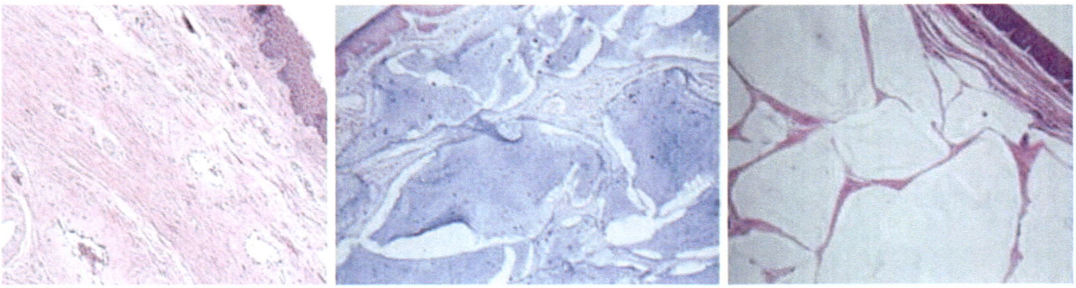

Fig. 12.3 Histological section of the canine glans penis at 6 months post-injection of hyaluronic acid gel. The image demonstrates basophilic, amorphous material retained within the lamina propria, indicating long-term stability and biocompatibility (x200). Surrounding tissue shows no signs of inflammation, confirming the biocompatibility and stability of the injected gel

Left: normal control glans tissue

Middle: implanted basophilic amorphous material

Right: Alcian blue staining after hyaluronidase treatment confirmed the digestibility and biocompatibility of HA gel (x200)

12.3 Human Studies: Aesthetic Indications

12.3.1 Study Design and Patient Groups

A total of 187 patients were studied: Group I ($n = 100$): men with subjective small glans penis. Group II ($n = 87$): men dissatisfied with relative glans size after PGE with dermofat grafts. All patients received 2 mL of Perlane® injected subcutaneously into the glans penis.

12.3.2 Evolution of Injection Techniques

Linear threading technique: Initially employed but involved multiple punctures, leading to uneven distribution. Fan technique: Later adopted, allowing uniform filler dispersion through a single puncture site and reducing procedural discomfort [9]. Figures 12.4 and 12.5 illustrate these injection techniques.

12.3.2.1 Injection Technique Evolution

12.3.3 Results and Patient Outcomes

At 1-year follow-up: Maximal glandular circumference increased significantly in both groups. Patient-reported residual volume estimated by visual analogue scale (VAS) results: Gr 3 (50–75% retention): 38% in Group I, 29.9% in Group II; Gr 4 (>75% retention): 57% in Group I, 70.1% in Group II. Satisfaction rates: 77% in Group I and 69% in Group II reported Gr 3 or 4 satisfaction levels [10]. No major adverse events; transient swelling and discoloration resolved within 2 weeks. Table 12.1 and Figs. 12.6, 12.7, and 12.8 provide detailed data and representative pre/post images.

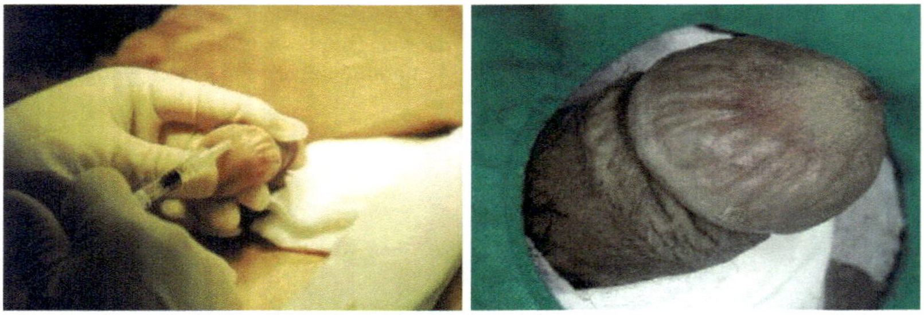

Fig. 12.4 Linear threading technique for glans penis augmentation. This technique involves multiple punctures along the proximal one-third of the glans, extending to the coronal sulcus, to deliver hyaluronic acid gel in a linear fashion. While effective in achieving localized volume enhancement, this method requires refinement for more uniform filler distribution and patient comfort

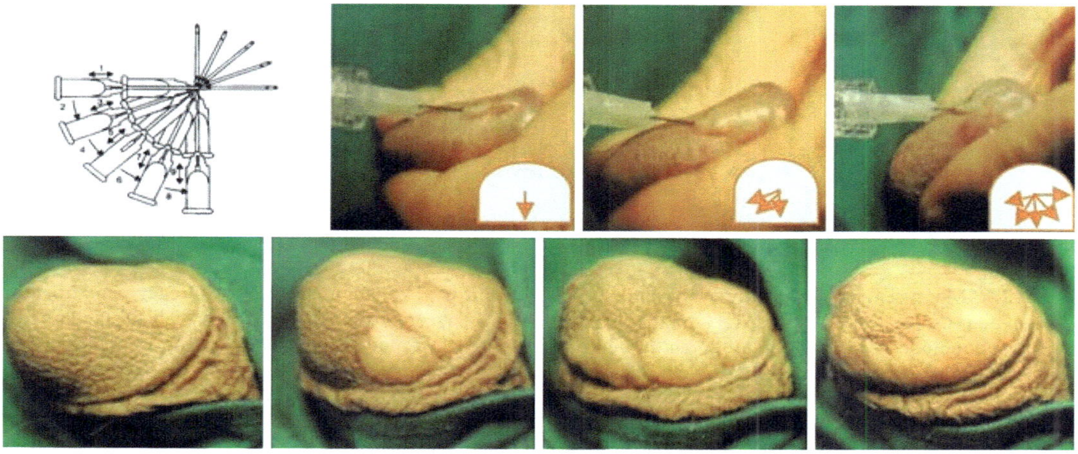

Fig. 12.5 The fan technique for glans penis augmentation
Left: A schematic representation of the fan technique, illustrating the radial pattern of filler injection with a single puncture site at the proximal glans.
Middle and right panels: Sequential clinical images demonstrating the fan technique in practice. The needle is inserted subcutaneously, and filler is distributed evenly in multiple radial directions from a central entry point. The fan technique ensures uniform filler distribution with minimal punctures, enhancing procedural efficiency and aesthetic outcomes.

Table 12.1 Results of glandular augmentation by injectable hyaluronic acid gel

		Group I	Group II	
No. of patients		100	87	
Mean age (year)		42.22 (30–70)	42.13 (28–61)	
Basal circumference (cm)		9.13 ± 0.64	9.49 ± 1.05	
Net circumference (mm)*		14.93 ± 0.80	14.73 ± 0.89	
Patient's estimation	Gr 0	0 (0%)	0 (0%)	
	Gr 1	0 (0%)	0 (0%)	
	Gr 2	5 (5%)	0 (0%)	
	Gr 3	38 (38%)	26 (29.9%)	
	Gr 4	57 (57%)	61 (70.1%)	
Mean		3.52	3.70	$P = 0.01$
Patient's satisfaction	Gr 0	0 (0%)	0 (0%)	
	Gr 1	1 (1%)	0 (0%)	
	Gr 2	22 (22%)	27 (31%)	
	Gr 3	50 (50%)	53 (61%)	
	Gr 4	27 (27%)	7 (8%)	
Mean		3.03	2.77	$P = 0.003$

Group I: Subjective small glans penis, Group II: Relative small glans after augmentation phalloplasty with girth enhancement by dermofat graft. A net increase of maximal glandular circumference 1 year after augmentation compared to before augmentation

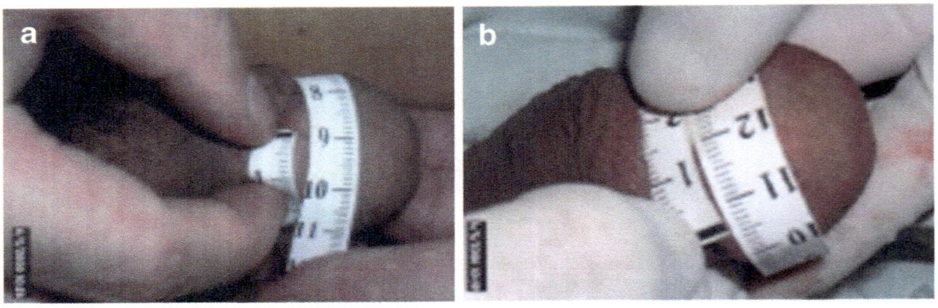

Fig. 12.6 Measurement of glandular circumference post-injection using a tapeline. The image demonstrates the method used to evaluate the net increase in maximal glandular circumference, 1 year after hyaluronic acid gel augmentation. (**a**) Preaugmentation and (**b**) 1 year after augmentation. This standardized approach provided objective data for assessing procedural outcomes

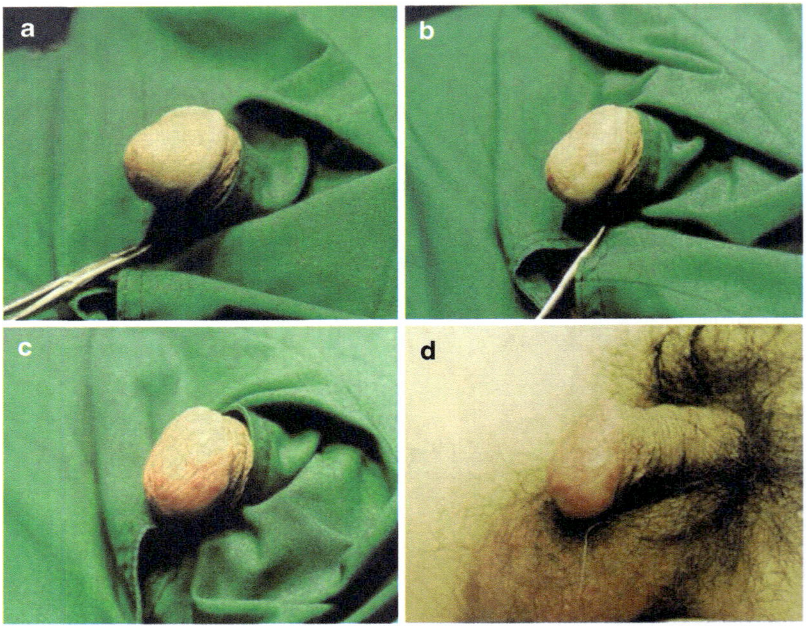

Fig. 12.7 Representative images from Group I patients with subjective small glans penis. (**a**) Preaugmentation baseline appearance. (**b**) During the augmentation procedure. (**c**) Immediate post-augmentation result showing enhanced glans volume. (**d**) Appearance at 1 year post-augmentation, demonstrating sustained volume and natural contour

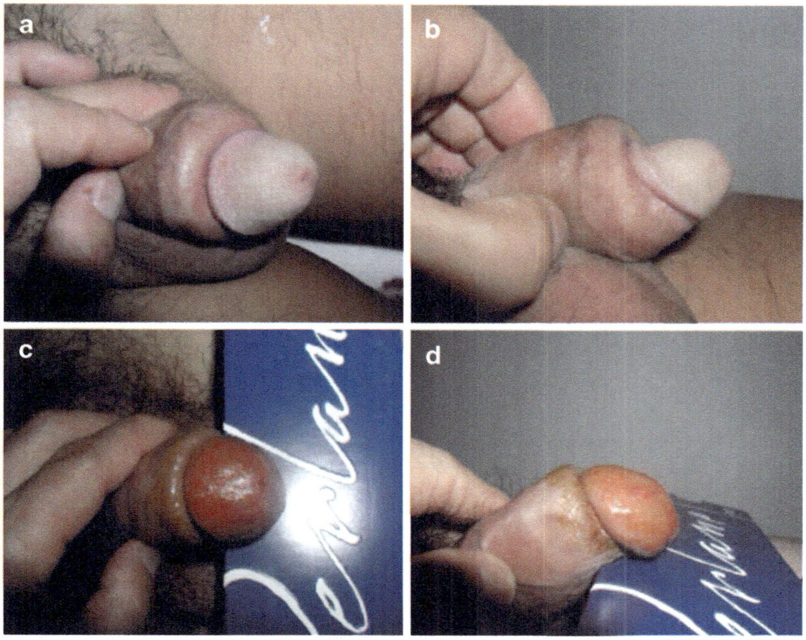

Fig. 12.8 Representative images from Group II patients with iatrogenic relative small glans penis after penile girth enhancement using dermofat graft. (**a**) Dorsal view before augmentation, showing multiple tiny skin folds and smooth indentations extending from the tip to the proximal glans. (**b**) Lateral view before augmentation, illustrating the disproportionate morphology of the glans. (**c**) Dorsal view after augmentation with hyaluronic acid gel, showing the elevation of indentations and disappearance of skin folds. (**d**) Lateral view after augmentation, demonstrating restored balance and smooth contours of the glans.

12.4 Discussion

This pioneering work demonstrated that GPA with HA gel is technically feasible and well-tolerated in humans. The elastic nature of the glans facilitated filler placement, while patient-reported outcomes highlighted high satisfaction rates and natural appearance post-procedure. Minor surface irregularities observed early often resolved during erection.

Compared to surgical alternatives, GPA using HA gel offers significant advantages, minimally invasive and reversible, no risk of scarring or permanent deformity, and suitable for patients with subjective small glans syndrome and post-PGE disproportion. Other researchers have supported these findings. Shaeer et al. introduced a modified technique for indirect GPA, further expanding options for glans augmentation [11]. International studies have emphasized the psychological and relational benefits of addressing penile morphology concerns, reinforcing the relevance of GPA in clinical practice [12, 13]. These findings laid the groundwork for extending GPA applications to functional disorders such as PE, discussed in the next chapter.

12.5 Conclusion

The development of GPA using HA gel represents a milestone in male sexual medicine. Its minimally invasive nature, biocompatibility, and high patient satisfaction underscore its role as a primary option for glans augmentation. Future directions include the use of more durable fillers and ultrasound-guided techniques to enhance precision and safety.

References

1. Perovic S, Djordjevic M. Penile lengthening. BJU Int. 2000;86(9):1028–33.
2. Alter GJ. Augmentation phalloplasty. Urol Clin North Am. 2007;34(4):593–9.
3. Ebbehøj J, Metz P. Lacking tumescence of glans during penile erection. J Urol. 1985;134(6):1220.
4. Montague DK. Penile prosthesis implantation: size matters. Eur Urol. 2007;51(4):887–8.
5. Chew K, Stuckey B. Use of transurethral alprostadil (MUSE)(prostaglandin E1) for glans tumescence in a patient with penile prosthesis. Int J Impot Res. 2000;12(3):195–6.
6. Bae YD, Park MG, Oh MM, Moon DG. Endoscopic subureteral injection for the treatment of vesicoureteral reflux in children: polydimethylsiloxane (Macroplastique®) versus dextranomer/hyaluronic acid copolymer (Deflux®). Korean J Urol. 2010;51(2):128–31.
7. Lee TW, Oh MM, Jin MH, Moon DG. Efficacy of the modified STING procedure for the treatment of high grade vesicoureteral reflux. Korean J Urol. 2008;49(11):1024–8.
8. Moon D, Kwak T, Cho H, Bae J, Park H, Kim J. Augmentation of glans penis using injectable hyaluronic acid gel. Int J Impot Res. 2003;15(6):456–60.
9. Kim J, Kwak T, Jeon B, Cheon J, Moon D. Human glans penis augmentation using injectable hyaluronic acid gel. Int J Impot Res. 2003;15(6):439–43.
10. Kwak T, Jin M, Kim J, Moon D. Long-term effects of glans penis augmentation using injectable hyaluronic acid gel for premature ejaculation. Int J Impot Res. 2008;20(4):425–8.
11. Shaeer O. Shaeer's glans augmentation technique: a pilot study. J Sex Med. 2012;9(12):3264–9.
12. Mondaini N, Ponchietti R, Gontero P, Muir G, Natali A, Caldarera E, et al. Penile length is normal in most men seeking penile lengthening procedures. Int J Impot Res. 2002;14(4):283–6.
13. Veale D, Miles S, Read J, Troglia A, Carmona L, Fiorito C, et al. Phenomenology of men with body dysmorphic disorder concerning penis size compared to men anxious about their penis size and to men without concerns: a cohort study. Body Image. 2015;13:53–61.

Glans Penis Augmentation for the Treatment of Premature Ejaculation

13

Contents

13.1 Introduction

Premature ejaculation (PE) remains the most prevalent male sexual dysfunction, with pharmacotherapy established as the primary treatment modality in the 2010 International Society for Sexual Medicine (ISSM) guidelines and reaffirmed in subsequent updates [1]. While selective serotonin reuptake inhibitors (SSRIs) and topical desensitizing agents have demonstrated efficacy, their clinical utility is limited by recurrence of symptoms upon cessation of therapy and varying patient compliance [2].

Emerging evidence suggests that penile hypersensitivity, particularly of the glans penis, plays a significant role in the pathophysiology of lifelong PE. This sensory hypersensitivity provides an organic basis for alternative therapeutic strategies targeting peripheral mechanisms [3]. Topical agents aimed at reducing glans sensitivity have been explored; however, their effects are often transient and inconsistent [4].

D. G. Moon, *Penile Augmentation with Injectable Hyaluronic Acid*,
https://doi.org/10.1007/978-981-95-5385-3_13

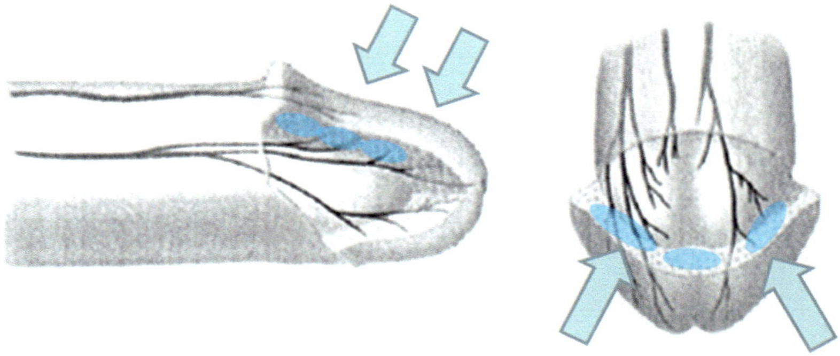

Fig. 13.1 Conceptual mechanism of GPA in reducing glans sensitivity for PE treatment

Surgical interventions, such as dorsal neurectomy, were developed to address this hypersensitivity by selectively excising branches of the dorsal nerve to decrease sensory input [5, 6]. Despite reports of improved intravaginal ejaculatory latency time (IELT) in select patients, dorsal neurectomy has not gained widespread acceptance due to its invasiveness, uncertain long-term outcomes, and potential complications—including glans numbness, paresthesia, neuroma formation, Peyronie's disease, and erectile dysfunction [7]. Nevertheless, it remains an option for carefully selected patients refractory to medical treatment.

The sensory characteristics of the glans penis are influenced by the distribution of the dorsal nerve, receptor density and thresholds, and accessibility of external stimuli to these receptors [8]. Based on this anatomical and physiological understanding, the introduction of a physical barrier using a biocompatible bulking agent such as hyaluronic acid (HA) gel has been proposed. By interposing HA gel between external stimuli and the sensory receptors, glans penis augmentation (GPA) can effectively reduce tactile sensitivity in a minimally invasive manner. This approach offers the potential to achieve symptom relief comparable to dorsal neurectomy while mitigating the risks and complications inherent to surgical procedures [9].

To investigate this hypothesis, we conducted clinical studies evaluating the efficacy and safety of GPA using injectable HA gel for PE management. This chapter further presents two key investigations: a comparative study assessing GPA alone, dorsal neurectomy alone, and their combination, followed by a 5-year longitudinal study evaluating the long-term durability, functional outcomes, and patient satisfaction with GPA (Fig. 13.1).

A schematic illustration showing the anatomical placement of HA filler beneath the glans surface. The figure highlights (1) external tactile stimuli, (2) HA gel layer acting as a physical barrier, and (3) dampened transmission of stimuli to dorsal nerve endings. This visualizes the hypothesized mechanism by which GPA reduces sensory input and prolongs ejaculatory latency.

13.2 Effects of Glans Penis Augmentation Using Hyaluronic Acid Gel for Premature Ejaculation

13.2.1 Patients

A total of 139 men with lifelong premature ejaculation (PE) were enrolled in this study. Patients were divided into three groups: Group I ($n = 25$) underwent dorsal neurectomy alone; Group II ($n = 49$) received a combined procedure of dorsal neurectomy with glans penis augmentation (GPA) using injectable hyaluronic acid (HA) gel; and Group III ($n = 65$) underwent GPA alone.

13.2.2 Procedures

Dorsal neurectomy was performed under local anesthesia using 1% lidocaine. A circumferential incision was carefully made approximately 2 cm proximal to the coronal sulcus, providing optimal access for nerve identification. Under surgical magnification, selective excision of the dorsal nerve branches was carried out with precision. On one side, the dorsal branch was excised, while on the contralateral side, the lateral and ventral branches were targeted. This approach was chosen to reduce glans sensitivity effectively while preserving enough neural pathways to minimize the risk of excessive sensory loss and postoperative complications such as numbness or paresthesia [5].

For patients undergoing glans penis augmentation (GPA) with hyaluronic acid (HA) gel, a minimally invasive technique was employed. Prior to injection, topical anesthesia was applied using EMLA® cream (lidocaine 25 mg, prilocaine 25 mg; AstraZeneca) for 30 min to ensure patient comfort. Subsequently, 2 mL of cross-linked HA gel (Perlane®, Q-Med, Uppsala, Sweden) was administered subcutaneously via a 27-gauge needle. The needle was inserted at the proximal third of the glans and advanced toward the coronal sulcus to achieve even filler distribution along the subdermal layer. After the primary augmentation, minor irregularities in the glans contour were corrected with supplementary injections of a finer HA gel (Restylane®) using a 30-gauge needle for enhanced precision and surface smoothing [7].

This dual approach, combining surgical and minimally invasive techniques, allowed for targeted modulation of glans sensitivity with the potential for synergistic effects in managing premature ejaculation (PE).

13.2.3 Evaluation

The efficacy and safety of these interventions were systematically assessed at 6 months post-treatment. Primary outcomes included measurement of intravaginal ejaculatory latency time (IELT) and vibratory threshold (VT) of the glans. VT assessments were conducted using a biothesiometer (Bio-Medical Instrument Co., USA), ensuring consistent and objective evaluation of glans sensitivity.

Secondary outcomes focused on both functional and patient-centered parameters. Changes in maximal glandular circumference were recorded using a flexible tape measure to quantify volumetric retention following GPA. Patients provided subjective assessments of residual implant volume through a five-grade visual analogue scale (VAS), ranging from 0 (no perceived volume) to 4 (near-complete retention). Satisfaction levels of both patients and their partners were also determined, with partners surveyed via telephone interviews when direct consultation was not feasible. All adverse events, including sensory changes, local inflammation, or other complications, were meticulously documented throughout the follow-up period.

This comprehensive evaluation strategy enabled a thorough understanding of both the objective and subjective benefits of GPA and dorsal neurectomy in the management of PE, providing critical insights into their comparative outcomes.

13.2.4 Results

The mean age was 43.2 years in Group I, 41.8 years in Group II, and 42.1 years in Group III (Table 13.1). All groups demonstrated significant improvements in ELT and VT at 6 months compared to baseline ($P < 0.01$). No significant differences in ELT or VT were observed between the three groups.

In Groups II and III, glans circumference increased significantly from a baseline of 9.16 ± 0.59 cm to 15.41 ± 0.82 mm (Group II) and 16.58 ± 0.85 mm (Group III) at 6 months ($P < 0.01$ for both). No significant difference was noted between these two groups.

Patients' visual estimation of residual implant volume showed that 26.5% (Group II) and 24.6% (Group III) perceived >50% retention (Grade 3), while 61.2% and 65.2%, respectively, perceived >75% retention (Grade 4). Mean residual volume grades were 3.49 and 3.55 for Groups II and III, respectively.

Patient satisfaction (Grade 3 or 4) was highest in Group II (80%), followed by Group

Table 13.1 Characteristics and parameters of all patients

	Group I	Group II	Group III
No. of pts	25	49	65
Age (y)	43.2 (25–67)	41.8 (28–70)	42.1 (27–66)
EL (s)			
Pre	89.2 (30–150)	101.5 (25–180)	96.5 (35–210)
Post	235.6 (210–430)*	324.2 (220–480)*	281.9 (250–420)*
VT (mA)			
Pre	4.14 (3–7)	4.38 (3–7)	4.54 (3–7)
Post	9.95 (8–12)*	9.80 (8–12)*	9.10 (8–12)*
GC (mm)	—	15.41 (13–16)	16.58 (12–17)
Pt's estimation (Gr)	—	3.49 (2–4)	3.55 (2–4)
Pt's satisfaction	68% (17/25)	80% (39/49)	75% (49/65)
Partner's satisfaction	44% (7/16)	66% (25/38)	62% (32/52)
Adverse reaction (%):	24% (5/25)	20% (9/45)	0% (0/65)
Numbness (6), paresthesia (4), pain for neuroma (3), Peyronie's disease (1)			

Data are expressed as mean and min/max range. Group I: dorsal neurectomy; Group II: dorsal neurectomy with glandular augmentation; Group III: glandular augmentation. *EL* ejaculatory latency, *VT* vibratory threshold; $*P = 0.01$. GC: net increase of maximal glandular circumference. Estimation of glans volume (Grades 0–4): Gr 0, 0%; Gr 1, less than 25%; Gr 2, 25–50%; Gr 3, 50–75%; Gr 4, 75–100% compared to initial volume

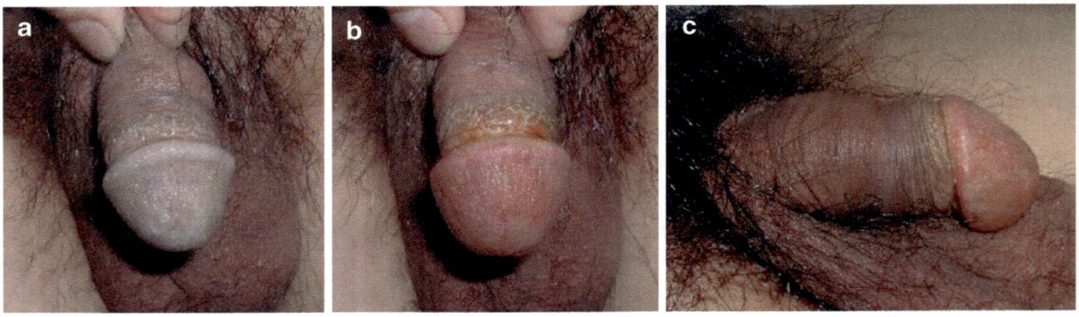

Fig. 13.2 Representative results of glans penis augmentation using injectable HA gel. (**a**) Pre-augmentation: Multiple fine skin folds and shallow indentations visible dorsally. (**b**) Post-augmentation (dorsal view): Elevated surface with smooth contour. (**c**) Post-augmentation (lateral view): Evenly distributed volume and disappearance of indentations

III (75%) and Group I (68%). Notably, satisfied patients had significantly longer postoperative ELT than dissatisfied patients in Groups II and III ($P < 0.01$). Partner satisfaction was 44% in Group I, 66% in Group II, and 62% in Group III.

Adverse events occurred in 24% of Group I (numbness, paresthesia, neuroma pain, Peyronie's disease), 20% of Group II, and none in Group III. Mild discoloration from swelling resolved within 2 weeks in Groups II and III, and no severe complications were observed (Fig. 13.2).

13.2.5 Discussion

The role of glans hypersensitivity in the pathophysiology of PE continues to generate debate. Anatomical studies confirm that the dorsal nerve of the penis (DNP) and its branches provide rich innervation to the glans, with nerve fibers running 3–6 mm beneath the epithelial surface [10]. In dorsal neurectomy, careful nerve excision is essential to minimize sensory loss; however, adverse effects such as numbness and paresthesia still occurred in 14% of patients in this study.

Conversely, GPA with HA gel offers a minimally invasive alternative. HA gel, when injected subdermally, acts as a barrier above nerve terminals, effectively dampening sensory input without compromising glans integrity. This study showed GPA alone produced comparable improvements in ELT and patient satisfaction to dorsal neurectomy, but without associated sensory complications. Moreover, GPA also contributed to enhanced self-esteem and confidence through glans enlargement—potentially amplifying functional outcomes.

Although dorsal neurectomy remains an option for refractory cases, its invasive nature and risk profile limit its appeal. GPA, as demonstrated here, may serve as a first-line intervention for men with PE and confirmed glans hypersensitivity.

13.3 Study Summary 1: Comparative Study (GPA Versus Dorsal Neurectomy)

This comparative study demonstrated that glans penis augmentation (GPA) using injectable hyaluronic acid (HA) gel provides a minimally invasive alternative to dorsal neurectomy for managing lifelong premature ejaculation (PE). GPA achieved comparable improvements in intravaginal ejaculatory latency time (IELT) and vibratory threshold (VT) with a significantly lower incidence of adverse events. Patient and partner satisfaction rates were high, particularly in the combined GPA and dorsal neurectomy group, but GPA alone showed favorable results without the complications associated with surgical nerve excision. These findings support GPA as a safe and effective therapeutic option, especially for patients seeking a reversible and less invasive intervention.

13.4 Long-Term Effects of Glans Penis Augmentation Using Injectable HA Gel for Premature Ejaculation

While the feasibility of glans penis augmentation (GPA) using injectable hyaluronic acid (HA) gel has been established, a major limitation of earlier studies was the lack of long-term efficacy and safety data. This prospective follow-up study evaluated the residual implant volume and clinical efficacy of GPA in managing premature ejaculation (PE) 5 years post-procedure [11].

13.4.1 Patients and Evaluation

Among the initial cohort of 65 patients who underwent glans penis augmentation (GPA) with hyaluronic acid (HA) gel for glans hypersensitivity, 38 patients completed a 5-year follow-up and were included in this long-term analysis. This subgroup provided an opportunity to assess both the durability of the implants and the sustained clinical efficacy of the procedure in managing premature ejaculation (PE).

The evaluation encompassed multiple dimensions of treatment outcome, ensuring a comprehensive assessment. Changes in maximal glandular circumference were measured using a flexible tape measure, allowing precise documentation of volume retention over time. Patients were also asked to provide subjective assessments of residual implant volume through a five-grade visual analogue scale (VAS), ranging from 0 (no perceptible volume) to 4 (nearly complete retention).

To evaluate functional outcomes related to PE, intravaginal ejaculatory latency time (IELT) and vibratory threshold (VT) of the glans were measured. VT was assessed using a biothesiometer

(Bio-Medical Instrument Co., USA), providing objective quantification of glans sensitivity.

Patient and partner satisfaction were key secondary outcomes. Patients rated their satisfaction on a graded VAS (0–4), while partner feedback was obtained via telephone interviews when joint clinical visits were not feasible. Finally, all adverse events—including changes in glans sensation, local inflammation, or other long-term complications—were meticulously documented throughout the follow-up period to establish the safety profile of the procedure.

13.4.2 Results

At the 5-year follow-up, the mean age of the patients was 37.7 years (range: 31–47 years), representing a relatively young cohort with glans hypersensitivity as a predominant concern. The net increase in maximal glandular circumference, which had been 16.58 ± 0.85 mm at 6 months post-procedure, showed a modest reduction to 14.10 ± 0.65 mm at 5 years—a decrease of approximately 15% that reached statistical significance ($P < 0.05$) (Table 13.2). Despite this measurable reduction in circumference, patients reported consistent satisfaction with implant volume. Subjective assessments using a visual analogue scale (VAS) revealed mean grades of 3.60 at 6 months and 3.56 at 5 years, indicating that the minor volume loss was not perceptible to most patients.

Functional outcomes demonstrated durable improvements in premature ejaculation parameters. The mean intravaginal ejaculatory latency time (IELT) increased markedly from a baseline of 84.2 s to 376.7 s at 6 months, with a slight decrease to 352.2 s at 5 years. This change remained statistically significant compared to baseline ($P < 0.05$). Similarly, the vibratory threshold (VT) of the glans increased from a baseline of 3.44 mA to 9.72 mA at 6 months and stabilized at 9.50 mA at 5 years, reflecting a sustained reduction in glans sensitivity consistent with the hypothesized barrier effect of the HA gel.

Patients' satisfaction levels remained high throughout the study period. At both 6 months and 5 years, 76% of patients rated their satisfaction as Grade 3 or 4 on the VAS, suggesting enduring psychological and functional benefits. Partner satisfaction followed a similar trend, with 68% reporting positive outcomes at 6 months and 63% at 5 years, a slight but not statistically significant decline.

Importantly, no significant adverse events were reported during the 5-year follow-up. There were no instances of sensory changes, local inflammation, or granulomatous reactions. The mild glandular swelling and discoloration observed immediately after augmentation resolved spontaneously within 2 weeks in all cases. Throughout the follow-up period, the glans maintained a natural consistency and appearance, further supporting the biocompatibility and long-term safety of the HA gel filler.

13.4.3 Discussion

This 5-year follow-up study underscores the durability and safety of GPA using injectable HA gel for PE management. While a modest 15%

Table 13.2 Results of long-term residual implants volume and efficacy for premature ejaculation

	Pre-op	6 months	5 years
Net increase of GC (mm)		16.58 ± 0.85	14.10 ± 0.65*
Pt's estimation (Gr)		3.60 (2–4)	3.56 (2–4)
IELT (s)	84.2 (45–170)	376.7 (270–470)	352.2 (220–410)*
VT (mA)	3.44 (2–6)	9.72 (8–11)	9.50 (8–11)*
Pt's satisfaction		76% (29/38)	76% (29/38)
Partner's satisfaction		68% (25/38)	63% (24/38)

GC net increase of maximal glans circumference, *EL* ejaculatory latency, *VT* vibratory threshold
*$p < 0.05$

reduction in glandular circumference was observed, this volume loss was largely imperceptible to patients, as reflected in stable VAS grades and satisfaction rates. The cross-linked structure of HA gel contributes to its extended tissue residence and isovolemic degradation, maintaining implant stability and avoiding visible deformities [12, 13].

Compared to 6-month outcomes, slight decreases in IELT and VT were noted at 5 years; however, these parameters remained significantly improved relative to baseline. The persistence of these effects supports GPA's role in sustained reduction of glans hypersensitivity and PE symptom control.

The absence of severe long-term complications, including sensory loss and inflammatory responses, reaffirms HA gel's excellent biocompatibility and safety profile [14]. Furthermore, GPA's psychological benefits, such as enhanced self-esteem and sexual confidence, likely contributed to maintained patient and partner satisfaction despite minor decreases in IELT and VT.

Although manufacturers and different publications claim that HA fillers are nontoxic and non-immunogenic, unwanted side effects have been reported with various compounds [15–17]. However, no severe adverse reactions were observed in this 5-year study, supporting the long-term safety of GPA.

13.5 Study Summary 2: Long-Term Follow-Up (5-Year Study)

The 5-year follow-up study underscored the durability and safety of GPA using HA gel for PE management. Despite a modest 15% reduction in glandular circumference over 5 years, subjective assessments of implant volume remained stable, and patient satisfaction levels were maintained. Functional outcomes, including IELT and VT, showed sustained improvements compared to baseline, with only minor declines from 6 months to 5 years. Importantly, no severe adverse events or delayed complications were observed, reaffirming HA gel's biocompatibility and long-term safety. These results highlight GPA as a reliable and enduring treatment option for PE, with the added advantage of easy supplementation through reinjection if necessary.

13.6 Chapter Conclusion

The findings presented in this chapter highlight glans penis augmentation (GPA) using hyaluronic acid gel as a novel, safe, and effective intervention for managing premature ejaculation. Comparative data show GPA achieves similar functional benefits to dorsal neurectomy while avoiding the invasiveness and potential complications of surgical nerve excision. Long-term follow-up further confirms the durability of GPA, with minimal volume loss, sustained functional improvements, and high patient and partner satisfaction persisting over 5 years. Together, these studies establish GPA as a promising minimally invasive alternative for patients with glans hypersensitivity, supporting its potential role in future clinical guidelines for PE management.

References

1. McMahon CG, Althof SE, Waldinger MD, et al. An evidence-based definition of lifelong premature ejaculation: report of the International Society for Sexual Medicine Ad Hoc Committee for the Definition of Premature Ejaculation. J Sex Med. 2008;5(7):1590–606.
2. Waldinger MD. Premature ejaculation: state of the art. Urologia. 2011;78(Suppl 18):1–8.
3. Serefoglu EC, McMahon CG, Waldinger MD, et al. An evidence-based unified definition of lifelong and acquired premature ejaculation: report of the second Ad Hoc International Society for Sexual Medicine Committee for the Definition of Premature Ejaculation. J Sex Med. 2014;11(6):1423–41.
4. Carson C, Gunn K. Premature ejaculation: definition and prevalence. Int J Impot Res. 2006;18(1):S5–S13.
5. Liu Q, Li S, Zhang Y, Cheng Y, Fan J, Jiang L, et al. Anatomic basis and clinical effect of selective dorsal neurectomy for patients with lifelong premature ejaculation: a randomized controlled trial. J Sex Med. 2019;16(4):522–30.
6. Tullii R, Guillaux C, Vaccari R, Ferreira R. Premature ejaculation-selective neurectomy: a new therapeutic technique-base, indications and results. Int J Impot Res. 1994;6:109–13.

7. Moon DG, Kim JJ, Bae JH, et al. Glans penis augmentation using injectable hyaluronic acid gel for premature ejaculation: a novel treatment. Int J Impot Res. 2003;15(5):456–60.
8. Halata Z, Munger BL. The neuroanatomical basis for the protopathic sensibility of the human glans penis. Brain Res. 1986;371(2):205–30.
9. Kim J, Kwak T, Jeon B, Cheon J, Moon D. Effects of glans penis augmentation using hyaluronic acid gel for premature ejaculation. Int J Impot Res. 2004;16(6):547–51.
10. Sundaram H, Cassuto D. Biophysical characteristics of hyaluronic acid soft-tissue fillers and their relevance to aesthetic applications. Plast Reconstr Surg. 2013;132(4 Suppl 2):5S–21S.
11. Signorini M, Liew S, Sundaram H, De Boulle KL, Goodman GJ, Monheit G, et al. Global aesthetics consensus: avoidance and management of complications from hyaluronic acid fillers—evidence-and opinion-based review and consensus recommendations. Plast Reconstr Surg. 2016;137(6):961e–71e.
12. Porst H, Montorsi F, Rosen RC, et al. The Premature Ejaculation Prevalence and Attitudes (PEPA) survey: results from a multinational patient survey. J Sex Med. 2007;4(6):1498–507.
13. Lafaille P, Benedetto A. Fillers: contraindications, side effects and precautions. J Cutan Aesthet Surg. 2010;3(1):16–9.
14. Kwak T, Jin M, Kim J, Moon D. Long-term effects of glans penis augmentation using injectable hyaluronic acid gel for premature ejaculation. Int J Impot Res. 2008;20(4):425–8.
15. Narins RS, Bowman PH. Injectable skin fillers. Clin Plast Surg. 2005;32(1):151–62.
16. Lemperle G, Morhenn VB, Charrier U. Human histology and persistence of various injectable filler substances for soft tissue augmentation. Aesth Plast Surg. 2003;27(5):354–66.
17. Christensen L, Breiting V, Janssen M, et al. Adverse reactions to injectable soft tissue permanent fillers. Aesth Plast Surg. 2005;29(1):34–48.

Is There a Place for Surgical Treatment of Premature Ejaculation?

14

Contents

14.1 Introduction

Premature ejaculation (PE) is one of the most common male sexual dysfunctions, with a prevalence estimated at 20–30% in adult men worldwide [1–3]. Over the past two decades, considerable advances have been made in understanding its epidemiology, pathophysiology, and management. These developments include an evidence-based definition of PE and international guidelines for diagnosis and treatment published by the International Society for Sexual Medicine (ISSM) [4, 5].

Pharmacotherapy, particularly with selective serotonin reuptake inhibitors (SSRIs) and topical local anesthetics, currently forms the cornerstone of PE management according to these guidelines. Shindel et al. [6] found in a nationwide US survey that 71% of urologists prescribed SSRIs as first-line therapy, while 35% employed other treatments initially, and 50% used alternative therapies as second-line options. Despite their effectiveness in many patients, these pharmacological treatments have limitations. SSRIs are associated with recurrence of symptoms upon discontinuation, and topical anesthetics—though effective—can cause local irritation, hypoesthesia, and inconvenience during sexual activity [7–9].

Before the introduction of ISSM guidelines, surgical interventions such as selective dorsal neurectomy (SDN) and glans penis augmentation (GPA) using hyaluronic acid (HA) gel were developed to reduce penile hypersensitivity, an

D. G. Moon, *Penile Augmentation with Injectable Hyaluronic Acid*,
https://doi.org/10.1007/978-981-95-5385-3_14

identified contributing factor in lifelong PE [10, 11]. However, ISSM guidelines published in 2010 and updated in 2014 recommend against surgical treatment, citing concerns over potential permanent sensory loss and insufficient reliable data [5, 12]. This position was reaffirmed in the 2021 AUA/SMSNA guidelines, which categorized surgical management as experimental and advised its use only within ethically approved clinical trials [13].

Despite these recommendations, SDN and GPA remain popular in Asian countries, particularly Korea and China, where they are employed for patients refractory to pharmacological treatment or with proven hypersensitivity to tactile stimuli. A nationwide Korean survey reported that 72.9% of urologists had prior experience with SDN in such patients, and 54.3% utilized GPA with HA gel [14]. These findings highlight a discrepancy between guideline recommendations and clinical practice.

In this chapter, we examine the evolution of surgical approaches for PE, with a focus on technical developments, reported efficacy, and safety profiles. We also discuss the controversies surrounding their place in current guidelines and consider the potential for these interventions to serve as viable options for select patients.

14.2 Current Guidelines and Recommendation Status

The pathophysiology of premature ejaculation (PE) includes biological and psychological components, with penile hypersensitivity recognized as a significant contributing factor [14]. Based on this, surgical interventions such as selective dorsal neurectomy (SDN) and glans penis augmentation (GPA) with hyaluronic acid (HA) gel have been proposed to reduce glans sensitivity. However, major professional societies remain cautious about recommending surgical options.

The 2004 American Urological Association (AUA) and European Association of Urology (EAU) guidelines focused mainly on pharmacological management of PE and did not address surgical interventions [15, 16]. The first ISSM guidelines in 2010 defined lifelong PE as an intravaginal ejaculatory latency time (IELT) of less than 1 min and acquired PE as IELT less than 3 min and emphasized pharmacotherapy and behavioral therapy as first-line treatments [5]. In their 2014 update, the ISSM reinforced this position, explicitly advising against SDN and GPA because of the potential for permanent sensory loss and the lack of large-scale, reliable data supporting their efficacy [9, 12, 17].

This cautious stance created controversy, particularly in countries where surgical treatment was already established. In Korea, the 2013 nationwide survey conducted by the Korean Society for Sexual Medicine and Andrology (KSSMA) revealed that 91.5% of urologists considered SSRIs the primary treatment, while 72.9% reported experience with SDN in patients who either responded to topical anesthetics or exhibited glans hypersensitivity [14]. Moreover, 54.3% of urologists had performed GPA using HA gel for PE management.

The 2021 AUA/SMSNA guidelines maintained a conservative view, recommending that clinicians inform patients that surgical management—including injection of bulking agents—should be considered experimental and only performed in the context of an ethically approved clinical trial [13]. Similarly, they expressed concern over invasive treatments potentially causing permanent loss of penile sensation.

However, the 2024 International Consultation on Sexual Medicine (ICSM) consensus introduced a more nuanced position. For patients with lifelong or acquired PE, ICSM allowed clinicians to offer GPA using HA gel in high-volume centers under strict informed consent. Conversely, SDN and other nerve ablation techniques were still classified as experimental and restricted to institutional ethical committee-approved clinical trials.

These divergent positions underscore the tension between guideline recommendations prioritizing safety and real-world practices in regions where surgical treatments remain prevalent. This chapter further explores the evidence supporting and contesting these recommendations.

14.3 Reported Efficacy of Selective Dorsal Neurectomy (SDN)

Selective dorsal neurectomy (SDN) was first introduced as a surgical option for patients with PE who were refractory to conventional pharmacological and behavioral therapies. The rationale for SDN lies in reducing penile hypersensitivity by excising specific branches of the dorsal penile nerve while preserving enough sensory input to maintain sexual function.

In Korea, SDN has been performed for over two decades and remains widely practiced in private clinics. A landmark study by You [18] reported on 143 patients with primary PE and documented that 81.8% were satisfied with increased IELT and decreased vibratory threshold postoperatively. Complications were noted in 11.8% of patients and included glans pain or discomfort (4.9%), penile edema (4.2%), wound dehiscence (2.1%), and delayed ejaculation (0.6%). Importantly, no permanent sensory loss was reported.

Kim et al. [19] further evaluated SDN in 74 patients, performing selective excision of the dorsal branch on one side and lateral and ventral branches on the other. They reported a threefold increase in IELT and a twofold decrease in vibratory threshold, with patient satisfaction around 70%. Numbness occurred in 8.1% of patients but was transient in most cases.

The Korean Society for Sexual Medicine and Andrology (KSSMA) conducted a nationwide survey of 527 urologists, reporting on 4400 SDN cases [13]. According to this survey, 56% of patients expressed satisfaction with SDN, while only 3.4% were dissatisfied. Recurrence of PE occurred in approximately 10% of cases. Reported complications included glans pain or paresthesia (3.8%) and erectile dysfunction (0.4%), both of which were rare.

Recent Chinese studies have also contributed to the growing body of evidence supporting SDN. Zhang et al. [8] and Shi et al. [20] documented significant improvements in IELT without reports of permanent sensory loss. Zhang's study increased IELT from 1.1 to 3.8 min and noted no complications aside from postoperative wound pain. Prologo et al. [21] reported on a minimally invasive variation using CT-guided cryoablation of the dorsal penile nerve in 24 patients, which significantly increased IELT but caused temporary penile flaccidity in four patients. The flaccidity resolved with phosphodiesterase type 5 inhibitor treatment and time.

Despite these encouraging findings, SDN has not been without controversy. Critics highlight the variability in procedural techniques and patient selection, as well as the lack of large-scale randomized controlled trials. Moreover, the ISSM guidelines' concerns about potential permanent sensory loss and rare erectile dysfunction remain relevant. However, published evidence from Korea and China suggests that when performed selectively and with careful patient selection, SDN can achieve significant symptom relief with a low complication rate.

14.4 Establishment of a Standard SDN Procedure

The dorsal penile nerve, responsible for glans sensation, plays a crucial role in the neurophysiology of ejaculation. Selective resection of its branches can decrease glans sensitivity and prolong IELT, but excessive excision risks permanent sensory loss and erectile dysfunction. Establishing a standardized surgical approach is critical for optimizing therapeutic outcomes while minimizing complications.

Anatomical studies have demonstrated considerable variability in the number and distribution of dorsal penile nerve branches. Yang and Bradley [22] described the peripheral distribution of these branches, noting 2–5 main trunks that further divide at the coronal sulcus level. Zhang et al. [23] reported an abnormal increase in dorsal nerve branches in patients with primary PE, identifying a mean of 7.16 branches compared to 3.55 in cadaveric specimens. This finding supports the hypothesis of penile hypersensitivity as an organic basis of PE and suggests that targeted nerve excision may normalize sensory input.

Korean surgeons typically perform limited excisions, targeting 2–3 lateral branches bilaterally or combining dorsal branch excision on one side with lateral and ventral branch excisions on the other. Kim et al. [19] reported favorable outcomes with this approach, achieving a threefold increase in IELT and a low incidence of numbness (8.1%), which was transient in most patients.

In contrast, Chinese surgeons have adopted more aggressive techniques. Shi et al. [20] resected 3–10 branches while preserving only two main trunks in 483 patients, achieving a 2.5-fold increase in IELT without reported changes in sexual function. Zhang et al. [8] performed segmental resection near the coronal sulcus, removing approximately half of the distributed dorsal nerve branches and reporting similar improvements in IELT and patient satisfaction.

Despite these promising results, procedural variation remains a significant limitation. There is no consensus on the optimal number of branches to resect or the precise level of nerve excision. Over-resection may result in hypoesthesia or erectile dysfunction, particularly in older patients with declining erectile reserve. Conversely, under-resection may lead to insufficient symptom relief.

To address these issues, patient selection and preoperative counseling are paramount. Candidates for SDN should include younger men with lifelong PE and documented glans hypersensitivity, especially those with positive responses to topical anesthetics but poor outcomes with SSRIs. Patients with mild erectile dysfunction or advanced age should generally be excluded due to higher risks of sensory impairment exacerbating erectile difficulties.

The KSSMA survey highlighted that SDN is predominantly performed in private clinics rather than hospital settings, where urologists tend to favor nonsurgical treatments. This disparity underscores the need for collaborative, multicenter studies that can refine surgical techniques, establish clear procedural guidelines, and provide high-level evidence to inform future recommendations.

14.5 Glans Penis Augmentation (GPA) Using HA Gel

Glans penis augmentation (GPA) was initially developed as a cosmetic procedure to increase glans size [24], but its potential therapeutic benefit in premature ejaculation (PE) emerged serendipitously when some patients reported improved ejaculatory control after augmentation [19]. The theoretical basis for GPA in PE lies in its ability to act as a physical barrier that reduces glans sensitivity by dampening tactile stimuli before they reach nerve endings.

Anatomical studies by Yang and Bradley [22] and Halata and Munger [25] have shown that free nerve endings and genital corpuscles are concentrated in the dermal layers of the glans. Injecting a filler such as cross-linked hyaluronic acid (HA) gel into the dermis just above these nerve terminals creates a subcutaneous cushion that reduces mechanical stimulation without affecting the integrity of the dorsal penile nerve itself. This contrasts with the more invasive approach of selective dorsal neurectomy (SDN), making GPA an attractive alternative for patients seeking a reversible, minimally invasive treatment.

Kim et al. [19] conducted a comparative study evaluating SDN alone, SDN with GPA, and GPA alone in patients with lifelong PE. They found that GPA alone achieved a threefold increase in intravaginal ejaculatory latency time (IELT) with a patient satisfaction rate of approximately 70%. Importantly, no patients in the GPA group experienced numbness, paresthesia, or erectile dysfunction, highlighting its favorable safety profile.

A long-term follow-up study by Kwak et al. [7] further evaluated GPA's durability. In 38 patients followed for 5 years, the net increase in maximal glans circumference decreased by only 15% (from 16.58 mm at 6 months to 14.10 mm at 5 years; $P < 0.05$). Patient-reported satisfaction remained high, with 76% rating their outcomes as "good" or "excellent." No cases of sensory loss or erectile dysfunction were reported, and the procedure's reversibility was underscored by the ability to dissolve residual HA gel using hyaluronidase if overcorrection or aesthetic concerns arose—even years after augmentation.

While GPA offers a less invasive approach, its limitations include potential long-term volume loss due to HA biodegradation, occasional surface irregularities resulting from uneven filler distribution, and the high cost of HA gel. Additionally, multicenter studies and randomized controlled trials are needed to confirm its efficacy and establish standardized protocols.

Despite these limitations, GPA's minimally invasive nature, safety profile, and reversibility position it as a promising treatment option for patients with PE and documented glans hypersensitivity, particularly those unwilling to undergo nerve surgery. The 2024 ICSM guidelines recognized this by suggesting that GPA may be offered in high-volume centers with appropriate patient consent and counseling.

14.6 Minimally Invasive Techniques

In addition to traditional surgical methods such as selective dorsal neurectomy (SDN) and glans penis augmentation (GPA), several minimally invasive techniques have emerged as alternative approaches for managing premature ejaculation (PE). These methods aim to reduce glans sensitivity without the risks associated with permanent nerve resection or filler-based augmentation.

One such approach is computed tomography (CT)-guided cryoablation of the dorsal penile nerve, reported by Prologo et al. [21]. In their study involving 24 patients with lifelong PE, cryoablation significantly increased intravaginal ejaculatory latency time (IELT). However, four patients experienced temporary penile flaccidity post-procedure, which resolved with phosphodiesterase type 5 (PDE5) inhibitor treatment and time. Cryoablation offers the advantage of precise targeting and temporary nerve desensitization, allowing for potential reversibility if complications occur.

Another promising technique is neuromodulation of the dorsal penile nerve using pulsed radiofrequency (PRF). Basal et al. [26] evaluated this approach in patients with PE resistant to conventional therapies. PRF application resulted in increased IELT without any cases of erection problems, penile hypoesthesia, or pain. This method appears to induce transient alterations in nerve conduction, leading to reduced glans sensitivity without causing structural nerve damage.

Both techniques are appealing because they avoid permanent sensory loss and offer the possibility of repeat treatment if necessary. However, these approaches remain experimental, and their long-term safety and efficacy have yet to be established through large-scale, randomized controlled trials.

As technology advances, such minimally invasive methods could provide a middle ground between pharmacotherapy and traditional surgery, especially for patients seeking temporary or reversible solutions. Future research should focus on defining optimal treatment parameters, patient selection criteria, and comparative studies with established therapies like SDN and GPA (Table 14.1).

Table 14.1 Comparison of surgical and minimally invasive techniques for PE

Technique	Mechanism	Invasiveness	Reported efficacy	Complications	Reversibility
Selective dorsal neurectomy (SDN)	Excision of selected dorsal nerve branches to reduce sensitivity	Moderate (surgical)	Two- to threefold increase in IELT (Korean/Chinese studies)	Numbness (8–2%), paresthesia (3–5%), rare ED (0.4%)	Irreversible
Glans penis augmentation (GPA)	Subcutaneous HA gel injection forming barrier to stimuli	Minimally invasive (injection)	Threefold increase in IELT; 70% satisfaction; sustained for 5 years	Mild surface irregularity, potential volume loss over time	Reversible (hyaluronidase can dissolve HA)
Cryoablation of dorsal nerve	CT-guided freezing of dorsal nerve for temporary desensitization	Minimally invasive (needle-based)	Significant IELT improvement; temporary flaccidity in 16%	Temporary flaccidity, requires PDE5 inhibitors post-procedure	Reversible (nerve regrowth after cryoablation)
Pulsed radiofrequency (PRF)	Application of PRF to dorsal nerve altering conduction temporarily	Minimally invasive (needle-based)	Improved IELT; no reported sensory loss or erectile dysfunction	No significant complications reported in small studies	Reversible (no structural nerve damage)

14.7 Conclusions

The management of premature ejaculation (PE) has evolved considerably over the past two decades, with pharmacotherapy remaining the cornerstone of treatment according to international guidelines. However, for patients refractory to medical therapy or those with documented glans hypersensitivity, surgical interventions such as selective dorsal neurectomy (SDN) and glans penis augmentation (GPA) using hyaluronic acid (HA) gel continue to attract interest.

SDN has demonstrated clear efficacy in increasing intravaginal ejaculatory latency time (IELT) and improving patient satisfaction, particularly in Korean and Chinese studies. Despite concerns outlined in ISSM and AUA/SMSNA guidelines regarding potential sensory loss and rare erectile dysfunction, reported complication rates have been low in experienced hands. Yet, the absence of standardized surgical protocols and the lack of high-level evidence from multicenter trials remain significant barriers to broader acceptance.

GPA with HA gel represents a less invasive alternative with distinct advantages. By forming a subcutaneous barrier that attenuates glans sensitivity, GPA offers a reversible, safe, and effective solution. Long-term data over 5 years show sustained efficacy with minimal adverse effects. The 2024 ICSM guidelines cautiously acknowledge GPA as an option in specialized centers with informed patient consent, reflecting growing recognition of its potential.

Emerging minimally invasive techniques such as CT-guided cryoablation and pulsed radiofrequency neuromodulation further expand the therapeutic landscape. These approaches provide temporary desensitization without structural nerve damage, suggesting a promising middle ground between pharmacotherapy and permanent surgical interventions.

Ultimately, the place of surgical treatment in PE management should not be dismissed outright. Instead, it warrants careful reevaluation, guided by well-designed studies, standardized protocols, and stringent patient selection. For appropriately selected patients—particularly those with proven glans hypersensitivity and poor response to medical treatment—surgical interventions may offer durable relief and improved quality of life. As with all evolving practices, robust scientific evidence and collaboration between clinicians and guideline committees will be critical in defining their role in future PE management paradigms.

14.8 Future Directions

The evolution of surgical treatments for premature ejaculation (PE) underscores the dynamic interplay between clinical innovation and evidence-based medicine. Moving forward, the focus should be on:

Standardizing surgical techniques such as selective dorsal neurectomy (SDN) to ensure reproducibility and minimize complications across diverse patient populations.

Expanding multicenter, randomized controlled trials to provide robust data on both SDN and glans penis augmentation (GPA) using hyaluronic acid (HA) gel.

Evaluating minimally invasive technologies like cryoablation and pulsed radiofrequency neuromodulation for their potential to offer reversible, low-risk interventions.

Integrating patient-reported outcomes into clinical studies to capture psychosocial and quality-of-life benefits beyond ejaculatory latency metrics.

Revisiting guideline recommendations in light of emerging evidence, ensuring that clinicians and patients have access to a broader spectrum of safe and effective therapies.

The reappraisal of surgical options, coupled with technological advancements, may eventually pave the way for their inclusion in future PE management algorithms, particularly for well-selected patients unresponsive to medical therapy.

References

1. Laumann EO, Paik A, Rosen RC. Sexual dysfunction in the United States: prevalence and predictors. JAMA. 1999;281(6):537–44.
2. Porst H, Montorsi F, Rosen RC, Gaynor L, Grupe S, Alexander J. The Premature Ejaculation Prevalence and Attitudes (PEPA) survey: prevalence, comorbidities, and professional help-seeking. Eur Urol. 2007;51(3):816–24.
3. Lee S, Lee J, Sung H, Park H, Park J, Choi S, et al. The prevalence of premature ejaculation and its clinical characteristics in Korean men according to different definitions. Int J Impot Res. 2013;25(1):12–7.
4. Saitz TR, Serefoglu EC. Advances in understanding and treating premature ejaculation. Nat Rev Urol. 2015;12(11):629–40.
5. Althof SE, Abdo CH, Dean J, Hackett G, McCabe M, McMahon CG, et al. International Society for Sexual Medicine's guidelines for the diagnosis and treatment of premature ejaculation. J Sex Med. 2010;7(9):2947–69.
6. Shindel AW, Nelson CJ, Brandes SB. Urologist practice patterns in the management of premature ejaculation: a nationwide survey. J Sex Med. 2008;5(1):199–205.
7. Kwak T, Jin MH, Kim JJ, Moon DG. Long-term effects of glans penis augmentation using injectable hyaluronic acid gel for premature ejaculation. Int J Impot Res. 2008;20(4):425–8.
8. Zhang GX, Yu LP, Bai WJ, Wang XF. Selective resection of dorsal nerves of penis for premature ejaculation. Int J Androl. 2012;35(6):873–9.
9. Althof SE, McMahon CG, Waldinger MD, Serefoglu EC, Shindel AW, Adaikan PG, et al. An update of the ISSM guidelines for the diagnosis and treatment of premature ejaculation. J Sex Med. 2014;11(6):1392–422.
10. Schapiro B. Premature ejaculation: a review of 1130 cases. J Urol. 1943;50(3):374–9.
11. Morales A, Barada JH, Wyllie MG. A review of the current status of topical treatments for premature ejaculation. BJU Int. 2007;100(3):493–501.
12. Serefoglu EC, McMahon CG, Waldinger MD, Althof SE, Shindel AW, Adaikan PG, et al. An evidence-based unified definition of lifelong and acquired premature ejaculation: report of the second ISSM ad hoc committee. Sex Med. 2014;2(2):41–59.
13. Yang DY, Ko K, Lee WK, Park HJ, Lee SW, Moon KH, et al. Urologists' practice patterns including surgical treatment in the management of premature ejaculation: a Korean nationwide survey. World J Mens Health. 2013;31(3):226–31.
14. Xin ZC, Chung WS, Choi YD, Seong DH, Choi YJ, Choi HK. Penile sensitivity in patients with primary premature ejaculation. J Urol. 1996;156(3):979–81.
15. Montague DK, Jarow JP, Broderick GA, Dmochowski RR, Heaton JP, Lue TF, et al. AUA guideline on the pharmacologic management of premature ejaculation. J Urol. 2004;172(1):290–4.
16. Colpi GM, Weidner W, Jungwirth A, Pomerol JM, Papp GK, Hargreave TB, et al. EAU guidelines on ejaculatory dysfunction. Eur Urol. 2004;46(5):555–8.
17. Serefoglu EC, McMahon CG, Waldinger MD, Althof SE, Shindel AW, Adaikan PG, et al. An evidence-based unified definition of lifelong and acquired PE: ISSM second ad hoc committee report. Sex Med. 2014;2(2):41–59.
18. You HS. The partial neurectomy of the dorsal nerve of the penis for patients with premature ejaculation. Korean J Androl. 2000;18(2):143–8.
19. Kim JJ, Kwak TI, Jeon BG, Cheon J, Moon DG. Effects of glans penis augmentation using hyaluronic acid gel for premature ejaculation. Int J Impot Res. 2004;16(6):547–51.

20. Shi WG, Wang XJ, Liang XQ, Liu ZQ, Huang MJ, Li SQ, et al. Selective resection of branches of the dorsal penile nerves for primary premature ejaculation. Zhonghua Nan Ke Xue. 2008;14(5):436–8.
21. Prologo JD, Snyder LL, Cherullo EA, Passalacqua M, Pirasteh A, Corn D. CT-guided cryoablation of the dorsal penile nerve for symptomatic PE. J Vasc Interv Radiol. 2013;24(2):214–9.
22. Yang CC, Bradley WE. Peripheral distribution of the human dorsal nerve of the penis. J Urol. 1998;159(6):1912–6.
23. Zhang CY, Li XH, Yuan T, Zhang HF, Liu JH, Ye ZQ. Regional anatomy of the dorsal penile nerve and its clinical significance. Zhonghua Nan Ke Xue. 2009;15(2):130–3.
24. Moon DG, Kwak TI, Cho HY, Bae JH, Park HS, Kim JJ. Augmentation of the glans penis using injectable hyaluronic acid gel. Int J Impot Res. 2003;15(6):456–60.
25. Halata Z, Munger BL. The neuroanatomical basis for the protopathic sensibility of the human glans penis. Brain Res. 1986;371(2):205–30.
26. Basal S, Goktas S, Ergin A, Yildirim I, Atim A, Tahmaz L, et al. Neuromodulation of dorsal penile nerves by pulsed radiofrequency for PE resistant to conventional treatment. J Androl. 2010;31(2):126–30.

General Principle of GPA by Injectable HA Gel

15

Contents

15.1 Introduction

Glans penis augmentation (GPA) is a topic as intriguing as it is still debated. The lack of high supporting evidence and its technically challenging aspects seem to be the main limits to the widespread adoption of GPA. However, the growing demand for GPA makes it a "hot topic" in the field of andrological surgery.

A thorough understanding of the glans anatomy, with its uniqueness and differences from the penis shaft, is the basis for safe and effective management of the patient's needs.

Before use of HA filler in Urology, STING for VUR (vesicoureteral reflux) [1, 2], and recnet penile augmenation by the author [3], HA mostly used in fascial esthetics. It is essential and useful to learn the knowledge and tips from esthetic plastic

D. G. Moon, *Penile Augmentation with Injectable Hyaluronic Acid*,
https://doi.org/10.1007/978-981-95-5385-3_15

surgery. Promising results of various fillers are mostly from cosmetic surgery. To achieve optimal results without adverse effects, it is crucial to understand facial anatomy, the effects of aging on skin tissue, and appropriate correction methods. Effective use of fillers requires selecting the most suitable injection techniques tailored to the procedure's purpose [4]. These techniques vary based on the type and size of needles or cannulas, injection volume, angle, and number of entry points and must be chosen according to the treatment area, injection layer, and the physicochemical properties of the filler [5, 6].

GPA means the volumetric increase of the glans size, with a medical or surgical approach [7]. It is suitable to manage both cosmetic and functional issues. GPA by HA has two objectives, making barrier to interrupt tactile stimuli to the receptor and general enlargement of glans surface, glans augmentation that increases patient's confidence, and necessary for small glans penis or glans deformity. In patients of glans penis deformity, focal injection maybe enough. In patients of premature ejaculation with glans penis hypersensitivity, focal injection into the sensitive is maybe enough, but unnatural appearance maybe dissatisfied in premature ejaculation patient. In most patients, global GPA with even distribution of HA filler would be the optimal goal.

By thoroughly understanding various injection techniques, practitioners can select the most appropriate technique for each dermal area and the specific needs of the patient. The choice of technique should consider not only the purpose of the procedure but also the physical properties of the filler and the required volume. Selecting the appropriate injection layer and technique ensures optimal results, achieving the desired aesthetic improvements while minimizing complications. Understanding the anatomical and structural differences of glans area is crucial in tailoring the treatment to each patient's unique needs.

15.2 Glans Penis Anatomy

The glans forms the distal end of the penis and the penis can't do anything without the glans. Historically considered as the anterior bulge of the corpus spongiosum of the urethra, it covers the tip of the corpora cavernosa. The conical shape of the glans is functional to its role in sexual intercourse, which consists of promoting penetration [8]. The arterial vascularization is supported by the internal pudendal artery, via the dorsal artery of the penis [9]. The structure of the arterial tree is manifestly terminal, an aspect not to be underestimated during invasive maneuvers on the glans. The venous system is ensured by the tributary branches of the deep dorsal vein, which after passing the root of the penis disappears into the dorsal vascular plexus of Santorini [9]. The glans mucosa has a great wealth of sensitive nerve branches [10]. The glans mucosa is rich in sensitive nerve branches. Underneath a stratified squamous epithelium, the dermis is made up of a dense layer of connective tissue as in typical skin. The innervation comes mainly from the branches of the genitofemoral nerve and the internal pudendal nerve and continues as the dorsal nerve of the penis. Nerve endings are predominantly corpuscular.

15.2.1 Feasibility in Human Application

15.2.1.1 Location

Existence of potential space: the presence of histological space within the glans to accommodate filler material.

The authors proved potential space at lamina propria of glans penis in both animal and human study and technical feasibility to inject HA filler submucosally into the glans penis.

Due to the narrow depth of lamina propria layer, too deep injection may induce perforation into underlying corpus spongiosum of glans and resultant leakage of filler into the cavernosal vascular space. Too superficial injection may induce superficial bullae or mucosal tearing. Too deep or too superficial injections cannot make proper augmentation and can induce complication. Given the relatively larger and more elastic structure of the human glans penis compared to animal models, these results suggested that submucosal HA injection is feasible in humans. The findings from these animal studies demon-

Table 15.1 Causes of injectable filler complications

Type	Description
Technical errors	(a) Volume (too much or too little)
	(b) Depth (too superficial or too deep)
	(c) Location (wrong location)
	(d) Product choice (inappropriate product)
Inflammatory	(a) Infectious agent (bacterial, fungal, viral, or biofilm mediated)
	(b) Immune mediated (not related to infectious agent)

strated that HA gel is safe, biocompatible, and capable of achieving sustained augmentation effects. Furthermore, the versatility of HA fillers in other fields of soft tissue augmentation underscored their potential as a new material for GPA.

Despite the proven lamina propria of glans penis for GPA [11], penile skin, especially glans penis, is different from the skin of the other part of the body. Even penile skin layer for penile girth enhancement is different from dermis of glans penis for GPA. The learning from dermal esthetics should be applied to GPA with proper selection. No procedure is free from complications and dermal fillers are no exception. Every filler can cause complication and the causes of injectable filler complication can be classified as technical and inflammatory [12]. Technical errors are improper volume, improper depth, improper location and implants property is much important [13]. Successful GPA requires attention to detail, including proper depth, volume, and filler selection, to ensure optimal results and minimize risks (Table 15.1).

15.3 Preoperative Preparation

15.3.1 Patient Selection

Despite of normal sized penis, SPS (small penis syndrome) patients need a larger penis to compensate for their lack of self-confidence, mainly for themselves not for their partners. GPA can be applied small glans penis or glans penis deformity after hypospadias repair, penile reconstruction for congenital micropenis, or secondary micropenis resulting from trauma, infection, or iatrogenic causes. However, careful explanation and patient's consent should be for headed before the application of GPA for subjective cases, such as perceived small glans size during erection, sexual inferiority, or premature ejaculation.

The choice to perform a GPA approach can be shared with the patient to address a spectrum of clinical conditions, from purely esthetic, but no less worthy reasons, to otherwise functional ones. The need for in-depth counseling remains pivotal, which, if properly addressed, can be decisive in many cases [14]. Sexual problems intimately affect the psychological sphere of patients and cause profound stress, in a vicious circle that is difficult to overcome. Among the cosmetic reasons that lead the patient to medical observation, the subjective dimensional perception distorted by conditions of clear glans-shaft penis asymmetry should be distinguished. The internet and social media have significantly influenced mass culture by offering wrong models and stereotypes to imitate. Consequently, it is an ethical need to dissuade clinically inappropriate requests. On the other hand, medical or surgical correction is appropriate for the management of various unsightly conditions. Asymmetries between the glans and the shaft of the penis can result from penile enlargement procedures or penile prosthesis implantation. In prosthetic surgery for the treatment of erectile dysfunction or penile curvatures, glans management remains an unmet medical need [15]. The lack of firmness and the relatively smaller size are a source of functional and esthetic dissatisfaction for patients. The functional issue in these cases is the difficult promotion of penetrative sexual intercourse. Other situations worthy of correction are congenital asymmetrical and malformative conditions. Moreover, acquired micropenis can result from infections and trauma or present an iatrogenic etiology [7]. A clinical indication to GPA by fillers is the management of patients with premature ejaculation (PE) [14]. However, its indication remains still controversial. In ISSM guideline for PE [16], pharmacotherapy must be considered as the first-line management option for patients with lifelong PE. The main limitation of pharmacotherapy is the relapse after withdrawal of medication. Decreasing glans sensitivity by injecting hyaluronic acid (HA) into the dermis of the glans was initially proposed by Korean researchers in 2004 and since then has gained popularity mainly in Asian countries [17].

15.3.2 Informed Consent

It is advisable not to address patients' requests indiscriminately, but to screen cases worthy of treatment through in-depth counseling. Here more than elsewhere, it is suitable to share with patients the supporting literature, the range of management options available, advantages and disadvantages, as well as the expected results and possible complications. Surgical options, while promising for specific cases, require careful counseling regarding risks, benefits, and potential for chronic complications. Before operation, operative principles, characteristics of filler, postoperative conditions, and patient's expectation should be discussed with the patient to avoid legal problems. The operation should be done after patient's consent by himself. Postoperative complications should be managed properly.

15.3.3 Preparations

Local anesthesia is typically sufficient for GPA. Thirty minutes after applying a topical anesthetic cream (e.g., EMLA containing lidocaine 25 mg and prilocaine 25 mg), submucosal injection of the filler can be performed. For patients requiring additional pain control, a penopubic root block with 3–5 mL lidocaine can be administered. GPA does not need canula, but 27G needle is better for controlled injection manually without injector. Historically, techniques such as the linear and serial threading injection technique or the serial puncture injection technique were commonly used, where the needle is inserted along the wrinkle line, and the filler is injected parallel to the wrinkle direction. However, for deeply embedded wrinkles, a slight misplacement of the needle can result in the filler being injected into the tissues adjacent to the wrinkle rather than directly underneath it. Any kind of monophasic HA 1 ml can be injected via 27G–30G into submucosa of glans penis manually, but 30G needle is better for fine injection. The most shortcoming of submucosal injection of HA for GPA is undulation glans surface, multiple tiny fold originating from the underlying rete ridge. At the beginning, biphasic Perlanes were injected 27G needle and undulation of glandular surface was supplemented by injection of small particle biphasic Restylane via 30-guage needle. It was inevitable but much relieved with recent development of fine monophasic HA filler and injectability with 30G needle manually (Table 15.2).

Table 15.2 Recommended HA filler properties for GPA

Parameter	Recommendation	Rationale
Filler type	Monophasic HA	Smoother surface, reduced undulations
Particle size	Medium (fine particle preferred for superficial layers)	Easier injection, better surface finish
Viscosity	Medium viscosity	Balances durability and injectability
Needle gauge	30G for superficial layers; 27G for deeper correction	Minimizes trauma and improves precision
Volume per session	4–6 mL total	Adequate for global glans coverage without overfilling risks
Retouch interval	1–2 weeks for minor correction; 6–12 months for booster	Maintains long-term aesthetic and functional outcomes

15.4 Injection Techniques for Filler Procedures

To achieve optimal results without adverse effects, it is crucial to understand glans anatomy and appropriate correction methods. Effective use of fillers requires selecting the most suitable injection techniques tailored to the procedure's purpose. These techniques vary based on the type and size of needles or cannulas, injection volume, angle, and number of entry points and must be chosen according to the treatment area, injection layer, and the physicochemical properties of the filler [5, 6]. By thoroughly understanding various injection techniques, practitioners can select the most appropriate technique for GPA and the specific needs of the patient. Among the basic injection techniques commonly used for different facial areas, the choice of technique should consider not only the purpose of the procedure but also the physical properties of the filler and the required volume for GPA. Selecting the appropriate injection layer and technique ensures optimal results, achieving the desired aesthetic improvements while minimizing complications. Understanding the anatomical and structural differences of each facial area is crucial in tailoring the treatment to each patient's unique needs.

To utilize fillers effectively, it is necessary to select the most suitable injection techniques according to the procedure's purpose. A thorough understanding of the basic injection techniques is essential for selecting the appropriate method.

In addition to basic injection technique, several injection techniques for GPA have been described, but none have been proven to be better than the others (Figs. 15.1 and 15.2) [18, 19]. To develop a simple and effective injection technique, the linear threading approach was initially introduced (Fig. 15.1a). Despite its ease of use and more uniform distribution of the injected material, this technique requires more punctures with an increased risk of bleeding and leaking from injection sites. The fan technique (Fig. 15.1b), on the other hand, allows fewer needle punctures. In both techniques, the injection needle was indwelled subcutaneously at one-third of

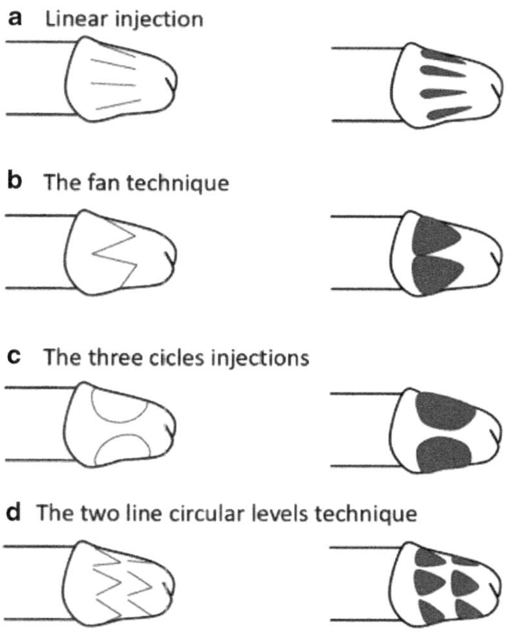

Fig. 15.1 Different injection techniques. Injection techniques: (**a**) the linear threading, (**b**) the fan, (**c**) the three-circle, (**d**) the circular two level

the distance proximally from the tip of the glans to the coronal sulcus. The three-circle technique involves dividing the glans surface into three circular areas at a distance of 1 cm from each other (Fig. 15.1c). The circles are then divided into quadrants, each of which needs to be filled with the injected material. Finally, the circular two-level technique was described (Fig. 15.1d). The limit between the two circular levels passes through the midway between the corona of the glans and the urethral meatus. The approach involves more injections at the proximal (coronal) level than in the distal circle. Regardless of the technique used, to avoid overfilling, the appropriate injection volume is approximately 4–6 ml [8].

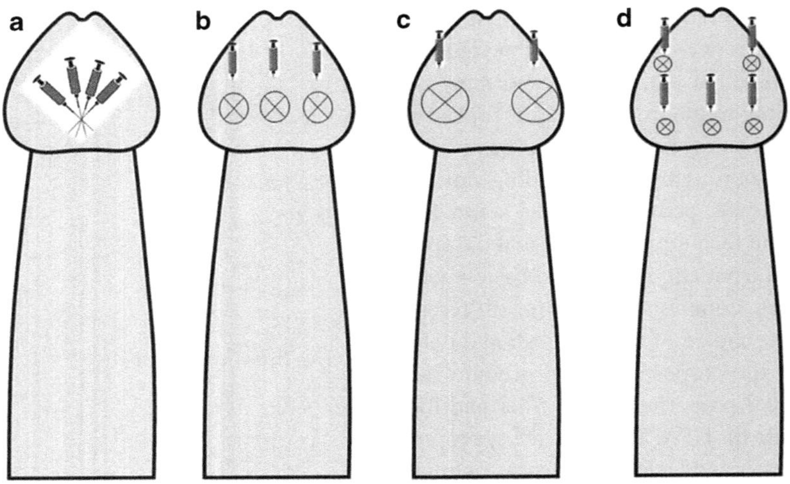

Fig. 15.2 GPA techniques by Muslim Dogan Deger [19]. (**a**) The fan technique; injection needle was indwelled subcutaneously at proximal one-third from tip of glans to coronal sulcus. (**b**) The one-third technique; injection needle indwells subcutaneously at proximal one-third from tip of glans to coronal sulcus. (**c**) The three circles technique; the circumference of the glans penis was divided into three circles, from the base of the glans at a 1-cm distance from each other. The circles were then divided into quarter circles. (**d**) The two circular levels technique: this technique was developed to allow more uniform distribution of the injected material. Multiple points of entry were created starting from the proximal one-third of the glans along the coronal sulcus together with the frenulum

15.5 Various Injection Method Adopted for GPA

Injection needle was indwelled subcutaneously at distal one-third from tip of glans to coronal sulcus; thereafter, HA gel was injected. To address any residual undulations or irregularities in the glandular surface after the Perlane® injection, Restylane® (Hyaluronic acid gel, Q-Med, Uppsala, Sweden) was administered via a 30G needle for surface refinement.

15.5.1 Dr. Moon's Initial Technique [11]

Linear Threading Technique Initially, the filler was delivered via linear threading, with 27G needle inserted subcutaneously at the proximal one-third of the glans, extending to the coronal sulcus. Due to the large size of 27G needle, Fan technique was difficult and not a true Fan technique but multiple linear threading. Moreover, this method required multiple punctures, leading to suboptimal efficiency (Fig. 12.4).

Fan Technique To overcome the challenges of the linear threading method, the fan technique was adopted with 30G needle. This approach allowed for more even distribution of the filler with fewer punctures, improving patient outcomes (Fig. 12.5).

Injection needles were indwelled subcutaneously at the distal one-third from the tip of the glans to the coronal sulcus. Thereafter, HA gel was injected. To address residual undulations or irregularities in the glandular surface after the Perlane® injection, Restylane® (Hyaluronic acid gel, Q-Med, Uppsala, Sweden) was administered via a 30G needle for surface refinement.

Both Restylanes and Perlanes are injectable HA gel and have the same composition of 20 mg/mL of stabilized HA gel. The difference between the products is the size of the gel particles. Approximate number of gel particles is 100,000/mL in Restylanes and 1000/mL in Perlanes. The suppliers recommend 30-gauge needle to inject Restylanes into the mid to upper part of dermis and 27-gauge needle to inject Perlanes into the deep layer of the dermis (Figs. 15.3, 15.4, and 15.5).

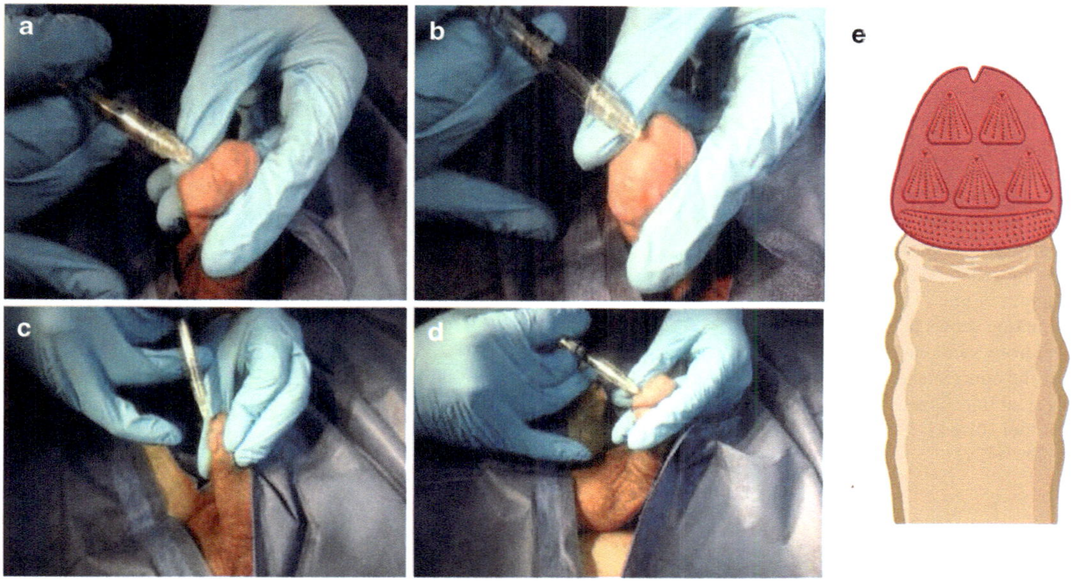

Fig. 15.3 Glans penis augmentation with hyaluronic acid gel; (**a**, **b**) injection mid-way between the corona and urethral meatus, (**c**) injection under the frenulum, d injection in corona glandis, e illustration of injection sites in glans penis. An informed consent was obtained from the patient for publishing the photos of the procedure. Dr. Alahwany's technique [20]

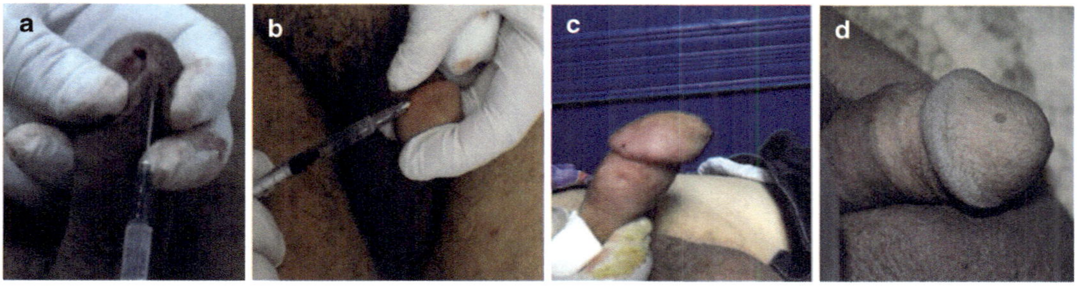

Fig. 15.4 Injection technique of hyaluronic acid in the glans penis. (**a**) Injection of the frenulum by Hyaluronic acid. (**b**) Injection of coronal sulcus. (**c**) Appearance of the glans after immediate injection. (**d**) Appearance of the glans after 3 months. Dr. Shebl's deep dermal injection technique [21]

15.5.2 Current Moon's Injection

The injection technique evolved over the course of the study. Among various injection techniques, the author does not use only one technique but combines multiple techniques. At the beginning, biphasic Perlanes was injected 27G needle and undulation of glandular surface was supplemented by injection of small particle biphasic Restylanes via 30-guage needle. Initial injection method was linear threading and back and forth technique. After some trial, I added Fan Technique to initial techniques. It was inevitable but much relieved with recent development of fine monophasic HA filler and injectability with 30G needle manually. Recently the authors favored two-layer injection similar to Dr. Alahwany method [20] and usually four punctures at distal layer and additional four punctures at second layer. At distal coronal circular area usually requires 4 ml of HA through four puncture sites. From mid to distal tip, 1.5 ml of two

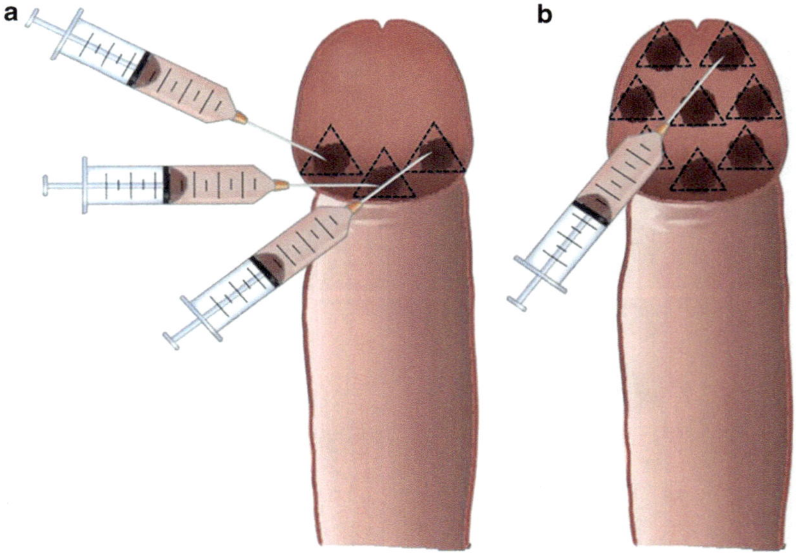

Fig. 15.5 (**a**) The diagrammatic presentation of coronary sulcus injection shows that hyaluronic acid is only located in the coronary sulcus area after injection, and the glans penis will not be significantly enlarged. (**b**) The schematic diagram of Fan technique shows that the hyaluronic acid nodule fills the entire glans after regional injections. Coronal sulcus injection by Chen [22]

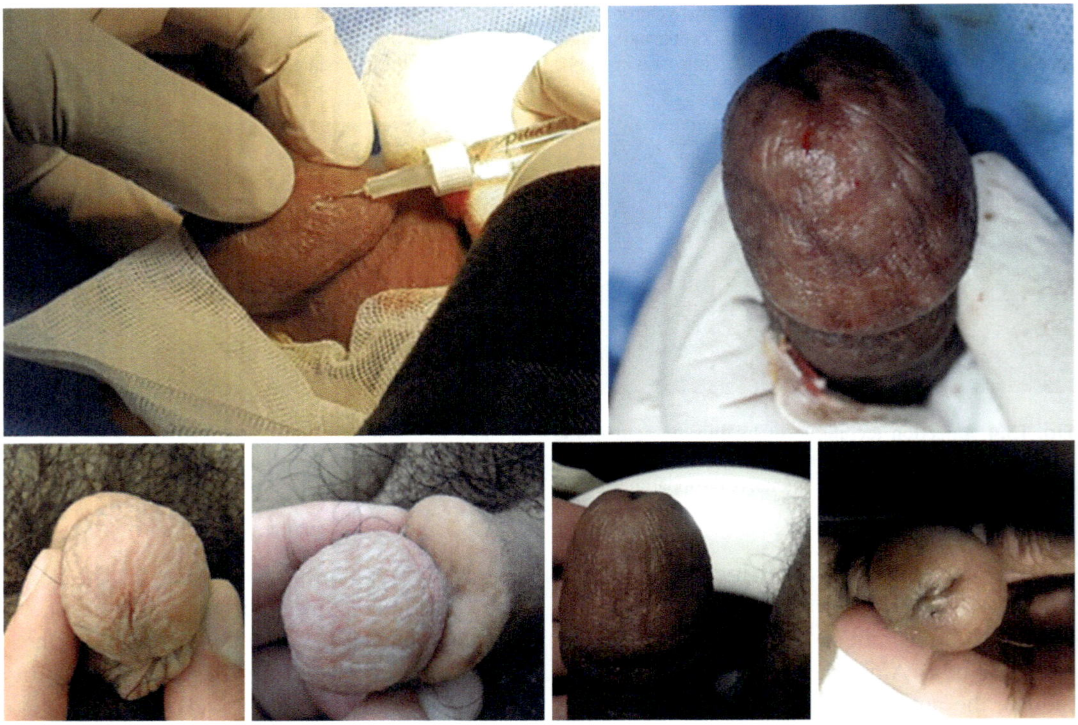

Fig. 15.6 Current Moon's technique above, comparison of surface undulation from biphasic vs monophasic HA filler, below

puncture sites and 0.5 ml of each frenula site can cover almost whole glans. Compared to the surface undulations induced biphasic Perlane in the beginning of 2003, this combined approach ensures comprehensive coverage and optimal aesthetic and functional outcomes for patients with recent monophasic HA fillers (Figs. 15.6 and 15.7).

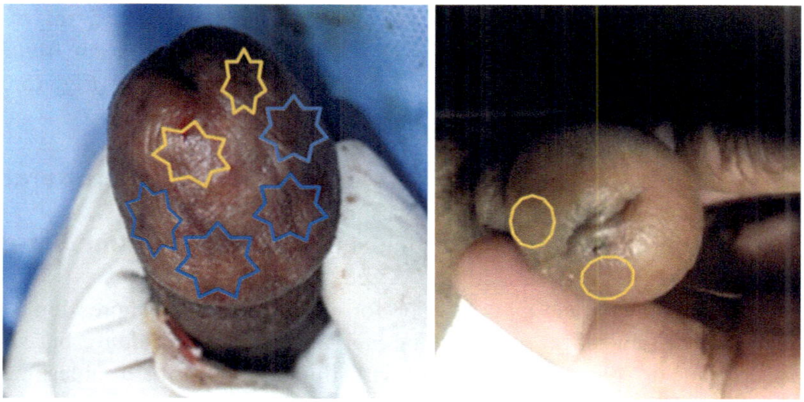

Fig. 15.7 Current Moon's technique of injection site and volume

Table 15.3 Summary of key principles and injection techniques for GPA with HA fillers

Technique	Key features	Advantages	Limitations	Preferred use
Linear threading	27G needle; filler injected along straight submucosal tracts	Simple; predictable tract creation	Requires multiple punctures; uneven distribution; higher risk of bleeding	Early GPA applications with biphasic fillers
Fan technique	Single entry point; multiple radial submucosal injections using 30G needle	Fewer punctures; broader area coverage	Potential for filler pooling at pivot points; requires skill for even distribution	Modern practice with monophasic fillers
Three-circle technique	Glans divided into three concentric circles; quadrants injected sequentially	Systematic; ensures comprehensive coverage	Time-intensive; requires multiple punctures; potential for surface irregularities	Selected cases requiring precise volume distribution
Circular two-level	Two concentric levels: Proximal (coronal) and distal; larger volume in proximal area	Mimics natural glans contour; good for volumetric symmetry	Technically demanding; increased risk of ecchymosis with multiple punctures	Advanced GPA applications; correction of asymmetries
Combination (Moon's current)	Hybrid of fan + linear + two-level; monophasic HA; four distal and four proximal punctures	Even distribution; minimal surface irregularity; fewer touch-ups	Requires advanced skill; filler properties critical (favor monophasic, fine particle size for injectability)	Preferred current technique for most patients
Coronal sulcus injection	Targeted submucosal injection limited to coronal sulcus	Simple; minimal volume needed	Does not enlarge entire glans; limited utility in cosmetic GPA	Focal correction of deformities; supplementary technique
Deep dermal injection	Filler placed within deeper dermal layer using 27G needle	Durable volume; useful for larger defects	Risk of mucosal tearing; uneven surface; possible deep vascular compromise	Rarely used; reserved for post-reconstruction deformities

Usually inject total 6 cc of HA gel; 4 injection of each 1 cc lower level and 2 injection at upper level of each 0.5 cc and 2 ventral of each 0.5 cc (Table 15.3).

15.6 Volume of Injection

At the beginning, the authors injected 2 mL of injectable hyaluronic acid gel (Perlane®, Q-Med, Uppsala, Sweden) using a 27G needle at one circular level. Perlane is initial biphasic HA and large volume injection was risk of mucosal tearing. According to the initial report [8], most researchers inject only 2 cc [18]. Some physicians inject more volume for multi-puncture or multilayer rather than Fan technique. Due to recent evolution of HA fillers usually to monophasic, personally, I prefer to inject 6 ml at whole glans evenly at initial visit and retouch at empty by absorbed area. At distal coronal circular area usually requires 4 ml of HA through four puncture sites. From mid to distal tip, 1.5 ml of two puncture sites and 0.5 ml of each frenula site can cover almost whole glans (Fig. 15.6).

15.7 Postoperative Care

15.7.1 Immediate Care

Gentle compression is enough for small bleeding from puncture, but small size adhesive strip is better for troublesome bleeding. Application of liquid adhesive (e.g., Liquid Medifoam®) for 1–2 days enhances waterproofing, allowing patients to shower. Preventive antibiotics should be administered for 3 days to minimize the risk of infection (Fig. 15.8).

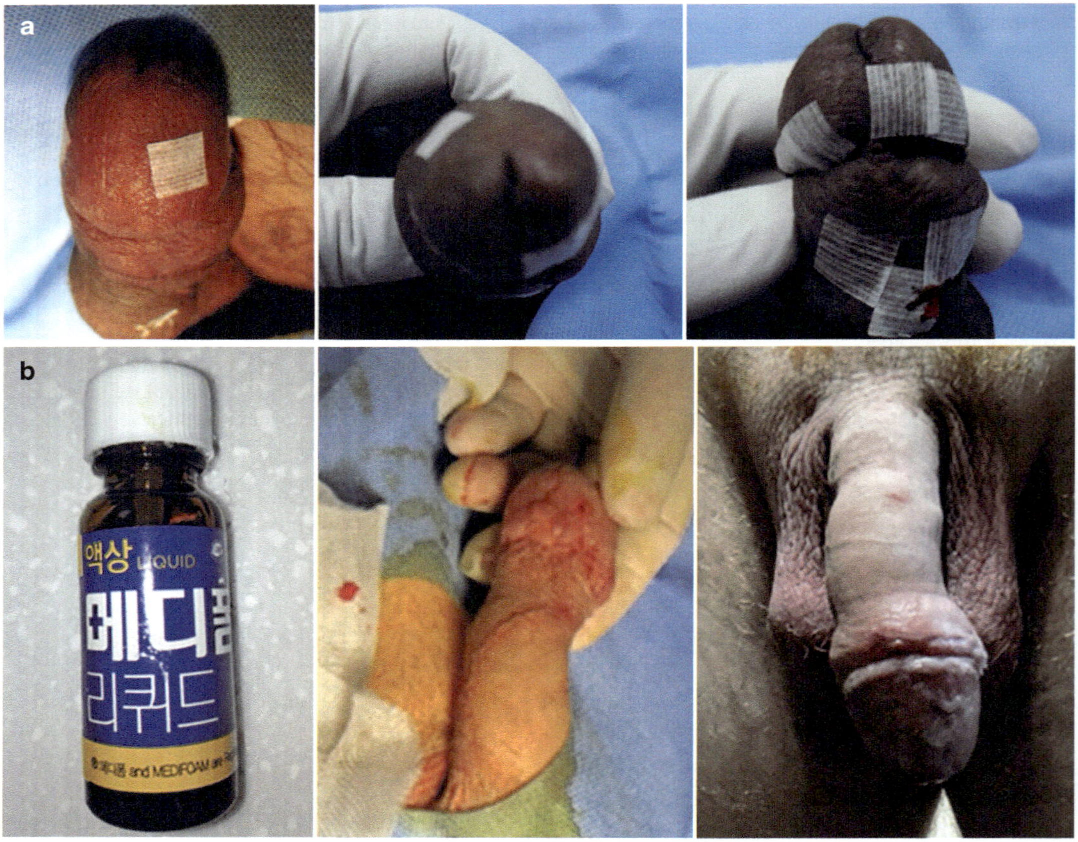

Fig. 15.8 (**a**) Gentle compression and small size adhesive strip for mucosal bleeding. (**b**) Application of liquid adhesive (e.g., Liquid Medifoam)

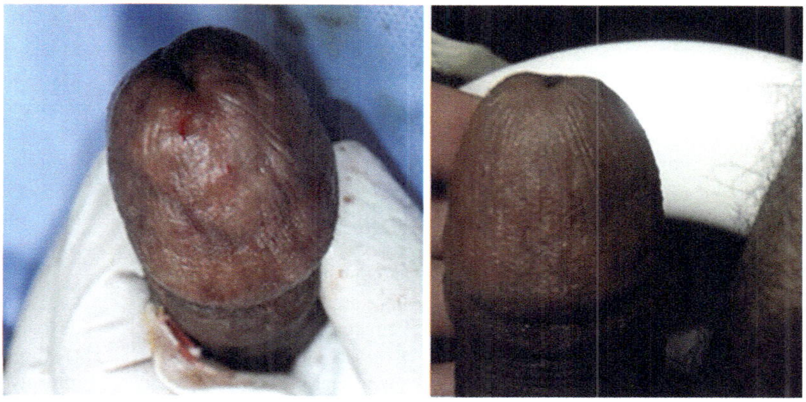

Fig. 15.9 Retouch 1 week later and gross appearance at 3 months later

15.7.2 Retouch

At the beginning, Restylane® (Hyaluronic acid gel, Q-Med, Uppsala, Sweden) was administered via a 30G needle for surface refinement to address any residual undulations or irregularities in the glandular surface after the Perlane® injection,

Nowadays, supplementary injections at 1–2 weeks later can prevent complications such as ischemic necrosis and reduce the need for initial over-injection. It's better to optimize long-term outcomes and minimize risks (Fig. 15.9):

Timed supplementation can be done several months or years later. As with esthetic fascial plasty, periodic touch-ups ensure sustained volume and efficacy over several years. In cases of glans necrosis, complications predominantly arose from the use of non-HA fillers or impure materials, as well as a lack of knowledge about proper management protocols. Hyaluronidase can effectively manage immediate complications or correct uneven results [23, 24]. With the aid of hyaluronidase, HA gel remains a superior filler for GPA due to its safety, biocompatibility, and effectiveness.

15.8 Complication

The popularity of fillers is related to the ease of application, significantly improved appearance, and low complication rates. Filler-related complications can be classified as those related to filler properties, those related to an improper technique, and those related to inflammation [12, 13]. The selection of proper fillers is important (based on the target tissue) to avoid AEs after PA using fillers. Technical errors are classified into three types as follows: volume-related errors (too much or too little filler injected), inappropriate depth of injection (too superficial injections cause an unnatural appearance or pressure necrosis, and too deep injections cause a no-augmentation effect or deep vascular compromise), and wrong placement. Infection and an immune-mediated response cause inflammation.

The mechanism to explain why some fillers cause a greater degree of vascular compromise than others when similar volumes of both are administered remains unclear. This observation may be attributed to the filler's specific tendency to promote inflammation or, alternatively, may be secondary to arterial compromise because vascular complications involve tissue anoxia and possible progression to necrosis [7]. Accidental intra-arterial filler injections may obstruct the arterial blood supply. Outcomes of differing severity occur depending on the nature and quantity of the filler, which is based on the particle size and their ability to reach the area of obstruction. PMMA microsphere-based fillers precipitate extensive facial necrosis with subsequent need for flap reconstruction secondary to concomitant collagen-induced activation of the clotting system.

Filler-related complications are categorized as early and late events and as minor and major

Table 15.4 Common complications of GPA with HA fillers and management strategies

Complication	Timing	Cause	Management
Surface undulations	Early (days–weeks)	Uneven distribution, biphasic filler properties	Massage, early retouch with fine monophasic HA
Ecchymosis and minor bleeding	Immediate	Multiple punctures, fragile mucosa	Gentle compression, adhesive strips, liquid adhesive (Medifoam®)
Mucosal tearing	Immediate	Large needle gauge (27G), overfilling, poor technique	Conservative management, avoid large volumes in one session
Filler leakage	Early (days–weeks)	Too deep injection into corpus spongiosum	Monitor; hyaluronidase if persistent
Infection	Early (within 1 week)	Poor aseptic technique, hematoma formation	Oral antibiotics; drainage if abscess develops
Ischemic necrosis	Early (rare)	Excessive filler pressure, superficial injection, vascular compromise	Hyaluronidase injection, topical nitroglycerin, hyperbaric oxygen if severe
Granuloma formation	Late (months–years)	Immune-mediated reaction, especially with non-HA fillers	Intralesional steroids, surgical excision if refractory
Volume loss (reabsorption)	Late (6–12 months)	Isovolemic degradation of HA	Booster injection or retouch
Psychological dissatisfaction	Variable	Unrealistic expectations, insufficient counseling	Preoperative counseling, possible retouch or reversal if appropriate

complications [12]. Usually, temporary fillers cause complications immediately after injections and these are easily treated, or they resolve spontaneously. Biodegradable fillers including collagen and HA are less likely to cause late complications because the filler disappears spontaneously over a period. Although most complications are transient and mild, serious AEs causing irreversible functional and aesthetic deficits may occur [13]. Complications of non-reabsorbable or permanent fillers may occur several years after implantation and often cause severe permanent reactions. Significant complications include overcorrection, surface irregularities, filler visibility, the Tyndall effect, and granuloma formation. Severe complications include visual impairment, skin necrosis, and anaphylaxis. Currently, numerous filler agents are available commercially (Table 15.1). Although a few are less risky than others, all can induce AEs [14, 15].

New techniques using various fillers are constantly developed and refined. Promising results of various fillers are mostly from cosmetic surgery. These fillers not only differ with respect to chemical composition, dynamics, and interaction with the surrounding host tissue but also show different patterns regarding adverse reactions. Firm evidence of safety and efficacy of each technique and materials should be offered (Table 15.4).

15.9 Limitations

Previously, the author stated the limitations of GPA with HA. In this Chap. 15, the updated information for the last 20 years and answer from the author to the queries of the researchers and reviewers of following publications.

In humans, HA injection into the dermis of the glans penis was associated with delay in ejaculation, eventually leading to restricting its use to males with premature ejaculation where it would serve both purposes of delaying ejaculation and augmentation [25]. Originally, GPA with HA was developed for small glans penis and injectable fillers showed efficiency in correction of glans defect after penile surgery [7, 26].

The primary limitations of GPA include the challenging injection technique required for even distribution of the gel throughout the glans penis and the minor surface undulations that arise from the underlying rete ridge structure [17]. However, although this undulation sometimes looks unnatural, it does often disappear during glans erection and as a result most patients are still satisfied [27]. Compared to the surface undulations induced biphasic HA filler in the beginning of 2003, the current combined approach ensures comprehensive coverage and optimal aesthetic and functional outcomes for patients with recent monophasic HA fillers (Fig. 15.7).

The second challenge of this procedure is the absence of a precise measure for the needed volume of HA to inject in order to achieve satisfactory, effective but nonexaggerated results [14]. Successful GPA requires proper volume of filler injection [13]. Due to biphasic large HA filler and large needle, the author injected 2 cc initially and currently maximal 6 cc first time for whole glans and retouch as needed.

The third concern is the depth of injection [14]. Too superficial injections can exaggerate these surface undulations and might even cause pressure necrosis due to the lack of elasticity of the glandular skin, while deep injections may not lead to an adequate size augmentation or effective sensory inhibition, and most importantly can lead to deep vascular compromise. In my patients of GPA with HA gel, no case of pressure necrosis occurred. Every filler can cause complication and proper depth is important [13].

Another challenge is the choice of the size and the consistency of the HA gel particles. Medium molecular weight and medium viscosity HA are preferable in terms of ease to inject and esthetic appearance. Large molecular weight and viscous HA are logically less esthetically and practically acceptable considering the small surface and space as well as the low elasticity present within the glandular area. The author tried to inject large filler deeply and small filler superficially. In many cases of the author, pure HA never induced mucosal necrosis, which means implants property is much more important.

Taken together, successful GPA requires attention to detail, including proper depth, volume, and filler selection, to ensure optimal results and minimize risks.

Finally, the number and the distribution of injection sites remains to be tailored according to each glans anatomical appearance and surgeons' experience while considering the risk/benefit ratio [14]. The main risk of multiple injections is the increased incidence of injections sites complications (ecchymosis, pain, local infection, etc.), while the main benefit is esthetically more adequate and homogenous repartition of the filler material throughout the glandular surface. The statement of harmful multiple injections at the beginning should be revised. First, I recommend reducing the number of needle punctures to minimize the potential risks including mucosal tearing, bleeding, and leakage through the needle site. Nowadays, most fillers are fine monophasic and use fine needles at least six punctures for double layers. Additionally, postoperative strip bands or liquid adhesives are better to control mucosal bleeding and healing of mucosal tearing.

The reason behind performing a prior circumcision in the setting of glans penis augmentation is probably purely esthetic [14]. Circumcision is not always required before GPA but for PGE (penile girth enhancement) by HA gel. However, some studies had shown that distal circumcision itself may be an effective surgical treatment of lifelong PE in patients with an excessive prepuce [28, 29], while others rejected this theory [30].

It is noteworthy to mention that most of these studies (except that of Kwak et al. [31]) lack long-term follow-up [14]. Although HA fillers are considered nontoxic and non-immunogenic, unwanted side effects can occur. Early cosmetic applications of HA reported no significant bioincompatibility. However, recent evidence highlights the potential for major local or systemic, immediate, or delayed adverse effects. Despite these concerns, the author's study [31] reports no serious adverse reactions after 5 years of follow-up, such as delayed or recurrent chronic inflammatory and granulomatous reactions.

Another limitation is patient satisfaction assessment. In fact, two studies only reported the patient satisfaction rate and this was done using a non-validated tool [14]. It is important to note, in these studies, the small samples size, the extremely variable and different patient-related inclusion criteria (Primary PE, secondary PE, etc.) and exclusion criteria (circumcision, previous medical treatment for PE, chronic psychiatric or systemic diseases, alcohol or substance abuse, etc.), as well as the postoperative evaluation criteria (intervals, patient satisfaction, partner satisfaction, etc.). However, proper patient selection is crucial. In fact, the use of glans penis augmentation seems more logical in patients when pharmacotherapy has failed or if there was a good response to topical treatment [32].

Finally, HA fillers undergo shrinkage over time due to degradation in the fashion of isovolemic degradation and time-dependent reabsorption, which leads to potential deformities, necessitating additional injections for correction. In most approval studies and clinical studies, most researchers estimate the longevity of implants as the best property of filler [33], but we should change the concept. As stated in the ideal characteristics of fillers, ideal filler should be biodegradable and ultimate requirement of reinjection. Retouch immediately after injection or reinjection several months or years after initial injection is very important in esthetics. It's the same for GPA and GPE by filler. Hence correction of irregularity by retouch and booster injection to maintain volume, e.g., girth in PGE, is prerequisite to determine long-term efficacy. According to the property of each filler, easy retouch and reinjection should be considered in the selection of filler to use.

Although feasible, the relatively decreased adoption of glans penis augmentation is probably related to its yet unproven outcomes but also to its technically challenging aspects [14]. The author's reply would be helpful in helping to solve the limitations.

15.10 Conclusion

The growing demand for GPA makes it a hot topic in the field of andrological surgery, albeit still widely debated. Glans penis augmentation (GPA) using hyaluronic acid (HA) fillers is an innovative approach addressing both aesthetic and functional concerns. The technique requires a deep understanding of glans anatomy, careful patient selection, and mastery of advanced injection techniques. Despite challenges such as surface irregularities, reabsorption, and technical complexities, HA fillers remain the gold standard due to their biocompatibility, safety, and effectiveness. Continued advancements in filler technology and techniques have significantly enhanced outcomes, making GPA a viable option for patients with diverse needs.

References

1. Läckgren G, Wåhlin N, Stenberg A. Endoscopic treatment of children with vesico-ureteric reflux. Acta Paediatr. 1999;88:62–71.
2. Bae YD, Park MG, Oh MM, Moon DG. Endoscopic subureteral injection for the treatment of vesicoureteral reflux in children: polydimethylsiloxane (Macroplastique®) versus dextranomer/hyaluronic acid copolymer (Deflux®). Korean J Urol. 2010;51(2):128–31.
3. Lee TW, Oh MM, Jin MH, Moon DG. Efficacy of the modified STING procedure for the treatment of high grade vesicoureteral reflux. Korean J Urol. 2008;49(11):1024–8.
4. Hong G-W, Kim S-B, Yoon SE, Wan J, Felice F, Velthuis PJ, et al. Injection techniques for filler procedures with illustration: narrative review. J Craniofac Surg. 2025;36:10.1097.
5. Heydenrych I, Kapoor KM, De Boulle K, Goodman G, Swift A, Kumar N, et al. A 10-point plan for avoiding hyaluronic acid dermal filler-related complications during facial aesthetic procedures and algorithms for management. Clin Cosmet Investig Dermatol. 2018;11:603–11.
6. Yi KH, Oh W, Kim HM, Ahn HS, Hu H, Kim HJ. Anatomical proposal for hyaluronic acid filler injection in subzygomatic arch depression: a dual-plane injection technique. Clin Anat. 2023;36(5):737–41.
7. Ahn ST, Il Kwak T, Park KS, Kim JJ, Moon DG. Complications of glans penis augmentation. Int J Impot Res. 2019;31(4):245–55.
8. Moon DG, Kwak TI, Kim JJ. Glans penis augmentation using hyaluronic acid gel as an injectable filler. World J Mens Health. 2015;33(2):50.
9. Campbell MF, Walsh PC, Wein AJ, Kolon TF, Partin AW, Dmochowski RR, et al. Campbell-Walsh-Wein urology twelfth edition review. (No Title).
10. Yang. Neuroanatomy of the penile portion of the human dorsal nerve of the penis. Br J Urol. 1998;82(1):109–13.
11. Moon D, Kwak T, Cho H, Bae J, Park H, Kim J. Augmentation of glans penis using injectable hyaluronic acid gel. Int J Impot Res. 2003;15(6):456–60.
12. DeLorenzi C. Complications of injectable fillers, part 2: vascular complications. Aesthet Surg J. 2014;34(4):584–600.

13. DeLorenzi C. Complications of injectable fillers, part I. Aesthet Surg J. 2013;33(4):561–75.
14. Kosseifi F, Chebbi A, Raad N, Ndayra A, El Samad R, Achkar K, et al. Glans penis augmentation using hyaluronic acid for the treatment of premature ejaculation: a narrative review. Transl Androl Urol. 2020;9(6):2814.
15. Shaeer O. Supersizing the penis following penile prosthesis implantation. J Sex Med. 2010;7:2608.
16. Althof SE, McMahon CG, Waldinger MD, Serefoglu EC, Shindel AW, Ganesan Adaikan P, et al. An update of the International Society of Sexual Medicine's guidelines for the diagnosis and treatment of premature ejaculation (PE). J Sex Med. 2014;11(6):1392–422.
17. Kim J, Kwak T, Jeon B, Cheon J, Moon D. Effects of glans penis augmentation using hyaluronic acid gel for premature ejaculation. Int J Impot Res. 2004;16(6):547–51.
18. Califano G, Arcaniolo D, Ruvolo CC, Manfredi C, Smarrazzo F, Cilio S, et al. Glans penis augmentation: when, how, and why? Int J Impot Res. 2022;34(4):343–6.
19. Deger MD, Gül M, Serefoglu EC. Surgical treatment of premature ejaculation: a narrative review. Int J Impot Res. 2024;36(5):474–9.
20. Alahwany A, Ragab MW, Zaghloul A, Abdallah H, Mostafa T. Hyaluronic acid injection in glans penis for treatment of premature ejaculation: a randomized controlled cross-over study. Int J Impot Res. 2019;31(5):348–55.
21. Shebl SE, Ali S, Shokr M. Hyaluronic acid injection in the glans penis for the treatment of refractory premature ejaculation: a prospective, controlled study. Andrologia. 2021;53(7):e14084.
22. Chen K, Li Q, Xu T, Zhang X. Hyaluronic acid injection to coronal sulcus of the penis for the treatment of premature ejaculation: a retrospective observational study. BMC Urol. 2023;23(1):55.
23. Brody HJ. Use of hyaluronidase in the treatment of granulomatous hyaluronic acid reactions or unwanted hyaluronic acid misplacement. Dermatologic Surg. 2005;31(8):893–7.
24. Hirsch RJ, Brody HJ, Carruthers JD. Hyaluronidase in the office: a necessity for every dermasurgeon that injects hyaluronic acid. J Cosmet Laser Ther. 2007;9(3):182–5.
25. Shaeer O. Shaeer's glans augmentation technique: a pilot study. J Sex Med. 2012;9(12):3264–9.
26. Perovic SV, Radojicic ZI, Djordjevic ML, Vukadinovic VV. Enlargement and sculpturing of a small and deformed glans. J Urol. 2003;170(4 Part 2):1686–90.
27. Gul M, Carvajal A, Serefoglu EC, Minhas S, Salonia A. European association of urology guidelines for sexual and reproductive health 2020: what is new? Int J Impot Res. 2020;32(5):477–9.
28. Gao J, Xu C, Zhang J, Liang C, Su P, Peng Z, et al. Effects of adult male circumcision on premature ejaculation: results from a prospective study in China. Biomed Res Int. 2015;2015(1):417846.
29. Gallo L. The prevalence of an excessive prepuce and the effects of distal circumcision on premature ejaculation. Arab J Urol. 2017;15(2):140–7.
30. Yang Y, Wang X, Bai Y, Han P. Circumcision does not have effect on premature ejaculation: a systematic review and meta-analysis. Andrologia. 2018;50(2):e12851.
31. Kwak T, Jin M, Kim J, Moon D. Long-term effects of glans penis augmentation using injectable hyaluronic acid gel for premature ejaculation. Int J Impot Res. 2008;20(4):425–8.
32. Jeong HG, Ahn ST, Kim JW, Seo KK, Lee DS, Uh HS, et al. Practice patterns among Korean urologists for glans penis augmentation using hyaluronic acid filler in the management of premature ejaculation. Sex Med. 2018;6(4):297–301.
33. Kim DW, Jeong HC, Ko K, Yang DY, Kim JK, Lee SH, et al. Which dermal filler is better for penile augmentation for aesthetic purposes? A prospective, single-surgeon study based on real-world experience. World J Mens Health. 2024;42.

16 Current Publications on Glans Penis Augmentation (GPA)

Contents

D. G. Moon, *Penile Augmentation with Injectable Hyaluronic Acid*,
https://doi.org/10.1007/978-981-95-5385-3_16

16.1 Introduction

The management of premature ejaculation (PE) has undergone significant evolution over the past two decades, with glans penis augmentation (GPA) using hyaluronic acid (HA) gel emerging as a novel therapeutic strategy. Originally introduced by Moon and colleagues in 2003 [1], GPA has attracted attention as a minimally invasive alternative to pharmacological therapies, particularly for patients with lifelong PE attributed to penile hypersensitivity.

The rationale for GPA lies in its capacity to attenuate sensory input by forming a subdermal layer of HA within the glans penis. This barrier reduces tactile stimulation, thereby modulating the ejaculatory reflex and prolonging intravaginal ejaculation latency time (IELT) [2]. This mechanism addresses a key aspect of PE pathophysiology, offering a targeted solution beyond the scope of centrally acting medications such as selective serotonin reuptake inhibitors (SSRIs).

Since its inception, GPA with HA has progressed from an innovative concept to a subject of robust clinical investigation. Early studies demonstrated its feasibility, safety, and patient-reported benefits. Subsequent research has refined injection techniques, assessed long-term outcomes, and identified potential complications, while systematic reviews and meta-analyses have synthesized these findings to guide clinical decision-making.

This chapter provides a detailed overview of these publications, presenting the trajectory of GPA research from its foundational studies to its current recognition within international sexual medicine forums. Through this analysis, the chapter aims to contextualize GPA within the broader therapeutic landscape of PE, highlighting its role in addressing the unmet needs of patients inadequately served by conventional treatments.

16.2 Key Highlights of Initial GPA Publication

In the early 2000s, the author and colleagues pioneered a novel approach to glans penis augmentation (GPA) through the subcutaneous injection of hyaluronic acid (HA) gel. Prior to this innovation, GPA was not recognized as a clinical procedure, largely due to limited anatomical understanding of the glans penis, the absence of suitable filler materials, and technical constraints in achieving uniform augmentation.

To overcome these barriers, the author conducted a series of foundational studies encompassing both preclinical and clinical research. In preclinical studies, animal models demonstrated the technical feasibility of HA filler injections into the glans penis. These studies confirmed the presence of histological potential spaces within the glans tissue, enabling retention of the filler material over time [3].

Subsequent human studies validated the clinical efficacy and safety of GPA using HA gel. Three landmark clinical trials published in prominent urological journals systematically investigated the procedure's outcomes:

- Volume augmentation: The initial study documented the ability to achieve significant and safe glans volume enhancement through HA injections [1, 4].

- Impact on premature ejaculation (PE): Subsequent research demonstrated that GPA improved premature ejaculation symptoms, likely by desensitizing the glans and increasing ejaculatory control [2].
- Long-term outcomes: A 5-year follow-up study confirmed the durability of the augmentation, with stable patient satisfaction and minimal complications reported [5].

One pivotal study, titled "Effects of Glans Penis Augmentation Using Hyaluronic Acid Gel for Premature Ejaculation" and published in 2004, employed a comparative design among three patient groups: dorsal neurectomy alone, dorsal neurectomy combined with GPA, and GPA alone. This trial enrolled 139 men diagnosed with PE, all of whom exhibited glans hypersensitivity. Patients in the GPA groups received subcutaneous injections of 2 mL HA gel into the glans penis.

At 6 months post-procedure, the study reported substantial improvements across all groups. Intravaginal ejaculation latency times (IELT) significantly increased, with the greatest improvement observed in the combination group (dorsal neurectomy + GPA), rising from 101.5 ± 59.4 s preoperatively to 324.2 ± 107.6 s postoperatively ($P < 0.01$). Similarly, patient and partner satisfaction rates were highest in the combination group (80% and 66%, respectively). Glandular girth measurements demonstrated significant enhancement in the GPA groups, with maximal girth increasing from 8.95 ± 0.54 cm to 11.67 ± 0.71 cm in the GPA-only group.

The authors concluded that GPA with HA gel was a safe and effective treatment for PE, providing sensory modulation of the glans penis and prolonging ejaculation latency. They recommended further long-term studies to assess residual filler volume and sustained efficacy (Figs. 12.4 and 12.5).

Study/ publication	Design	Key findings	Impact/response
Kim JJ, et al. (2004) Initial GPA Study	Prospective cohort study with three groups (dorsal neurectomy, neurectomy + augmentation, augmentation alone); $n = 139$; 6-month follow-up	Significant improvement in ejaculation latency (highest in Group II: 324 s). High patient and partner satisfaction. Increased glans girth with HA gel.	Recognized in an editorial comment by Seftel AD in *J Urol*, noted as an innovative and effective approach for PE treatment.

16.3 Editorial Commentary by Seftel AD: J Urol. 2005 Jun;173(6):2077

The innovative nature of these initial publications attracted attention in the international urological community. In an editorial commentary published in The Journal of Urology (2005), Seftel AD highlighted the significance of GPA with HA gel as a novel treatment modality for PE [6]. He noted: "The authors suggest that glans penis augmentation with an injectable gel composed of hyaluronic acid is safe and an effective modality to decrease sensation of the glans penis, which would translate into increased ejaculatory latency. This is an intriguing topic and certainly an interesting and timely treatment for this interesting disease." This recognition underscored the potential of GPA to fill critical gaps in PE management, particularly in cases where pharmacological therapies may fail or be poorly tolerated. Moreover, it validated the procedure's innovative role in addressing the challenge of recurrence following medication withdrawal, offering patients a durable, mechanism-based alternative.

16.4 Clinical Studies of GPA with HA for the Treatment of PE

16.4.1 Key Highlights of the 2012 Study by Abdallah H. et al.

In 2012, Abdallah and colleagues performed one of the first studies to examine hyaluronic acid (HA) gel injections as a treatment for premature ejaculation (PE). This randomized pilot study aimed to assess not only the efficacy of HA-based glans penis augmentation (GPA) but also to compare two different injection techniques—the fan technique and the multiple puncture technique [3].

The study enrolled 60 men with self-reported PE, equally divided between the two techniques. Each participant received a single injection of 2 mL micronized HA gel into the glans penis. Results demonstrated a significant improvement in intravaginal ejaculation latency time (IELT), increasing from a baseline of 2.12 ± 1.16 min to 7.71 ± 7.86 min at 1 month postinjection. Although IELT declined slightly at subsequent follow-ups, it remained substantially above baseline levels (5.32 ± 3.52 min). Both techniques were effective, and no superiority of one method over the other was identified.

This pioneering study provided valuable early evidence supporting GPA with HA as a minimally invasive option for PE. The authors emphasized the need for larger-scale studies and longer follow-up to confirm the procedure's durability and safety profile.

Study/ publication	Design	Key findings	Impact/response
Abdallah H. et al. (2012)	Randomized pilot study; *n* = 60; Fan vs. multiple puncture techniques for HA injection	Significant increase in IELT: baseline 2.12 min → 7.71 min (1 month) → 5.32 min (later follow-up). Both techniques effective	Supported the feasibility of HA fillers for PE treatment. Suggested larger studies for validation

16.4.2 Key Highlights of the Clinical Study by Littara A. et al.

A year later, in 2013, Littara and colleagues presented a larger clinical study evaluating HA-based GPA in 110 men with PE [7]. This investigation focused on the efficacy of injecting HA into the deep dermis of the glans penis and assessing outcomes over a 6-month period. The findings were compelling. IELT increased dramatically from a pretreatment average of 88.34 ± 3.14 s to 293.14 ± 8.16 s at 6 months post-procedure. Additionally, maximal glans circumference grew from 98.51 ± 0.71 mm to 114.35 ± 0.66 mm. Both patient and partner satisfaction were notably high, with mean scores of 5.3 and 5.1 on a six-point scale, respectively. The study reinforced HA-based GPA as a promising intervention for PE. However, the authors highlighted the need for further studies with longer follow-up periods to establish the procedure's long-term benefits and refine technical aspects (Figs. 16.1 and 16.2).

Study/ publication	Design	Key findings	Impact/response
Littara et al. (2013)	Clinical study; *n* = 110; HA injections into the deep dermis of the glans penis	IELT: baseline 88.34 s → 293.14 s (6 months). Glans circumference increased significantly. High patient and partner satisfaction	Confirmed HA injections as a safe and effective method for PE treatment. Suggested further long-term studies

16.4.3 Key Highlights of a Randomized Controlled Crossover Study by Alahwany A. et al.

In 2019, Alahwany et al. conducted a well-designed randomized controlled crossover trial to further explore the utility of GPA with HA for PE [8]. Thirty men with PE were randomized to receive either 2 mL HA injections or saline placebo injections. After a washout period, the groups crossed over to the alternate treatment.

The results demonstrated that the HA group achieved a 2.6-fold increase in IELT at 1 month postinjection, compared to only a 1.1-fold increase in the placebo group. Improvements in

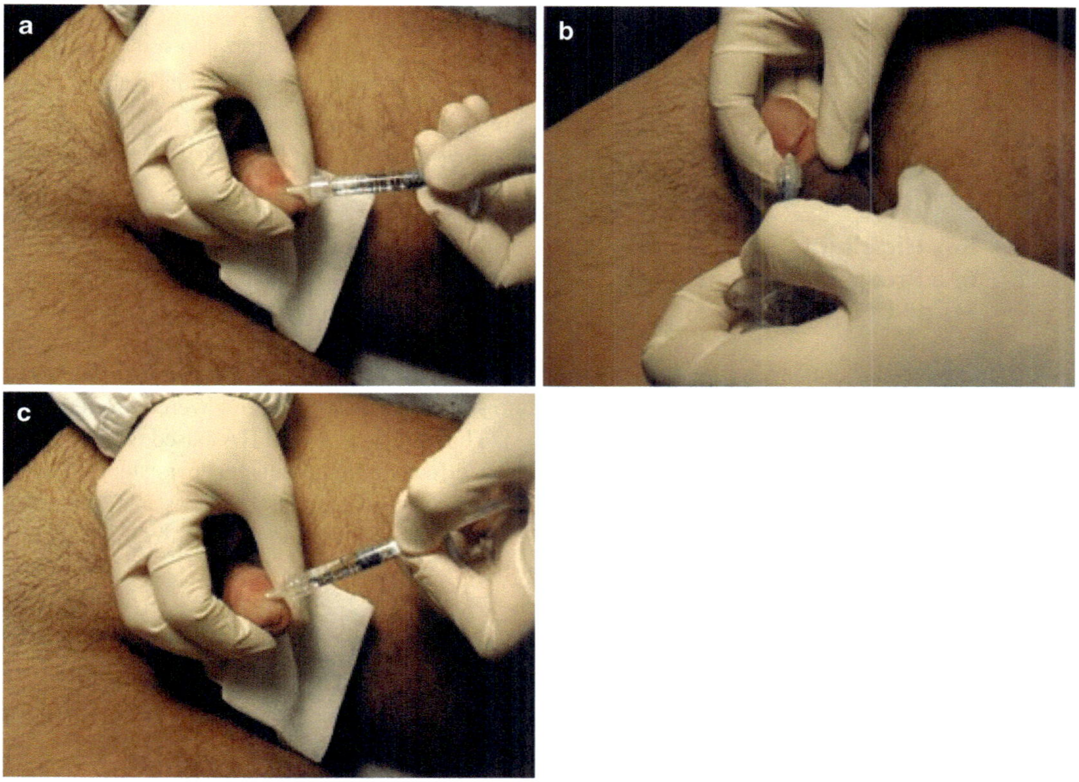

Fig. 16.1 (**a**, **b**) The circumference of the glans penis is virtually subdivided into three circles (starting from the base of the glans penis at a distance of 1 cm from each other). (**c**) Then, each circumference is further subdivided into quarter circles where 1 ml of hyaluronic acid is injected

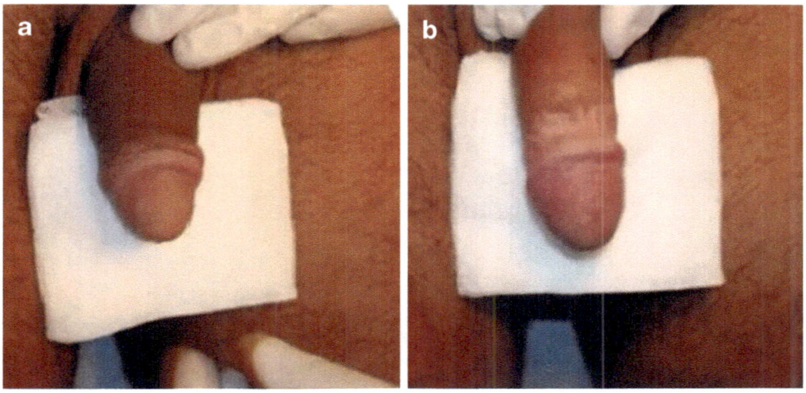

Fig. 16.2 Clinical situation (**a**) before and (**b**) after hyaluronic acid injection in the glans penis

the Arabic Index of Premature Ejaculation (AIPE) further supported the effectiveness of HA injections. Moreover, sustained IELT improvements were observed at 3, 6, and 9 months in responders. Adverse events were minimal and transient.

This study provided robust evidence of GPA's safety and efficacy, highlighting its potential to deliver meaningful benefits in PE management beyond placebo effects (Fig. 15.3).

Study/ publication	Design	Key findings	Impact/response
Alahwany et al. (2019)	RCT with crossover design; $n = 30$; HA vs. saline injection. Follow-up at 1 week, 1 month, and extended (3–9 months)	HA increased IELT by 2.6-fold (baseline to 1 month), vs. 1.1-fold for saline. AIPE scores improved significantly. Adverse effects minimal	Confirmed safety and efficacy of HA injection for PE. Highlighted sustained IELT improvement

16.4.4 Key Highlights of a Prospective, Controlled Study by Shebl SE et al.

In 2021, Shebl and colleagues reported a prospective controlled study involving 80 men with refractory PE—patients who had not responded to conventional therapies [9]. Participants were randomized to receive either HA injections or saline placebo using a four-inlet injection technique. At follow-up intervals of 1, 3, and 6 months, the HA group demonstrated sustained improvements in IELT and glans circumference. Patient satisfaction increased progressively, reaching 78.4% at 6 months, while partner satisfaction also showed improvement. Importantly, no significant adverse events were reported).

This study confirmed HA-based GPA as a safe and effective treatment for persistent PE and underscored its potential role as a mechanism-based therapy targeting glans hypersensitivity (Figs. 15.4 and 16.3).

Study/ publication	Design	Key findings	Impact/response
Shebl SE et al. (2021)	Prospective, controlled study; $n = 80$; HA vs. saline injection with four-inlet technique. 6-month follow-up	IELT improved significantly in HA group vs. baseline and control. Glans circumference increased at 1, 3, and 6 months. High patient and moderate partner satisfaction	Reinforced HA as a safe and effective treatment for persistent PE with sustained effects

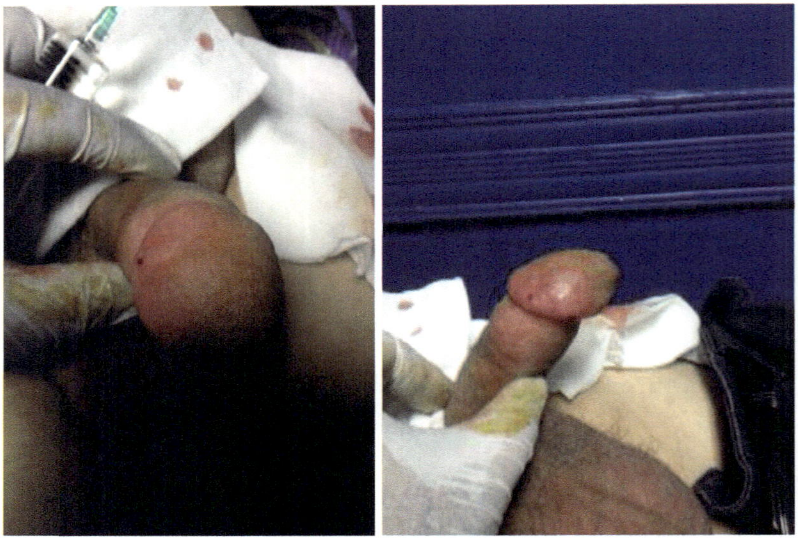

Fig. 16.3 Bleeding from injection site controlled by gentle compression

16.4.5 Key Highlights of a Retrospective Observational Study by Chen et al.

The most recent advancement in GPA research came in 2023 from Chen et al., who investigated a modified injection technique targeting the coronal sulcus rather than the glans body [10]. This retrospective study of 85 men compared traditional glans injection with the coronal sulcus method to determine whether the latter could reduce complications.

Both groups achieved significant IELT improvements, with baseline values of approximately 2 min increasing to over 8 min at 1 month post-procedure. At 6 months, IELT remained elevated at 280 ± 80.4 s. However, the complication rate was substantially lower in the coronal sulcus group (1.9%) compared to the glans group (25.8%).

The authors concluded that this modified technique might offer comparable efficacy while minimizing adverse effects, positioning it as a potentially safer alternative for HA-based GPA in PE treatment (Fig. 16.4 and Table 16.1).

This innovative technique offers a promising refinement to HA-based GPA, potentially reducing adverse effects while achieving comparable functional benefits (Fig. 15.5).

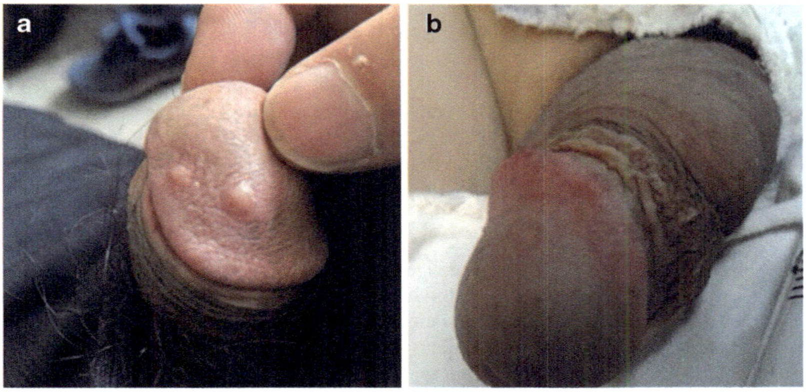

Fig. 16.4 Subcutaneous HA nodule at the penis. (**a**) The front view of a patients developed two subcutaneous HA nodules at the glans penis on the sixth day post intervention. (**b**) The front view of a patients developed fluctuation around coronal sulcus on the fifth day post intervention. HA gel is distributed more uniform by injecting around coronal sulcus. The HA nodules are revealed by nodes at the glans penis while fluctuation around coronal sulcus

Table 16.1 Combined summary of clinical studies (from initial GPA with HA study)

Study/ publication	Design	Key findings	Impact/response
Kim et al. (2004)	Prospective cohort study; $n = 139$; 3 groups: dorsal neurectomy, neurectomy + HA, HA alone.	IELT significantly increased across groups (e.g., Group II: +324 s). Glans circumference increased. High patient/partner satisfaction.	First evidence supporting glans augmentation with HA for PE. Editorial by Seftel AD highlighted its novelty and potential as a PE treatment.
Abdallah et al. (2012)	Randomized pilot study; $n = 60$; Fan vs. Multiple Puncture techniques.	IELT improved from baseline 2.12 min to 7.71 min (1 month) and 5.32 min (longer follow-up). Both techniques were effective.	Early evidence of efficacy; need for larger studies.
Littara et al. (2013)	Clinical study; $n = 110$; HA injections into the glans penis.	IELT increased from 88.34 s to 293.14 s (6 months). Glans circumference increased. High patient (5.3/6) and partner satisfaction (5.1/6).	Reinforced GPA as promising; suggested long-term studies.
Alahwany et al. (2019)	RCT with crossover design; $n = 30$; HA vs. saline injection.	IELT increased by 2.6-fold for HA group (baseline to 1 month), vs. 1.1-fold for saline. Significant AIPE score improvement. Adverse effects minimal.	Validated GPA efficacy; minimal adverse effects.
Shebl et al. (2021)	Prospective controlled study; $n = 80$; HA vs. saline injection using a four-inlet technique.	IELT and glans circumference improved significantly in HA group at 1, 3, and 6 months. Patient satisfaction: 78.4% (6 months). Minimal adverse effects.	Strong evidence for GPA in refractory PE cases.
Chen. K et al. (2023)	Retrospective observational study; $n = 85$; Glans vs. coronal sulcus injection (modified). Follow-up: 1, 3, 6 months.	IELT improved significantly across groups (1 month: 482.1 s; 6 months: 280 s). Complications significantly lower with coronal sulcus injection (1.9% vs. 25.8% for glans injection). No severe complications.	Introduced safer modified injection technique.

16.5 Review Articles of GPA with HA for the Treatment of PE

Premature ejaculation (PE) remains the most prevalent male sexual dysfunction globally, affecting approximately 5% of men [11]. Among proposed treatments, glans penis augmentation (GPA) using hyaluronic acid (HA) gel has garnered attention as a mechanism-based approach, particularly for cases of lifelong PE associated with penile hypersensitivity. The theoretical basis for HA's effectiveness lies in its ability to create a subcutaneous barrier within the glans, reducing tactile stimuli transmission to the dorsal nerve.

Although individual clinical studies have demonstrated promising outcomes, the role of HA-based GPA remains controversial and has yet to gain universal acceptance in clinical guidelines. Four key review articles—two narrative reviews and two systematic reviews—have analyzed the existing evidence, providing insights into its efficacy, safety, and practical considerations.

16.5.1 A Narrative Review of Kosseifi F, et al. (2020) Narrative Review [11]

In 2020, Kosseifi et al. published a narrative review assessing the application of HA injections for PE [11]. The authors identified five studies spanning two decades, which collectively demonstrated IELT increases ranging from 2.43- to 4.46-fold post-treatment. These effects persisted for up to 5 years in some cases.

Adverse events were minimal and transient, including mild discoloration and swelling of the glans. The review also described variations in injection techniques, though their relative efficacy remained uncertain.

Kosseifi et al. [11] concluded that HA augmentation shows considerable potential but stressed the importance of proper patient selection and technical expertise. They emphasized that surgical training and aesthetic precision are critical for achieving optimal outcomes.

16.5.2 A Narrative Review of Ambusaidi H, et al. (2023) Narrative Review [12]

Ambusaidi and colleagues' 2023 narrative review broadened the focus to include surgical interventions for PE, such as GPA, selective dorsal neurectomy (SDN), and neuromodulation [12]. The authors noted that while pharmaceutical therapies remain first line, surgical approaches have found wider acceptance in Asia, despite skepticism in Western medical practice.

GPA, in particular, was highlighted as a commonly performed procedure in Asian countries with promising early results. However, the authors cautioned that evidence quality varies and large-scale, high-quality studies are lacking. They emphasized the need for comprehensive patient counseling about the risks, benefits, and potential complications of surgical interventions. Focus: Evaluation of surgical management options for premature ejaculation (PE) as alternatives to medical therapy.

16.5.3 A Narrative Review of Zucchi A, et al. (2021) Narrative Review [13]

Zucchi and colleagues (2021) conducted a comprehensive narrative review of hyaluronic acid (HA) applications in andrology, covering Peyronie's disease, penile enlargement, and premature ejaculation (PE). Regarding PE, HA injection into the glans was described as a localized treatment aiming to delay ejaculation by dampening tactile stimulus to afferent receptors.

The authors summarized evidence from five clinical studies: three single-arm trials [2, 5, 7], one randomized noncontrolled trial [3], and one randomized controlled trial [8]. Collectively, these studies demonstrated that HA glans augmentation significantly prolonged intravaginal ejaculatory latency time (IELT), with sustained though partially reduced effects at long-term follow-up. Across studies, adverse events were mild (e.g., glans numbness, ecchymosis, local discomfort) and resolved spontaneously in most cases.

Notably, the original study by Kim et al. [2] showed meaningful IELT improvements across three treatment arms: dorsal neurectomy, GPA with HA, and the combined approach . Additional studies using different injection techniques—fan vs. multiple puncture—reported similar efficacy.

Overall, the review concluded that HA glans injection is an effective and safe intervention for selected PE patients, supporting its adoption into clinical practice with appropriate patient counseling (Fig. 16.5).

16.5.4 A Systematic Review and Meta-Analysis by Culha MG, et al. (2024)

Culha et al. provided a comprehensive evaluation of HA-based GPA in a 2024 systematic review and meta-analysis [14]. Their analysis included 13 studies involving 706 patients, assessing short- and medium-term outcomes.

IELT improvements were significant, with a mean increase of 176.2 s at 1 month and 143.9 s at 6 months post-treatment. Glans circumference

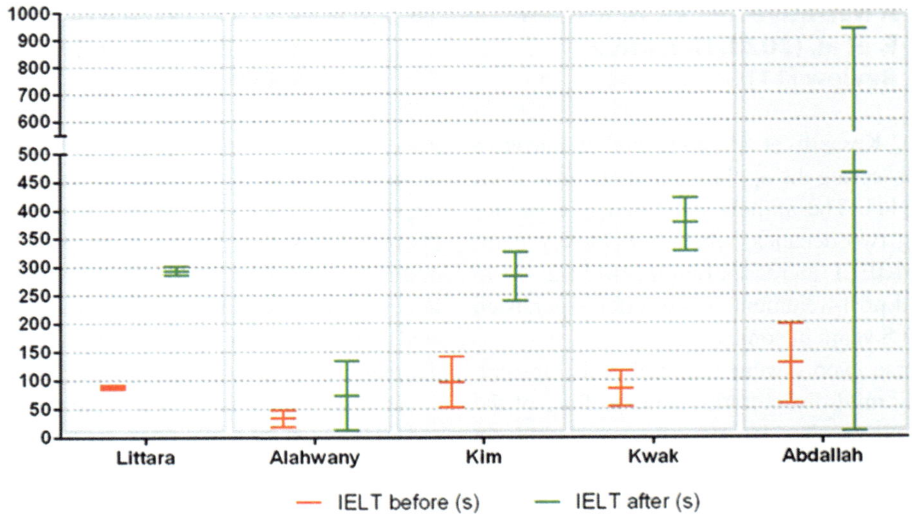

Fig. 16.5 Different results using hyaluronic acid in the treatment of premature ejaculation

also increased by an average of 14.8 mm. Adverse events were reported in 15.2% of patients, primarily pain, nodule formation, and ecchymosis—all of which were generally mild and self-limiting.

The authors concluded that GPA with HA is a promising, minimally invasive treatment for PE, but called for further studies to assess long-term efficacy and refine injection techniques.

16.5.5 Interventions to Treat Premature Ejaculation: A Systematic Review Short Report by Cooper K, et al. (2015)

In 2015, Cooper and colleagues conducted a systematic review encompassing a broad range of PE treatments, including pharmacologic, behavioral, and surgical options [15]. While their primary focus was not GPA, the review acknowledged surgical interventions like GPA and SDN but noted a lack of high-quality evidence to support their widespread use.

The review underscored the robust evidence supporting pharmacological treatments such as SSRIs and topical anesthetics while highlighting the need for more rigorous research into surgical techniques. Long-term safety and efficacy of procedures like GPA remained insufficiently explored.

Table 16.2 Combined summary of reviews (including Culha et al. meta-analysis)

Study/review	Type	Focus	Key findings
Kosseifi et al. (2020)	Narrative review	HA for glans augmentation in PE	IELT increase (2.43–4.46×) with effects persisting up to 5 years. Minimal adverse effects. Emphasized proper technique and patient selection.
Ambusaidi et al. (2023)	Narrative review	Surgical therapies for PE	GPA widely practiced in Asia; evidence limited; emphasized counseling and need for larger trials.
Cooper et al. (2015)	Systematic review	Comprehensive PE treatment options	Strong evidence for pharmacological therapies; insufficient data for GPA or other surgical options.
Culha MG et al. (2024)	Systematic review and meta-analysis	Efficacy and safety of HA-based GPA	IELT +176 s (1 month), +144 s (6 months); adverse events in 15%; promising but needs more research.

16.6 Key Highlights of the 2024 Systematic Review and Meta-Analysis by Culha MG et al. (Table 16.2)

Study/ publication	Design	Key findings	Impact/response
Culha MG et al. (2024)	Systematic review and meta-analysis; 13 studies; 706 patients. Outcomes: IELT, glans circumference, adverse events.	IELT: +176.18 s at 1 month, +143.93 s at 6 months. Glans circumference: +1.5 cm. Adverse events: 15.22% (most common: pain, bulla/nodule, ecchymosis)	Established HA as a safe and effective option for PE with evidence from diverse studies. Called for further research into mechanisms and long-term efficacy

16.7 Progress from Other Studies

The development of hyaluronic acid (HA) as a therapeutic option for premature ejaculation (PE) represents a decade-long trajectory of innovation, validation, and refinement. From its early conceptualization to its current status as a subject of systematic investigation, HA-based glans penis augmentation (GPA) has steadily evolved through key milestones in research and clinical practice.

16.7.1 Initial Validation (2004–2013)

The foundational work of Moon and colleagues between 2003 and 2004 established the feasibility of HA-based GPA for PE treatment. These pioneering studies demonstrated significant improvements in intravaginal ejaculation latency time (IELT), along with high levels of patient and partner satisfaction and minimal adverse events. This initial success sparked further interest in HA as a minimally invasive intervention targeting glans hypersensitivity—a key pathophysiological component of lifelong PE.

Building on this groundwork, subsequent studies such as those by Abdallah et al. [3] and Littara et al. [7] expanded the evidence base. Abdallah's randomized pilot trial compared injection techniques, demonstrating that both the fan and multiple puncture methods effectively improved IELT. Littara's larger prospective study reinforced these findings, highlighting sustained IELT gains and aesthetic benefits. Both studies emphasized the need for standardized injection protocols and long-term evaluations to optimize outcomes.

16.7.2 Expansion and Technique Refinement (2019–2023)

In the years that followed, researchers focused on strengthening the evidence base and refining injection techniques. Alahwany et al. [8] conducted a randomized controlled crossover trial that provided robust validation of HA's efficacy, showing significant IELT increases and sustained benefits in responders up to 9 months post-procedure.

Shebl et al. [9] contributed further by evaluating HA-based GPA in refractory PE cases using a four-inlet injection technique. Their prospective controlled study demonstrated significant improvements in IELT and patient satisfaction, reinforcing GPA's utility in patients unresponsive to conventional therapies.

A notable procedural innovation came from Kewei et al. [10], who introduced a modified injection approach targeting the coronal sulcus. This technique reduced complication rates dramatically—1.9% compared to 25.8% with traditional glans injections—while maintaining comparable efficacy. This modification marked a significant advancement in procedural safety and expanded the versatility of HA applications.

16.7.3 Systematic Evidence Base (2015–2024)

Alongside these clinical studies, systematic reviews have synthesized and quantified the growing body of evidence. Cooper et al. [15] provided a comprehensive overview of PE interventions, acknowledging the potential of surgical options like GPA but emphasizing the need for rigorous data.

More recently, Culha et al. [14] published a systematic review and meta-analysis that consolidated data from 13 studies involving 706 patients. Their findings revealed significant short- and medium-term IELT improvements and a low incidence of adverse events. With a mean IELT gain of 176 s at 1 month and 144 s at 6 months, and an overall adverse event rate of 15.2% (mostly mild and transient), Culha's work reinforced the clinical utility of HA-based GPA and called for further multicenter trials to establish its place in international guidelines.

This progressive accumulation of evidence—from pioneering case studies to refined techniques and comprehensive reviews—illustrates the maturation of HA-based GPA as a promising mechanism-based therapy for PE. As research continues to address unanswered questions regarding long-term durability and optimal patient selection, GPA with HA stands poised to become a viable addition to the therapeutic armamentarium for lifelong PE.

16.8 Summary of Reviews

The collective insights from narrative reviews, systematic reviews, and meta-analyses provide a comprehensive understanding of hyaluronic acid (HA) injections for glans penis augmentation (GPA) in the treatment of premature ejaculation (PE). Across diverse studies, several critical themes have emerged regarding efficacy, safety, challenges, and GPA's evolving position within the therapeutic landscape.

16.8.1 Efficacy

HA injections consistently demonstrate significant improvements in intravaginal ejaculation latency time (IELT), with reported increases ranging from 2.4- to 4.4-fold over baseline. In addition to functional outcomes, glans circumference has been shown to increase by approximately 1.5 cm post-procedure. These effects often persist for up to 6 months and, in some cases, longer. Such findings reinforce GPA's potential as a minimally invasive intervention capable of addressing the sensory hypersensitivity underlying lifelong PE.

16.8.2 Safety

Adverse events associated with HA injections are generally mild and self-limiting. Common complications include pain, temporary discoloration, and swelling, with an overall incidence of approximately 15% as reported by Culha et al. [14]. Importantly, these reactions typically resolve within a few weeks without the need for intervention.

Innovations in technique have further improved safety profiles. For instance, Chen et al. [10] introduced a modified injection method targeting the coronal sulcus rather than the glans body. This approach reduced complication rates dramatically, lowering adverse events to just 1.9% while maintaining comparable efficacy. Such refinements highlight the ongoing evolution of procedural methods aimed at minimizing risks and enhancing patient comfort.

16.8.3 Challenges

Despite these encouraging findings, several challenges persist. Variability in injection techniques, filler types, and patient selection across studies has contributed to heterogeneity in outcomes. This underscores the need for standardized protocols and comprehensive practitioner training to optimize both functional and aesthetic results.

Additionally, long-term data on safety and efficacy remain limited. Questions regarding volume retention, potential late-onset complications, and recurrence of PE symptoms after filler degradation have yet to be fully addressed in large-scale, long-term studies.

16.8.4 Position in the Treatment Landscape

Currently, pharmaceutical therapies such as selective serotonin reuptake inhibitors (SSRIs) and phosphodiesterase-5 (PDE5) inhibitors remain the mainstay for PE treatment. However, HA-based GPA has emerged as a promising alternative, particularly for patients who are unresponsive to medications or who prefer non-pharmaceutical options.

While GPA and other surgical interventions are increasingly practiced in Asia, they remain controversial in Western medical guidelines due to a relative paucity of high-quality evidence. Broader acceptance will likely depend on future studies that establish robust safety and efficacy profiles, paving the way for integration into international treatment recommendations.

16.9 Conclusion

The journey from the author's initial studies on glans penis augmentation to the most recent innovations reflects significant progress in applying HA for PE management. Collectively, the evidence underscores HA's potential as a minimally invasive, effective, and safe treatment that offers lasting benefits for both patients and their partners.

However, important challenges remain, including the need for standardized techniques, clear patient selection criteria, and robust long-term follow-up data. Moving forward, the integration of HA-based GPA into global guidelines will hinge on well-designed, large-scale studies that address these gaps.

As techniques continue to evolve—particularly with innovations like the coronal sulcus approach—HA-based GPA is poised to secure its place as a valuable option in the multifaceted management of PE, complementing established pharmaceutical and behavioral therapies.

References

1. Moon D, Kwak T, Cho H, Bae J, Park H, Kim J. Augmentation of glans penis using injectable hyaluronic acid gel. Int J Impot Res. 2003;15(6):456–60.
2. Kim J, Kwak T, Jeon B, Cheon J, Moon D. Effects of glans penis augmentation using hyaluronic acid gel for premature ejaculation. Int J Impot Res. 2004;16(6):547–51.
3. Abdallah H, Abdelnasser T, Hosny H, Selim O, Al-Ahwany A, Shamloul R. Treatment of premature ejaculation by glans penis augmentation using hyaluronic acid gel: a pilot study. Andrologia. 2012;44:650–3.
4. Kim J, Kwak T, Jeon B, Cheon J, Moon D. Human glans penis augmentation using injectable hyaluronic acid gel. Int J Impot Res. 2003;15(6):439–43.
5. Kwak T, Jin M, Kim J, Moon D. Long-term effects of glans penis augmentation using injectable hyaluronic acid gel for premature ejaculation. Int J Impot Res. 2008;20(4):425–8.
6. Seftel AD. Effects of glans penis augmentation using hyaluronic acid gel for premature ejaculation. J Urol. 2005;173(6):2077.
7. Littara A, Palmieri B, Rottigni V, Iannitti T. A clinical study to assess the effectiveness of a hyaluronic acid-based procedure for treatment of premature ejaculation. Int J Impot Res. 2013;25(3):117–20.

8. Alahwany A, Ragab MW, Zaghloul A, Abdallah H, Mostafa T. Hyaluronic acid injection in glans penis for treatment of premature ejaculation: a randomized controlled cross-over study. Int J Impot Res. 2019;31(5):348–55.
9. Shebl SE, Ali S, Shokr M. Hyaluronic acid injection in the glans penis for the treatment of refractory premature ejaculation: a prospective, controlled study. Andrologia. 2021;53(7):e14084.
10. Chen K, Li Q, Xu T, Zhang X. Hyaluronic acid injection to coronal sulcus of the penis for the treatment of premature ejaculation: a retrospective observational study. BMC Urol. 2023;23(1):55.
11. Kosseifi F, Chebbi A, Raad N, Ndayra A, El Samad R, Achkar K, et al. Glans penis augmentation using hyaluronic acid for the treatment of premature ejaculation: a narrative review. Transl Androl Urol. 2020;9(6):2814.
12. Ambusaidi H, Alshuaibi M, Zugail AS, Beley S. The role of surgical therapy in the management of premature ejaculation: a narrative review. Transl Androl Urol. 2023;12(10):1589.
13. Zucchi A, Scroppo FI, Capogrosso P, Salonia A, Durante J, Bini V, et al. Clinical use of hyaluronic acid in andrology: a review. Andrology. 2022;10(1):42–50.
14. Culha MG, Baran C, Erkoc M. Clinical efficacy and safety of hyaluronic acid gel injection in the glans penis for treatment of premature ejaculation: systematic review and meta-analysis. J Sex Med. 2024;21(10):878–88.
15. Cooper K, James M-S, Kaltenthaler E, Dickinson K, Cantrell A. Interventions to treat premature ejaculation: a systematic review short report. Health Technol Assess. 2015;19(21):1–180, v-vi.

Evolution of Guidelines for Premature Ejaculation (PE)

17

Contents

17.1 Introduction

Premature ejaculation (PE) remains one of the most prevalent male sexual dysfunctions, affecting approximately 20–30% of adult men worldwide [1–3]. Over the past two decades, significant progress has been made in understanding the epidemiology, pathophysiology, and management of PE. This evolution has been driven by studies highlighting its high prevalence, profound psychosocial impact, and the emergence of diverse therapeutic options [4, 5].

A range of interventions have been explored, including psychological counseling, behavioral therapy, topical anesthetics, and systemic pharmacotherapy. More recently, minimally invasive

D. G. Moon, *Penile Augmentation with Injectable Hyaluronic Acid*,
https://doi.org/10.1007/978-981-95-5385-3_17

surgical procedures such as selective dorsal neurectomy (SDN) and glans penis augmentation (GPA) using hyaluronic acid (HA) gel have gained attention, particularly in clinical settings where conventional medical approaches have failed [6–8].

17.2 Development of PE Guidelines

17.2.1 Early Guidelines and Pharmacotherapy

The 2010 International Society for Sexual Medicine (ISSM) guidelines marked a pivotal milestone in the management of premature ejaculation (PE), establishing evidence-based recommendations for diagnosis and treatment. This framework was later updated in 2014 to incorporate emerging data [5, 9]. Both editions emphasized pharmacotherapy—primarily selective serotonin reuptake inhibitors (SSRIs)—as the cornerstone of PE management while explicitly advising against surgical interventions such as selective dorsal neurectomy (SDN) and glans penis augmentation (GPA) using hyaluronic acid (HA) gel due to insufficient evidence and concerns over potential permanent loss of sexual function [5, 9].

Supporting this trend, a 2004 nationwide survey conducted by the American Urological Association (AUA) found that 71% of US urologists prescribed SSRIs as first-line therapy for PE. Notably, 35% of respondents reported using alternative first-line options, and nearly half resorted to other therapies as second-line strategies [10].

While SSRIs demonstrated efficacy, they were not without limitations. Recurrence of PE symptoms following discontinuation, partial response rates, and adverse effects such as nausea, fatigue, and delayed ejaculation diminished patient satisfaction. Similarly, topical anesthetics provided moderate benefit without systemic side effects but posed challenges including local irritation, potential transvaginal contamination, and interference with sexual spontaneity [11, 12].

Both the 2010 and 2014 ISSM guidelines reiterated a cautious stance against surgical approaches, categorizing them as not recommended due to safety concerns and a lack of high-quality clinical evidence [5, 9]. Despite these global recommendations, surgical treatments—particularly SDN and GPA with HA—have gained popularity in several Asian countries over the past decade. This trend was further fueled by the introduction of dapoxetine, as clinicians sought alternative or adjunctive options for patients dissatisfied with pharmacotherapy alone [8, 13].

17.2.2 Evolving Perspectives on Surgical Treatments

The penile dorsal nerve is the sensory nerve for the glans and penis. Patients with primary PE have penile hypersensitivity, which provides further evidence for an organic basis of PE [14]. Based on the neurobiological pathophysiology of PE, the principle of current surgical treatments is to decrease sensitivity of the glans penis.

Despite these recommendations, surgical treatments like SDN and GPA with HA have gained traction in regions such as Asia, particularly following the introduction of dapoxetine, the first FDA-approved SSRI for PE [8, 13]. Surgical approaches targeted reducing glans sensitivity, addressing the neurobiological basis of PE. SDN was first suggested for selective patients resistant to conventional PE treatments [15], and GPA using HA was developed as a less invasive surgical treatment to avoid possible permanent sensory loss due to SDN [16].

The ISSM guidelines graded local anesthetics as level 1 but do not recommend SDN or GPA with HA because of possible permanent loss of sexual function after SDN and insufficient reliable data [9]. This statement caused confusion among physicians and legal problems for unsatisfied patients after SDN in Korea. In 2013 Korean survey [13], 91.5% of Korean urologists considered SSRIs the primary treatment choice and 53.7% use local anesthetics, whereas 72.9% had prior experience with SDN for patients who benefitted from local anesthetics or who suffered from penile hypersensitivity.

In 2016, the author performed nationwide survey of urologist's practice pattern in surgical management of PE in Korea to assess the prevalence of the sensory loss and sexual dysfunction after local surgery by e-mail based survey with a specially designed questionnaire [17]. In the survey, 54 Korean urologists evaluated the efficacy and complications of SDN in 10,732 cases, HA GPA in 4344 cases, and autologous fat injection for glans augmentation in 1905 cases, respectively. Most complications had occurred in SDN, recurrence, pain, and erectile dysfunction. Fat injection usually induced scar and ischemic necrosis. HA is a rare complication and has no case of ED. GPA does not induce later sensory loss because the implanted HA gel eventually degrades and an injection of hyaluronidase dissolves the implants in cases of over correction even 10 years after the surgery. GPA is less harmful and safer for PE because it is a less invasive treatment that avoids the harmful complications of invasive SDN.

Besides the drawbacks of pharmacotherapy and debates about the ISSM guideline, recent development of PE increased the interest of PE for both patients and physicians. Surgical treatment for PE has increased continuously in Asian countries especially after launching of priligy.

A significant shift occurred in 2024, when the ISSM's guidelines recognized GPA with HA as an option for lifelong or acquired PE in specialized centers, provided that patients give informed consent.

17.2.3 Glans Penis Augmentation (GPA) Using Hyaluronic Acid (HA)

GPA with hyaluronic acid (HA) gel involves the subcutaneous injection of HA into the dermis of the glans penis. Originally developed as a cosmetic procedure to enhance glans size and aesthetics [18], subsequent clinical observations revealed its potential therapeutic benefit for patients with premature ejaculation (PE). The injected HA forms a physical barrier between external tactile stimuli and underlying nerve receptors, effectively reducing glans sensitivity without causing permanent sensory alteration [7, 16].

17.3 Advantages Over Selective Dorsal Neurectomy (SDN)

In contrast to SDN, which involves nerve resection and carries a risk of irreversible sensory loss, GPA is entirely nondestructive. The biodegradable nature of HA and its reversibility via hyaluronidase injection further enhance its safety profile. Reported complications are rare and generally minor, typically limited to temporary surface irregularities or mild discomfort.

17.4 Clinical Efficacy

Multiple studies have demonstrated significant clinical improvements with GPA. Patients commonly report a threefold increase in intravaginal ejaculatory latency time (IELT) and a satisfaction rate approaching 70%. Long-term follow-up studies confirm the durability of these benefits without significant adverse effects. A landmark 2008 study documented sustained improvements in IELT over 5 years in PE patients treated with GPA, with no reports of sensory loss [7].

17.5 Guideline Evolution and Current Status

The 2010 and 2014 ISSM guidelines grouped GPA with SDN, expressing caution due to limited reliable data and concerns regarding long-term safety [9]. However, accumulating evidence and expanding clinical experience have shifted perspectives. In 2024, the International Consultation on Sexual Medicine (ICSM) recognized GPA with HA as an optional intervention for lifelong or acquired PE within specialized centers, provided patients receive comprehensive counseling and give informed consent. This acknowledgment represents a significant paradigm shift in PE management.

17.6 Expanding Evidence Base

Recent years have seen growing global interest in GPA with HA as a treatment for PE, supported by an increasing number of high-quality publications [19–24].

This growing body of evidence underscores GPA's emergence as a safer, patient-centered alternative to traditional surgical options for PE. It highlights the need to consider GPA as a standard treatment option for patients refractory to pharmacotherapy or those who prefer a minimally invasive approach.

17.7 Selective Dorsal Neurectomy (SDN)

Selective dorsal neurectomy (SDN) involves targeted resection of sensory branches of the dorsal penile nerve to attenuate hypersensitivity in patients with premature ejaculation (PE). By partially severing these nerve fibers, SDN aims to diminish tactile stimulation of the glans penis, thereby prolonging intravaginal ejaculatory latency time (IELT).

17.8 Efficacy and Outcomes

Clinical studies have reported varying degrees of success with SDN. A 2013 nationwide survey conducted by the Korean Society for Sexual Medicine and Andrology (KSSMA), encompassing 4400 cases, demonstrated up to a threefold increase in IELT among carefully selected patients [13]. Reported patient satisfaction rates ranged from 56% to 81%, reflecting a potential therapeutic benefit for individuals refractory to conventional pharmacotherapy.

17.9 Complications and Limitations

Despite its efficacy in select populations, SDN carries notable risks. Reported complications include glans numbness, paresthesia, persistent penile pain, neuroma formation, and, in some cases, erectile dysfunction. The absence of standardized surgical protocols and variability in surgical expertise contribute to inconsistent outcomes and ongoing safety concerns. These issues have limited the widespread adoption of SDN and fueled the search for less invasive alternatives, such as glans penis augmentation (GPA) using hyaluronic acid.

17.10 Comparing SDN and GPA

Both selective dorsal neurectomy (SDN) and glans penis augmentation (GPA) with hyaluronic acid (HA) have been explored as surgical options for premature ejaculation (PE). While SDN has demonstrated efficacy in prolonging intravaginal ejaculatory latency time (IELT), it carries inherent risks due to its irreversible nature. In contrast, GPA offers a minimally invasive, reversible alternative with a favorable safety profile.

SDN effectively increases IELT by 2–3 times baseline values and reports patient satisfaction rates between 56% and 81.8%. However, complications such as glans numbness, paresthesia, and, in rare cases, erectile dysfunction have been documented, with overall complication rates ranging from 3% to 10% [25, 26].

GPA with HA provides comparable efficacy, achieving approximately a threefold increase in IELT and patient satisfaction rates near 70%. Importantly, the biodegradable nature of HA eliminates the risk of permanent sensory loss, and any overcorrection or irregularities can be safely addressed with hyaluronidase injection—even years after the procedure (Table 17.1).

Table 17.1 Key distinctions between SDN and GPA

Aspect	SDN	GPA with HA
Mechanism	Resection of dorsal nerve branches	Formation of a subdermal HA barrier reducing tactile sensitivity
Efficacy	2–3× increase in IELT	3× increase in IELT
Complications	Sensory loss, paresthesia, erectile dysfunction	Temporary surface irregularities, mild discomfort
Reversibility	Irreversible	Fully reversible with hyaluronidase
Patient satisfaction	56–81%	~70%

17.11 Current Guidelines and Recommendations

The development of guidelines is an evolutionary process that continually reviews data and incorporates the best new research. As recommended by the ISSM guidelines, SSRIs and topical anesthetics are insufficient, but the guidelines do not recommend surgical therapy. As described in the 2010 ISSM guidelines, the aim of the ISSM guidelines is to develop clearly worded, practical, evidenced-based recommendations for the diagnosis and treatment of PE by family practice clinicians and sexual medicine experts.

In the evolution of PE guideline, the AUA released the first guidelines in 2004 on the pharmacological management of PE [27] and the European Association of Urologists (EAU) released separate guidelines on ejaculatory dysfunction in 2004, which were updated in 2009 [28, 29]. The AUA and EAU guidelines mainly focused on medical treatments and did not consider surgical treatments because of the possible sensory loss and inadequate data for a recommendation.

Based on the 2004 AUA guidelines for treatment of PE, Shindel et al. [10] performed a nationwide survey to determine contemporary urologists' practice patterns for managing PE and reported no definitive treatment for PE.

From 2008, the ISSM proposed a comprehensive evidence-based definition of PE and pharmacotherapy, behavior, and psychotherapy are main treatments of PE in these new evidence-based guidelines. In 2008, the ISSM proposed a comprehensive evidence-based definition of lifelong PE and released PE guidelines in 2010 [30], which were updated with a definition in 2014 [5, 9, 31]. ISSM's guidelines for the diagnosis and treatment of PE in 2010 defined lifelong PE < 1 min of IELT in 2010 and acquired PE <3 min of IELT in an update of ISSM guideline in 2014.

The 2021 American Urological Association (AUA)/Sexual Medicine Society of North America (SMSNA) guidelines echo these sentiments [32], emphasizing the need for more robust evidence and cautioning against widespread adoption of surgical treatments outside research settings.

The 2024 ICSM guidelines now allow clinicians to offer GPA with HA for lifelong or acquired PE in high-volume centers with proper patient consent. However, SDN remains categorized as experimental and is recommended only within the context of ethical, board-approved clinical trials.

Continued updates from global organizations like ICSM and ISSM are expected to refine guidelines further, ensuring a balance between innovation and patient safety.

17.12 Future Directions and Recommendations

Glans penis augmentation (GPA) with hyaluronic acid (HA) has emerged as a minimally invasive, reversible option for managing premature ejaculation (PE), particularly in patients who are unresponsive to pharmacotherapy or reluctant to pursue invasive surgical procedures. Future studies should integrate patient-reported outcomes to better assess procedural success and quality of life. Additionally, data on the long-term safety and efficacy of repeated HA injections are needed to inform clinical practice and patient counseling.

The establishment of standardized techniques for both SDN and GPA is critical to ensuring consistent outcomes and minimizing complications. Variability in injection methods, filler selection, and procedural protocols currently poses challenges to reproducibility and global adoption. Multicenter, longitudinal studies with larger cohorts are essential to validate these approaches and refine best practices.

The growing global demand for GPA—including in Western societies—underscores the need for universally accepted, evidence-based guidelines. As additional high-quality data accumulate, surgical options such as GPA and SDN warrant reevaluation for their inclusion in international practice standards. The recognition of GPA with HA in the 2024 International Consultation on Sexual Medicine (ICSM) guidelines represents a pivotal step toward this goal, acknowledging the procedure as a viable option for select patients within specialized centers.

Continued collaboration between researchers, clinicians, and guideline committees will be vital in shaping the future of PE management, ensuring a balanced approach that embraces innovation while safeguarding patient safety.

17.13 Conclusion

Recent advances in premature ejaculation (PE) management underscore the emerging role of surgical interventions, particularly glans penis augmentation (GPA) with hyaluronic acid (HA). While pharmacotherapy remains the first-line treatment, GPA offers a promising, minimally invasive alternative for patients with refractory PE or those seeking options beyond conventional medical therapies. Its favorable safety profile, reversibility, and growing evidence base position GPA as a patient-centered complement to existing approaches.

As the field progresses, the development of standardized procedural protocols, robust multicenter studies, and long-term follow-up data will be pivotal in establishing GPA with HA as a recognized standard of care. Similarly, ongoing efforts to refine selective dorsal neurectomy (SDN) techniques and address associated safety concerns may contribute to its reevaluation as a viable option in carefully selected cases. Together, these advancements reflect a paradigm shift in PE management, fostering a more comprehensive and individualized treatment landscape.

References

1. Laumann EO, Paik A, Rosen RC. Sexual dysfunction in the United States: prevalence and predictors. JAMA. 1999;281(6):537–44.
2. Porst H, Montorsi F, Rosen RC, Gaynor L, Grupe S, Alexander J. The Premature Ejaculation Prevalence and Attitudes (PEPA) survey: prevalence, comorbidities, and professional help-seeking. Eur Urol. 2007;51(3):816–24.
3. Lee S, Lee J, Sung H, Park H, Park J, Choi S, et al. The prevalence of premature ejaculation and its clinical characteristics in Korean men according to different definitions. Int J Impot Res. 2013;25(1):12–7.
4. Saitz TR, Serefoglu EC. Advances in understanding and treating premature ejaculation. Nat Rev Urol. 2015;12(11):629–40.
5. Althof SE, Abdo CH, Dean J, Hackett G, McCabe M, McMahon CG, et al. International Society for Sexual Medicine's guidelines for the diagnosis and treatment of premature ejaculation. J Sex Med. 2010;7(9):2947–69.
6. McMahon CG, Jannini E, Waldinger M, Rowland D. Standard operating procedures in the disorders of orgasm and ejaculation. J Sex Med. 2013;10(1):204–29.
7. Kwak TI, Jin MH, Kim JJ, Moon DG. Long-term effects of glans penis augmentation using injectable hyaluronic acid gel for premature ejaculation. Int J Impot Res. 2008;20(4):425–8.
8. Zhang GX, Yu LP, Bai WJ, Wang XF. Selective resection of dorsal nerves of penis for premature ejaculation. Int J Androl. 2012;35(6):873–9.
9. Althof SE, McMahon CG, Waldinger MD, Serefoglu EC, Shindel AW, Adaikan GP, et al. An update of the International Society of Sexual Medicine's guidelines for the diagnosis and treatment of premature ejaculation (PE). J Sex Med. 2014;11(6):1392–422.
10. Shindel AW, Nelson CJ, Brandes SB. Urologist practice patterns in the management of premature ejaculation: a nationwide survey. J Sex Med. 2008;5(1):199–205.
11. Schapiro B. Premature ejaculation: a review of 1,130 cases. J Urol. 1943;50(3):374–9.
12. Morales A, Barada JH, Wyllie MG. A review of the current status of topical treatments for premature ejaculation. BJU Int. 2007;100(3):493–501.
13. Yang DY, Ko K, Lee WK, Park HJ, Lee SW, Moon KH, et al. Urologist's practice patterns including surgical treatment in the management of premature ejaculation: a Korean nationwide survey. World J Mens Health. 2013;31(3):226–31.

14. Xin ZC, Chung WS, Choi YD, Seong DH, Choi YJ, Choi HK. Penile sensitivity in patients with primary premature ejaculation. J Urol. 1996;156(3):979–81.
15. Tullii R, Guillaux C, Vaccari R, Ferreira R. Premature ejaculation-selective neurectomy: a new therapeutic technique—base, indications and results. Int J Impot Res. 1994;6:109–13.
16. Kim JJ, Kwak TI, Jeon BG, Cheon J, Moon DG. Effects of glans penis augmentation using hyaluronic acid gel for premature ejaculation. Int J Impot Res. 2004;16(6):547–51.
17. Jeong HG, Ahn ST, Kim JW, Seo KK, Lee DS, Uh HS, et al. Practice patterns among Korean urologists for glans penis augmentation using hyaluronic acid filler in the management of premature ejaculation. Sex Med. 2018;6(4):297–301.
18. Moon DG, Kwak TI, Cho HY, Bae JH, Park HS, Kim JJ. Augmentation of glans penis using injectable hyaluronic acid gel. Int J Impot Res. 2003;15(6):456–60.
19. Moon DG. Is there a place for surgical treatment of premature ejaculation? Transl Androl Urol. 2016;5(4):502–7.
20. Abdallah H, Abdelnasser T, Hosny H, Selim O, Al-Ahwany A, Shamloul R. Treatment of premature ejaculation by glans penis augmentation using hyaluronic acid gel: a pilot study. Andrologia. 2012;44:650–3.
21. Shebl SE, Ali S, Shokr M. Hyaluronic acid injection in the glans penis for the treatment of refractory premature ejaculation: a prospective, controlled study. Andrologia. 2021;53(7):e14084.
22. Chen K, Li Q, Xu T, Zhang X. Hyaluronic acid injection to the coronal sulcus of the penis for the treatment of premature ejaculation: a retrospective observational study. BMC Urol. 2023;23(1):55–60.
23. Kosseifi F, Chebbi A, Raad N, Ndayra A, El Samad R, Achkar K, et al. Glans penis augmentation using hyaluronic acid for the treatment of premature ejaculation: a narrative review. Transl Androl Urol. 2020;9(6):2814–21.
24. Shaeer O. Shaeer's glans augmentation technique: a pilot study. J Sex Med. 2012;9(12):3264–9.
25. You HS. The partial neurectomy of the dorsal nerve of the penis for patients with premature ejaculation. Korean J Androl. 2000;18:143–8.
26. Zhang CY, Li XH, Yuan T, Zhang HF, Liu JH, Ye ZQ. Regional anatomy of the dorsal penile nerve and its clinical significance. Zhonghua Nan Ke Xue. 2009;15(2):130–3.
27. Montague DK, Jarow JP, Broderick GA, Dmochowski RR, Heaton JPW, Lue TF, et al. AUA guideline on the pharmacologic management of premature ejaculation. J Urol. 2004;172(1):290–4.
28. Colpi GM, Weidner W, Jungwirth A, Pomerol J, Papp GK, Hargreave TB, et al. EAU guidelines on ejaculatory dysfunction. Eur Urol. 2004;46(5):555–8.
29. Hatzimouratidis K, Amar E, Eardley I, Giuliano F, Hatzichristou D, Montorsi F, et al. Guidelines on male sexual dysfunction: erectile dysfunction and premature ejaculation. Eur Urol. 2010;57(5):804–14.
30. McMahon CG, Althof SE, Waldinger MD, Porst H, Dean J, Sharlip ID, et al. An evidence-based definition of lifelong premature ejaculation: report of the ISSM ad hoc committee for the definition of premature ejaculation. J Sex Med. 2008;5(7):1590–606.
31. Serefoglu EC, McMahon CG, Waldinger MD, Althof SE, Shindel AW, Adaikan GP, et al. An evidence-based unified definition of lifelong and acquired premature ejaculation: report of the second ISSM ad hoc committee. Sex Med. 2014;2(2):41–59.
32. Shindel AW, Althof SE, Carrier S, Chou R, McMahon CG, Mulhall JP, et al. Disorders of ejaculation: an AUA/SMSNA guideline. J Urol. 2022;207(3):504–12.

Complications of Glans Penis Augmentation (GPA)

18

Contents

D. G. Moon, *Penile Augmentation with Injectable Hyaluronic Acid*,
https://doi.org/10.1007/978-981-95-5385-3_18

18.1 Introduction

Penile enlargement procedures are often pursued by younger men seeking a heightened sense of masculinity [1]. However, in recent years, increased life expectancy, greater partner engagement, higher sexual activity frequency, and the widespread use of phosphodiesterase type-5 inhibitors have driven a growing interest in penile size among older populations as well [2]. This trend has amplified concerns about perceived sexual inferiority and the demand for aesthetic and functional penile augmentation.

In 2003, we first reported the feasibility of glans penis augmentation (GPA) using injectable hyaluronic acid (HA) gel [3, 4], followed by a landmark 5-year follow-up study in 2008 [5] and subsequent work on penile girth enhancement (PGE) in 2011 [6]. Since then, multiple studies have demonstrated the efficacy of GPA in improving self-esteem, addressing aesthetic concerns, and managing premature ejaculation (PE) [7–9]. Despite these promising results, GPA remains a subject of debate, particularly in patients with a perceived small glans penis due to sexual inferiority, a disproportionate glans during erection, or PE. Many of these patients request GPA in combination with penile elongation and PGE to avoid secondary deformities caused by PGE-related disproportion between the penile body and glans [3].

Injectable fillers have become globally popular for aesthetic applications, from facial rejuvenation to body contouring, offering a less invasive alternative to surgery. However, warnings have been issued regarding their use due to adverse effects (AEs) such as infection, cutaneous necrosis, and even arterial embolism [10, 11]. Since the introduction of GPA using HA gel, various fillers have been applied for penile augmentation (PA). Unfortunately, not all have demonstrated favorable outcomes. Our experience and the existing literature reveal several complications associated with alternative fillers and different GPA techniques [12, 13].

While dermal filler complications in facial aesthetics are well documented [10, 14–18], reports on filler-related AEs in PA remain scarce. Negative outcomes are often underreported due to concerns about professional criticism or medicolegal implications. This lack of transparency risks propagating procedures that may result in serious complications. It is crucial to recognize that fillers demonstrating excellent long-term outcomes in facial applications may not be suitable for PA due to fundamental anatomical and functional differences in penile tissue.

Given the continuous introduction of new filler materials with varying safety profiles and longevity, careful consideration of filler properties and their interaction with penile tissues is essential. Drawing from our pioneering work in PGE and GPA using HA gel, this chapter presents an experience-based review of GPA complications and provides detailed analyses of complex cases referred to our center. While not the first review of dermal fillers, this is the first comprehensive evaluation of dermal fillers specifically for PA, with a focus on GPA-related complications.

18.2 Glans Penis Augmentation Using Injectable Fillers

The glans penis is a highly vascular, bulbous structure that protects the distal tips of the corpora cavernosa and serves as the spongy erectile end of the penis. It is covered by a thin layer of skin, which creates a unique challenge for augmentation procedures. Successful glans penis augmentation (GPA) using injectable fillers requires the presence of an adequate dermal space to accommodate the filler material without compromising vascular integrity or sensory function.

Previous animal studies have demonstrated the existence of a potential implant space within the lamina propria of the canine glans penis [4]. Building on these findings, human studies have confirmed the feasibility and clinical utility of GPA using injectable hyaluronic acid (HA) gel [3]. However, technical precision is paramount. The relatively thin dermis and dense vascular network of the glans mean that filler injection must be meticulously performed to avoid complications such as uneven distribution or vascular compromise.

Four representative dermal filler injection techniques have been described for GPA: serial puncture, linear threading, fanning, and cross-hatching. Each technique offers distinct advantages depending on the anatomical considerations and desired filler distribution (Fig. 8.5) [12, 19].

An overly superficial or excessively deep injection must be avoided to minimize the risks of mucosal tearing, bleeding, and filler leakage through the puncture site. Reducing the number of needle punctures further decreases the likelihood of these complications. Abdallah et al. [8] described a modified GPA technique using injectable HA gel for patients with premature ejaculation, employing multiple punctures to deliver a larger filler volume. However, undulations and embossing of the glans mucosal surface are common and typically resolve during erection. These fine, fold-like surface wrinkles are attributed to the underlying rete ridges, while embossing may result from augmentation of the basal crease and, in part, from the filler's particle size.

Combining HA fillers of varying particle sizes and carefully adjusting injection depth has been shown to mitigate the embossing effect. The application of dermal fillers for soft tissue augmentation represents both an art and a science [20]. Beyond technical proficiency and a thorough understanding of implantation techniques, a clinician must also consider the biochemical properties of the chosen filler. Scientifically, filler longevity is influenced by its concentration and cross-linking, whereas aesthetically, the durability of correction is highly dependent on injection technique and tissue integration.

Theoretically, HA gel begins to degrade approximately 6 months after the initial injection and is fully reversible over time or through hyaluronidase administration if needed. A 5-year follow-up study of patients who underwent GPA using subcutaneous HA injections showed a residual implant volume decrease of approximately 15% relative to the maximal glandular circumference in a subset of patients [5]. Interestingly, in some cases, HA gel injected into the lamina propria—a region with sparse vascularity—persisted for over 5 years.

Currently, several cost-effective HA fillers are available for retouch or refill procedures to address volume loss, offering patients and clinicians greater flexibility in maintaining aesthetic outcomes (Table 18.1) [21].

Table 18.1 Common fillers available for glans penis augmentation

Trade name	Manufacturer (Country)	Key component	Cost[a] ($)	KFDA approval[b]
Biodegradable products				
Restylane	Q-Med AB (Sweden)	Hyaluronic acid	100–140	Approved
Juvéderm	Allergan, Inc. (France)	Hyaluronic acid	100–140	Approved
Belotero	Merz Pharmaceuticals, LLC (United States)	Hyaluronic acid	100–140	Approved
Teosyal	Lifestyle Aesthetics (Switzerland)	Hyaluronic acid	100–140	Approved
Elravie	Humedix Co., Ltd. (Korea)	Hyaluronic acid	10–30	Approved
THE CHAEUM	Hugel, Inc. (Korea)	Hyaluronic acid	10–30	Approved
Lipen-D	Chunghwa Medipower Co., Ltd. (Korea)	Cross-linked dextran	70–90	Approved
MegaFill	L&C Bio Co., Ltd. (Korea)	Cross-linked human acellular dermal matrix	100–120	Approved
Non-biodegradable products				
Aquamid	Contura (Denmark)	97.5% sterile water and 2.5% polyacrylamide	130–150	Approved

KFDA Korea Food and Drug Administration
[a]Costs were based on Korea
[b]KFDA-approved fillers for soft tissue augmentation but not specifically approved for glans penis augmentation except Lipen-D®, which is approved for glans penis augmentation

18.3 Complications of Glans Penis Augmentation Using Fillers

The widespread popularity of injectable fillers in aesthetic medicine is attributed to their ease of application, immediate aesthetic improvements, and relatively low complication rates. However, complications in glans penis augmentation (GPA) can still occur and are generally classified into three categories: those related to filler properties, technical errors during injection, and inflammatory or immune-mediated responses [12, 17]. Careful selection of filler type, tailored to the target tissue, is critical to minimize adverse events (AEs) in penile augmentation (PA).

18.4 Technical Errors

Technical errors are among the most preventable causes of complications in glans penis augmentation (GPA). These errors can be classified into three primary categories based on their nature and impact:

1. Volume-related errors

The volume of filler injected plays a critical role in achieving aesthetically pleasing and functional results.

Overcorrection: Administering an excessive amount of filler may result in a bulbous, disproportionate appearance of the glans. This can lead to patient dissatisfaction and potential functional discomfort during intercourse.

Undercorrection: Conversely, insufficient filler volume may fail to produce the desired augmentation effect, often necessitating additional sessions to achieve an acceptable outcome.

2. Inappropriate depth of injection

The depth at which filler is deposited significantly influences both safety and aesthetic results.

Superficial injections: Placement too close to the mucosal surface increases the risk of visible lumps, undulations, and in severe cases, pressure-induced mucosal necrosis due to compromised vascularity.

Deep injections: Injecting filler too deeply can result in inadequate dermal support, leading to minimal or no visible augmentation. In rare instances, it may cause deep vascular compromise if critical penile vessels are affected.

3. Incorrect placement

Accurate placement within the dermal layer is crucial to prevent functional and aesthetic issues. Misplaced filler material can exacerbate surface irregularities, create asymmetry, or even interfere with penile sensitivity. Even distribution of the filler and meticulous injection technique are essential to optimize outcomes and minimize the need for corrective procedures.

18.5 Inflammation and Immune Responses

Post-procedural inflammation in glans penis augmentation (GPA) may result from infections or immune-mediated reactions. The underlying mechanisms by which certain fillers are more prone to induce vascular compromise remain poorly understood. Factors such as the filler's biochemical properties, its tendency to elicit inflammatory responses, and its potential to cause arterial obstruction are believed to contribute. Inflammatory reactions can lead to tissue hypoxia and, in severe cases, necrosis [18].

Accidental intra-arterial injection represents a critical risk during GPA. When filler material enters the arterial system, it may obstruct blood flow, with the severity of resulting ischemia determined by the filler's particle size and its capacity to migrate within the vascular network.

18.6 Vascular Complications

Vascular complications are among the most serious adverse events associated with injectable fillers. Polymethyl methacrylate (PMMA) microsphere-based fillers, in particular, have been implicated in cases of extensive tissue necrosis requiring complex reconstructive procedures, such as flap surgery. This phenomenon is thought to arise from collagen-mediated activation of the coagulation cascade, leading to thrombotic events within affected vessels.

Filler-related complications can be further categorized based on their timing and severity:

Early vs. late events: Temporary fillers such as collagen and hyaluronic acid (HA) are typically associated with early-onset complications, which are often mild and self-limiting or easily managed.

Minor vs. major complications: Minor adverse events include transient swelling, bruising, or localized discomfort. In contrast, major complications may involve irreversible functional or aesthetic deficits, including tissue necrosis, scarring, or sensory changes [22, 23].

Biodegradable fillers are less likely to cause late complications due to their resorption over time. However, serious adverse events—though rare—can result in lasting morbidity and underscore the importance of careful technique and filler selection.

18.7 Permanent Fillers and Severe Complications

Non-reabsorbable or permanent fillers carry a distinct risk profile compared to biodegradable agents. Complications associated with these materials often manifest several years after implantation and may result in severe, long-lasting adverse reactions. The inability of the body to metabolize these substances contributes to their tendency for chronic inflammatory responses and tissue integration issues.

18.8 Significant Complications

The most commonly reported complications of permanent fillers include:

Overcorrection: excessive volume leading to unnatural, disproportionate enlargement

Surface irregularities: palpable or visible unevenness of the glans surface

Filler visibility: particularly in areas with thin mucosal coverage, resulting in aesthetic dissatisfaction

Tyndall effect: a bluish discoloration when filler is placed too superficially

Granuloma formation: chronic inflammatory nodules due to foreign body reactions

18.9 Severe Complications

In rare but critical cases, permanent fillers have been associated with:

Visual impairment: Resulting from inadvertent vascular embolization in facial applications, underscoring the theoretical risk in penile use where vascular compromise could lead to glans necrosis

Skin necrosis: Secondary to vascular occlusion or inflammatory tissue damage

Anaphylaxis: Severe hypersensitivity reactions, although extremely rare, require immediate medical intervention.

Currently, a wide variety of filler agents are commercially available (Table 18.1) [21]. While some are perceived as safer due to their chemical composition and degradation profiles, all injectable fillers carry the potential for adverse events [14, 15, 24, 25]. The choice of filler should therefore be guided by a balance of efficacy, safety, and the clinician's familiarity with its handling characteristics. Complications of non-reabsorbable or permanent fillers may occur several years after implantation and often cause severe permanent reactions.

18.10 Complications of Other Fillers for GPA

During the early phase of glans penis augmentation (GPA) development, polyacrylamide hydrogel (PAAG) emerged as a seemingly promising filler for soft tissue augmentation [26]. PAAG consists of 2.5% polyacrylamide and 97.5% water for injection [27]. Since 1997, it was widely adopted for augmentation mammoplasty and other aesthetic applications [28–30].

However, post-market surveillance revealed a range of complications, including inflammation, infection, lump formation, tissue deformation, displacement, abnormal sensations, systemic toxicity, and immunological alterations. Reports in 2003 and 2004 highlighted these adverse events, raising concerns about the long-term safety of hydrogel injections [31, 32]. Consequently, regulatory authorities issued warnings regarding the use of PAAG for facial plastic surgery, and its application in breast augmentation was subsequently banned in many countries.

Following the successful introduction of penile girth enhancement (PGE) using injectable hyaluronic acid (HA) gel, various alternative fillers were trialed for GPA. In 2003, Dr. Perovic [26] reported his experience with submucosal hydrogel injections in nine patients presenting with glans deformities. While eight of these patients demonstrated satisfactory outcomes over a follow-up period of 12–26 months, the study emphasized the importance of careful patient selection and technique. Dr. Perovic noted that excessive hydrogel could be aspirated if necessary, as the thin, well-defined, permeable capsule surrounding the material allowed for its removal. The primary advantage of hydrogel at that time was its relatively low cost.

Nevertheless, subsequent studies and clinical experiences revealed that PAAG and similar hydrogels were unsuitable for soft tissue augmentation. Originally developed as a substitute for mammoplasty implants and correction of facial deformities, these materials were later associated with severe complications. By 2003 and 2004, cases of diffuse paranasal swelling and signs of cellulitis resulting from granulomatous inflammatory responses were documented. Regulatory agencies and professional societies issued warnings against the use of hydrogels in facial plastic procedures [31–33].

Despite the well-documented safety of hyaluronic acid (HA) fillers, attributed to their unique physicochemical properties and extensive clinical use, rare adverse events such as granulomatous foreign body reactions and ischemic necrosis have been reported. Granulomatous responses are thought to result from protein contaminants within the HA preparation, while ischemic complications typically arise from technical errors during injection.

Critical factors contributing to these complications include overly superficial placement of HA, excessive volume delivery within a single area, and inadvertent intravascular injection. Immediate postinjection signs, such as blanching or discoloration of the glans mucosa, may signal vascular compromise requiring urgent intervention.

Brody and colleagues [34] as well as Hirsh et al. [35, 36] described successful management of rare cases of impending necrosis following HA filler embolization. Their work emphasizes the importance of early recognition of vascular events and prompt administration of hyaluronidase as part of a standardized treatment algorithm. This intervention not only dissolves the obstructing HA material but also helps to restore perfusion and minimize tissue damage. In cases of immediate postinjection discoloration suggestive of vascular compromise, a systematic and timely intervention is critical to prevent tissue necrosis. The following management steps are recommended:

Cease injection immediately: Discontinue filler administration at the first sign of blanching or discoloration.

Apply gentle massage: This may help to disperse the filler material and alleviate localized vascular obstruction.

Initiate warm compress and vasodilation: Apply heat and a topical vasodilator such as nitroglycerine paste to promote blood flow and counteract vasospasm.

Administer hyaluronidase if necessary: If symptoms persist, inject intradermal hyaluronidase promptly. A typical regimen involves 75 units of Vitrase™ or 0.5 mL of a 150-unit hyaluronidase preparation at the affected site. Most cases of lumpiness resolve within 24 h, with

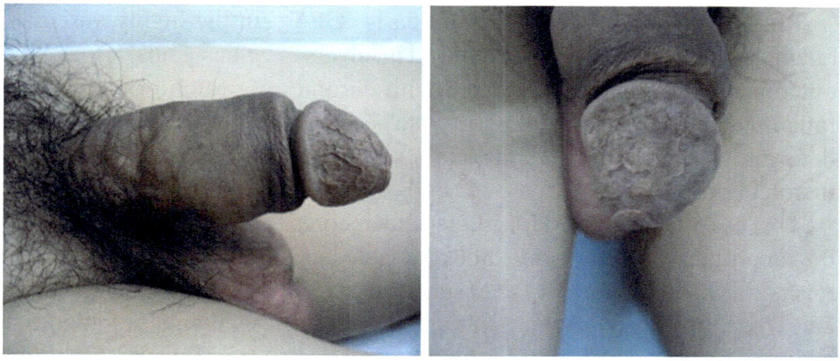

Fig. 18.1 The image shows asymmetrical enhancement of the penile body with some lumpiness and multiple healed scars from superficial ulcerative necrosis of the glans mucosa following polyacrylamide injection for penile girth enhancement. (Adapted with permission [12])

residual irregularities typically disappearing over the following days.

This algorithm, as proposed by Brody and Hirsh [34–36], underscores the importance of early recognition and intervention in mitigating potential ischemic injury.

18.11 Review of Referred Cases Presenting with Complications

Several previous studies have documented complications following glans penis augmentation (GPA), often linked to the use of inappropriate filler materials intended to enhance implant longevity. These issues have been particularly prevalent in cases where cheaper polyacrylamide products, such as polyacrylamide hydrogel (PAAG), were employed (Fig. 18.1) [12, 37].

While PAAG gained popularity in cosmetic applications due to its low cost, clinical experience has demonstrated that it is not an ideal material for soft tissue augmentation in the long term. Its non-biodegradable nature and tendency to elicit inflammatory responses have resulted in a range of complications, including chronic swelling, palpable nodules, and granulomatous reactions.

Our center has encountered numerous referred cases of GPA-related complications, most of which were associated with the use of non-HA fillers such as PAAG. These cases underscore the critical importance of filler selection and the need for heightened vigilance regarding off-label use of permanent or semipermanent agents in penile tissue.

18.12 Complications of Other Fillers: Bellagen and Rofilan

Among alternative fillers used for glans penis augmentation (GPA), products such as Bellagen and Rofilan have been notable for their association with significant complications.

Bellagen (Modified SureDerm®, Hans Biomed Corp., Korea) was developed as a convenient injectable suspension of cellular dermal fragments measuring 500–1000 μm in size. Packaged in a 1 cc/5 mL syringe and combined with 1.5 cc lidocaine and 0.3 cc gentamicin in a 3 mL syringe, Bellagen was intended to improve the longevity of hyaluronic acid (HA) gel augmentation. Although its primary indication was for soft tissue augmentation, it has been used off-label for GPA as a less invasive alternative to dermofat grafts or scaffold implantation in penile girth enhancement (PGE) [12, 38].

However, clinical experience has revealed significant drawbacks. Overinjection of Bellagen increases the risk of pressure-induced necrosis (Fig. 18.2). Furthermore, cellular dermal fragments within Bellagen are resistant to enzymatic degradation by hyaluronidase, making the correction of complications particularly challenging. Unlike HA-based fillers, which can be reversed with hyaluronidase in cases of overcorrection or irregularities, Bellagen's persistence and integration into tissue complicate both management and surgical removal.

Rofilan, another filler used in early GPA attempts, has similarly been implicated in adverse outcomes. Patients have presented with chronic inflammatory responses, nodularity, and aesthetic deformities requiring complex secondary interventions.

The use of such non-HA fillers underscores the importance of selecting biodegradable and reversible materials for GPA to ensure both safety and ease of management in the event of complications.

The characteristic well-elevated mound observed immediately after Bellagen injection is largely attributable to the presence of water in the aqueous lidocaine and gentamicin solutions mixed with the filler. This initial swelling typically subsides within a week as the excess water is absorbed by surrounding tissues.

However, complications associated with Bellagen extend beyond transient edema. The acellular collagen fragments within the suspension have been implicated in triggering inflammatory responses and vascular compromise, which can progress to glans necrosis in severe cases (Fig. 18.2). These adverse effects highlight the risks of using dermal fragment-based fillers in the highly vascular and delicate tissue of the glans penis.

Such outcomes emphasize the critical importance of selecting filler materials with predictable biodegradation profiles and minimal immunogenic potential when performing GPA.

Figures 12–15 Examples of complications, including autologous fat injection and other fillers, emphasize that unsatisfactory outcomes may require surgical intervention, often difficult even in "successful" cases.

Rofilan (Rofil, Netherlands), a mixture of polyacrylamide and a hyaluronic acid derivative, has also been associated with serious adverse events following its off-label use in glans penis augmentation (GPA). Clinical reports have described cases of suspected granulomatous reactions and mucosal necrosis linked to Rofilan injections (Fig. 18.3).

The polyacrylamide component is thought to contribute to chronic inflammatory responses, while the potential for vascular compromise may explain the development of multiple necrotic, ulcerative lesions observed on the glans mucosa.

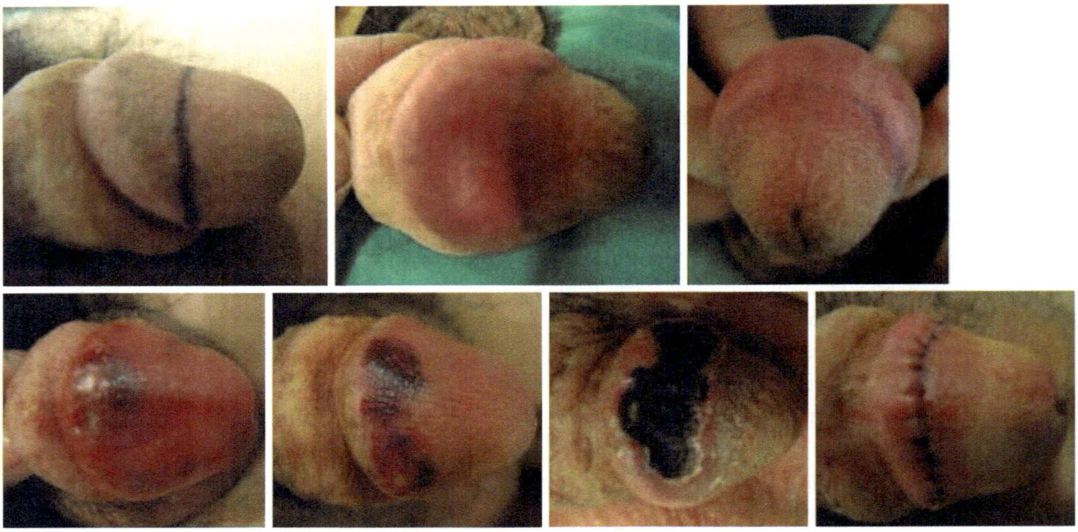

Fig. 18.2 The image shows injection of a suspension of acellular allogeneic dermal fragment, BellaGen (Modified SureDerm®, Hans Biomed Corp, Korea), leading to the development of gradual inflammation and deep necrosis of the glans penis: (Upper) before injection, 1 day after injection, (lower left) 1 week after injection, and (lower Rt.) 3 weeks after injection

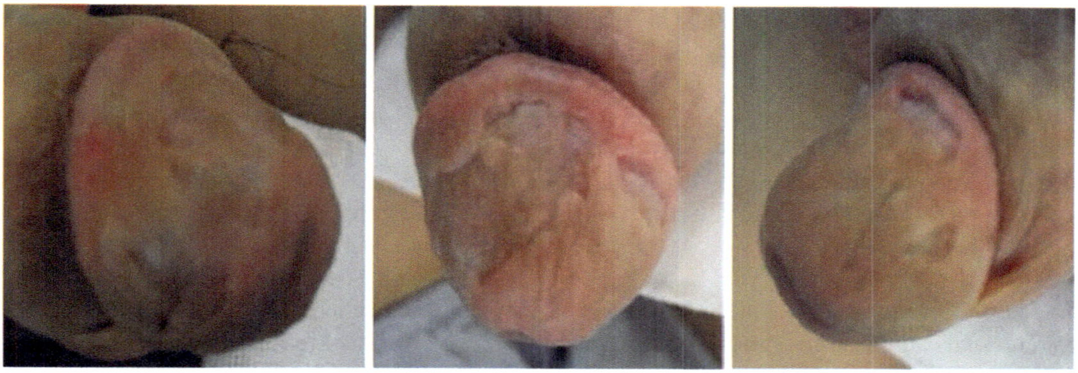

Fig. 18.3 The image shows multiple ulcerative necrotic lesions of the glans mucosa secondary to the injection of a mixture of polyacrylamide with hyaluronic acid derivative to increase the longevity of hyaluronic acid alone. (Adapted with permission [12])

These findings underscore the high risk associated with polyacrylamide-containing fillers when applied to sensitive, highly vascular tissues such as the glans penis.

The complications observed with Rofilan and similar permanent or semipermanent fillers reinforce the importance of restricting GPA procedures to materials with proven safety profiles, such as biodegradable hyaluronic acid gels.

18.13 Complications of Mixed and Semipermanent Fillers

In experimental efforts to enhance the longevity of temporary dermal fillers, combinations of different filler types have been tested. One such example is Dermalive® (DermaTech, Paris, France), a synthetic injectable product comprising 60% cross-linked hyaluronic acid (HA) gel as a viscoelastic carrier and 40% acrylic hydrogel particles—non-biodegradable microspheres of hydroxyethylmethacrylate and ethyl methacrylate with variable diameters [39]. This formulation was marketed as a "semipermanent" filler intended to remain intradermally for an undefined but prolonged duration [40].

However, the long-term safety of such mixed fillers has been called into question. Reports of severe adverse events, including granuloma formation and tissue necrosis, ultimately led to the withdrawal of Dermalive® and similar products such as Bio-Alcamid™ from the market. Their removal was associated with a notable decrease in the incidence of serious complications in clinical practice.

Non-absorbable filler particles, such as those in semipermanent products, are particularly unsuitable for injection into the shallow or deep mucosal layers of the glans penis. The delicate, highly vascular tissue of the glans is especially vulnerable to chronic inflammatory responses and vascular compromise when exposed to such materials.

Current guidelines recommend against injecting dermal fillers from chemically distinct categories into the same anatomical location. This precaution is due to the difficulty in determining which filler may have precipitated an adverse event when multiple materials coexist. Although clinical evidence supporting this hypothesis remains limited [40], there is concern that combining biodegradable HA fillers with irreversible agents like polymethyl methacrylate (PMMA) may exacerbate nodule formation.

Proposed pathomechanisms include the biofilm hypothesis, which suggests that bacterial biofilms formed around filler particles may trigger chronic inflammatory reactions and granuloma development [41–43]. Additionally, comparative histological studies have shown that polyacrylamide hydrogel (PAAG) tends to induce a more intense inflammatory infiltrate in granulomas than HA, further emphasizing the higher risk profile of non-biodegradable fillers [44].

18.14 Complications Associated with Cross-Linked Dextran Gel (Lipen-D®)

In an effort to address some of the limitations of traditional hyaluronic acid (HA) fillers, Yang et al. [7] recently reported on the use of a newly developed cross-linked dextran (CD) gel, Lipen-D® (Chunghwa Medipower Co. Ltd., Seoul, Korea), for glans penis augmentation (GPA). This CD gel was injected into the deeper layers of the glans tissue with the aim of minimizing surface undulations and achieving a more uniform aesthetic result. The study reported a mean increase of over 20% in glans surface area at 24 weeks postinjection and described no serious adverse events (AEs) during the follow-up period.

However, clinical experience from our center has revealed a different safety profile. Several patients presented with mucosal necrosis secondary to Lipen-D® injection and were referred to us for further management (Fig. 8). The mechanism behind these complications may involve localized ischemia due to deep filler placement or an inflammatory reaction unique to cross-linked dextran particles within the glans' highly vascular tissue.

These cases highlight the need for cautious evaluation of novel filler materials and techniques in GPA. Even when initial clinical trials report favorable outcomes, real-world use can reveal unforeseen complications, underscoring the importance of long-term surveillance and multicenter studies before widespread adoption. Recently, Yang et al. [7] reported the results of GPA using a newly developed cross-linked dextran (CD) gel, (Lipen-D®, Chunghwa Medipower Co. Ltd., Seoul, Korea). The CD gel was injected into the deep layer during GPA to avoid undulation of the glans surface and to increase the glans surface area by >20% 24 weeks after injection. Contrary to reports of no serious AEs, patients with mucosal necrosis secondary to Lipen-D® were referred to us for further management (Fig. 18.4).

Yang et al. [7] also acknowledged that cross-linked dextran (CD) gel injections may carry the risk of serious and persistent adverse events (AEs), including tissue necrosis—particularly in patients with underlying vasculopathy. This observation is supported by prior reports of complications associated with similar dextran-based materials. For instance, a case involving mucosal necrosis following intravesical injection of Deflux has been documented [45]. Unlike the bladder mucosa, where necrosis may not be immediately visible, necrotic changes of the glans penis are readily identifiable and amenable to prompt intervention.

To mitigate such risks, the use of safe and biocompatible fillers is essential. Supplementary injections performed 2 weeks postoperatively, rather than an initial overdose, may help avoid ischemic complications. Moreover, early administration of hyaluronidase in cases involving hyaluronic acid (HA) fillers has proven effective in reversing vascular compromise and preventing tissue loss [34, 35].

A critical factor contributing to complications may be the volume and depth of filler placement.

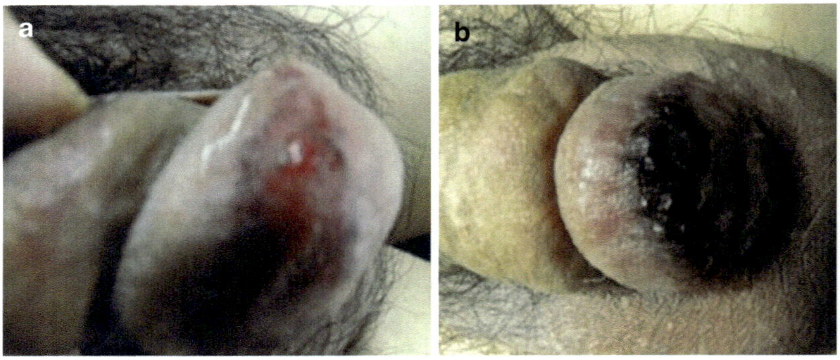

Fig. 18.4 The image shows glans penis necrosis after deep injection of Lipen-D® for glans penis augmentation. An erythematous painful swelling was observed 5 days after glans penis augmentation using Lipen-D® (**a**), partial necrosis was observed 2 weeks later (**b**)

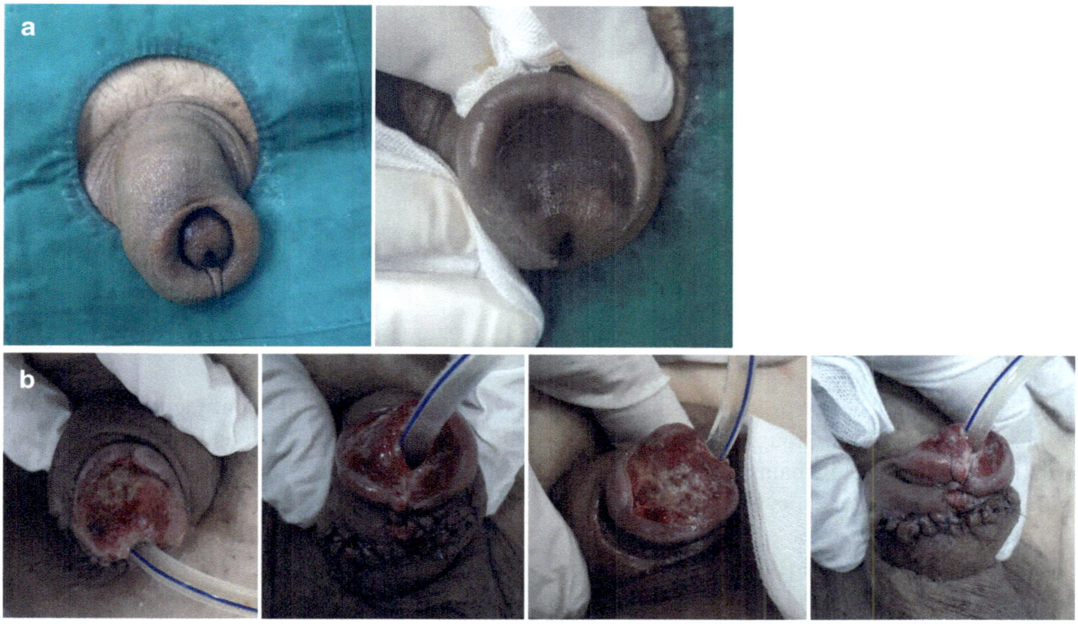

Fig. 18.5 HyaFilia (Cha Meditec, Korea) injection for PGE and GPA. (**a**) Penile discomfort and glans discoloration 1 day after PGE and GPA. (**b**) Surgical removal of injected filler and necrotic mucosa

Whereas Moon et al. [12, 13] advocated for a more conservative superficial injection of 2 mL HA gel, Yang's protocol involved a mean injection of 6.6 ± 0.9 mL (range: 4.9–8.8 mL) of CD gel into the deeper glans tissue. This substantial difference in both filler volume and depth may predispose to vascular compromise, ultimately leading to glans ulceration and necrosis.

Although CD gel has been approved by the Korean Food and Drug Administration (FDA) for use in GPA, physicians should exercise caution and ensure a thorough understanding of its properties, indications, and potential risks. Judicious application is paramount to maximizing benefits while minimizing severe complications (Fig. 18.5).

18.15 Autologuous Fat Injection

18.15.1 Autologous Fat Injection for GPA

In the 2024 5th International Consultation on Sexual Medicine (ICSM), biodegradable biopolymer fillers, such as hyaluronic acid (HA), and autologous fat injections were recognized as relatively safe options for penile augmentation. However, the panel noted that additional procedures are often necessary over time to maintain results. This recommendation was classified as Moderate with an Evidence Strength C, reflecting limited high-quality data and the need for further studies (currently unpublished).

Autologous fat transfer, involving liposuction and subsequent subcutaneous injection of fat for penile girth enhancement, has been extensively explored in the literature [46, 47]. Despite initial enthusiasm, clinical outcomes have been disappointing, with high rates of adverse effects and poor long-term durability.

Reports of glans penis augmentation (GPA) using autologous fat are rare. The primary challenges include fat atrophy and reabsorption, often attributed to inadequate vascularization of the transplanted adipose tissue, difficulty in immobilizing the injected area, and mechanical trauma from sexual activity. These factors contribute to volume loss and migration of the fat, resulting in deformities, asymmetry, and the loss of augmented girth over time.

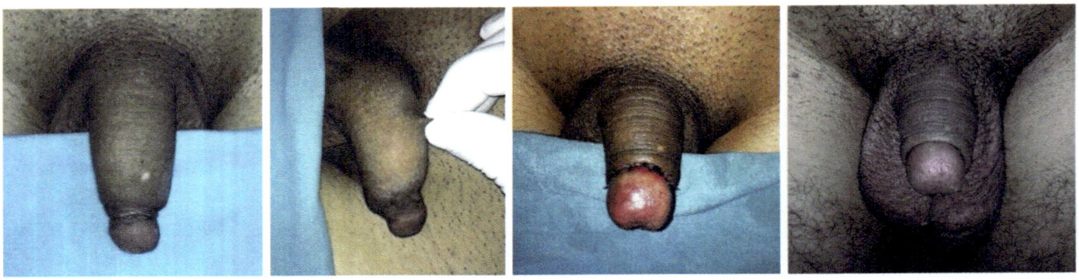

Fig. 18.6 Case report of successful GPA by fat injection [49]

The biological behavior of transplanted fat underscores these limitations. Revascularization occurs in a centripetal manner, with plasmatic imbibition supporting survival only within a 0.5–1.5 mm zone from the edges of the graft. To maximize viability, single threads of transplanted adipose tissue should not exceed 3 mm in diameter. Larger fat collections are prone to central necrosis, liquefaction, and cyst formation. These pathological changes, combined with technical imperfections, explain the high rates of resorption and the overall unpredictability of outcomes reported in the literature [48].

Consequently, autologous fat injection is not recommended as a primary technique for GPA and should be approached with caution even in experimental settings (Fig. 18.6).

18.16 Case Report: Autologous Fat Injection for Glans Penis Augmentation

A 22-year-old male presented with a complaint of penile deformity characterized by a hypoplastic glans and subglanular constriction, creating an exclamation mark appearance. His medical history revealed circumcision performed by an itinerant practitioner at the age of four. He denied any local pain, erectile dysfunction, ejaculatory problems, premature ejaculation, or urinary symptoms.

On physical examination, there was a noticeable subglanular stricture and hypoplastic glans without evidence of corporal tissue deficit or urethral fistula.

To address the deformity, autologous fat transfer was planned. Under local anesthesia, 10 cc of adipose tissue was harvested from the abdominal area using a 15-cm, two-hole blunt Coleman fat harvesting cannula and the wet technique. The harvested fat was centrifuged at 3000 rpm for 3 min and transferred into 1-mL syringes. Subsequently, 3 cc of processed fat was injected subcutaneously into the glans penis through a single puncture site using a blunt cannula.

Preoperative glans circumference measured 5.3 cm using a flexible tape measure. On the tenth postoperative day—after resolution of edema—the circumference increased to 9.2 cm. At the final follow-up visit 12 months postoperatively, the glans circumference measured 9.0 cm, reflecting a sustained ~70% increase in girth.

The patient reported no changes in erectile function, ejaculatory control, or glans sensation. International Index of Erectile Function-5 (IIEF-5) scores remained unchanged. Both objective and subjective evaluations suggested a satisfactory aesthetic and functional outcome, with no recurrence of deformity noted during the 1-year follow-up period (Fig. 18.7).

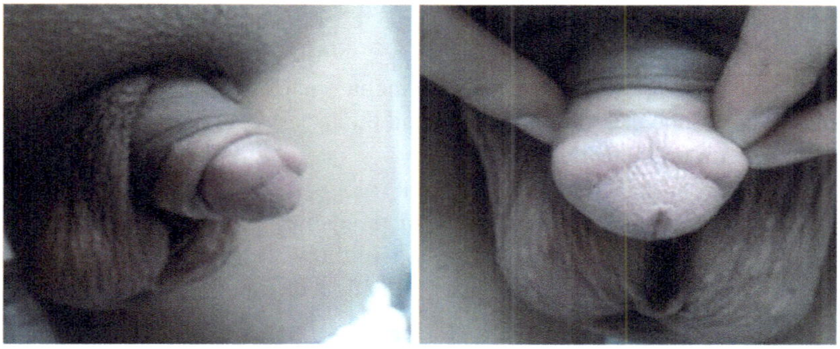

Fig. 18.7 Fat injection induced irregular volus in glans of young boy, 18 yrs

18.17 Case Report: Fatal Fat Embolism Following Penile Augmentation

In 2015, a 42-year-old male underwent penile augmentation with autologous fat injection. The procedure began with the injection of 15 cc of processed adipose tissue into the glans penis. During the subsequent injection of 10 cc into the penile girth, the patient developed a dry cough but reported no chest pain or other discomfort. Despite this, an additional 25 cc of fat was injected into the penile shaft.

Immediately after the procedure, the patient experienced worsening cough, chest tightness, and respiratory difficulty. Within 1 h, while in the recovery room, he became pale and developed severe respiratory distress, followed by sudden loss of consciousness. Cardiopulmonary resuscitation (CPR) was initiated, and the patient was transferred to a tertiary hospital. Unfortunately, he was pronounced dead en route. Autopsy findings confirmed fat embolism as the cause of death.

Fat embolism is an extremely rare but unpredictable and potentially fatal complication of fat transfer procedures. Unlike embolic events typically associated with large-volume fat harvesting sites, in this case, the embolism arose from localized fat injections into the penile tissues. This case underscores the importance of exercising caution with fat grafting techniques, especially in highly vascular areas such as the penis, where inadvertent intravascular injection may lead to catastrophic outcomes.

18.18 Complication of Indirect Glans Penis Augmentation

Since the introduction of hyaluronic acid (HA) fillers for glans penis augmentation (GPA), alternative techniques and materials have been explored in an effort to overcome the perceived drawbacks of HA, such as its relatively short longevity and high cost. Among these, indirect augmentation techniques have gained attention but carry significant risks.

Perovic et al. [50] described a method involving an incision at the coronal sulcus, followed by the creation of a potential space between the corpus spongiosum of the glans penis and the distal tip of the corpus cavernosum through blunt dissection. Careful preservation of the dorsal neurovascular bundle is crucial during this process. Into this prepared pocket, various implant materials—including prepared commercial dermal strips, silastic bars, or dermal matrices (autologous dermis, AlloDerm® [LifeCell Corporation, Branchburg, NJ, USA], Lyoplant)—can be inserted. Simple wound closure and standard postoperative wound care are typically performed.

Shaeer [51] introduced a similar grafting technique, termed Shaeer's glans augmentation, which involves the insertion of a dermofat graft harvested from the groin into the periurethral plane. This plane is developed by creating a glans flap through two incisions along the ventral aspect of the coronal sulcus. In a pilot study involving ten patients, promising results were reported, including retention of added volume at 1-year follow-up, preservation of glans sensitivity and engorgement, and no adverse events related to erectile function or ejaculatory control. However, limitations of the technique include its invasiveness due to groin harvesting and the lack of long-term outcome data.

More recently, a group of Korean andrologists developed an indirect GPA method inspired by Shaeer's technique (unpublished) [12]. Initially utilizing dermofat grafts, they later transitioned to collagen scaffolds such as AlloDerm® or Lyoplant to reduce procedural invasiveness. While early results suggested this method was simple and effective, longer follow-up studies revealed severe adverse events, including glans penis necrosis, painful hard lumps, and significant penile deformities (Figs. 18.8 and 18.9).

These findings underscore the risks inherent to indirect augmentation methods. Given their invasiveness and the potential for severe complications, such procedures should be reserved for major penile reconstruction in patients with significant anatomical deficits, such as inadequate penile length or partial loss of the corpora cavernosa [50].

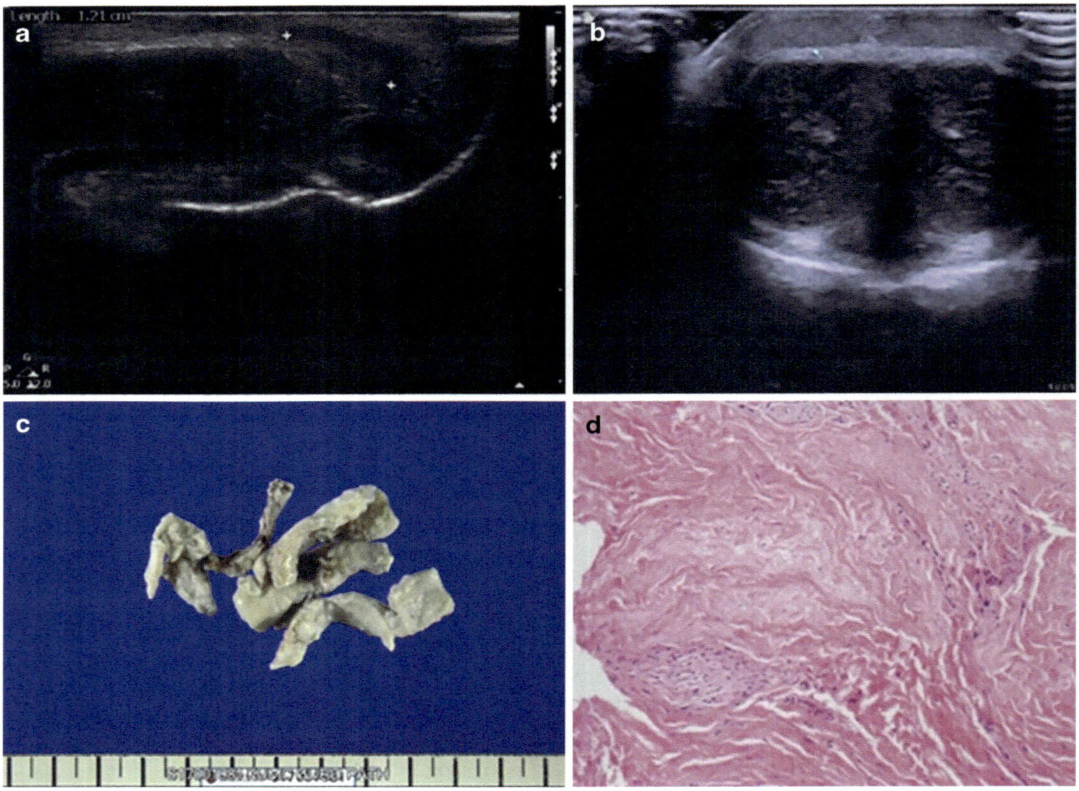

Fig. 18.8 A tender hard encircled mass is observed along the corpus cavernosum and the cavernosal tip beneath the corpus spongiosum of the glans penis following penile girth enhancement and indirect glans penis augmentation using Lyoplant (collagen scaffold) (**a**–**c**). After removal, plenty of pinkish thick collagen bundles and fibrosis with spindle-shaped fibroblast are observed (**d**)

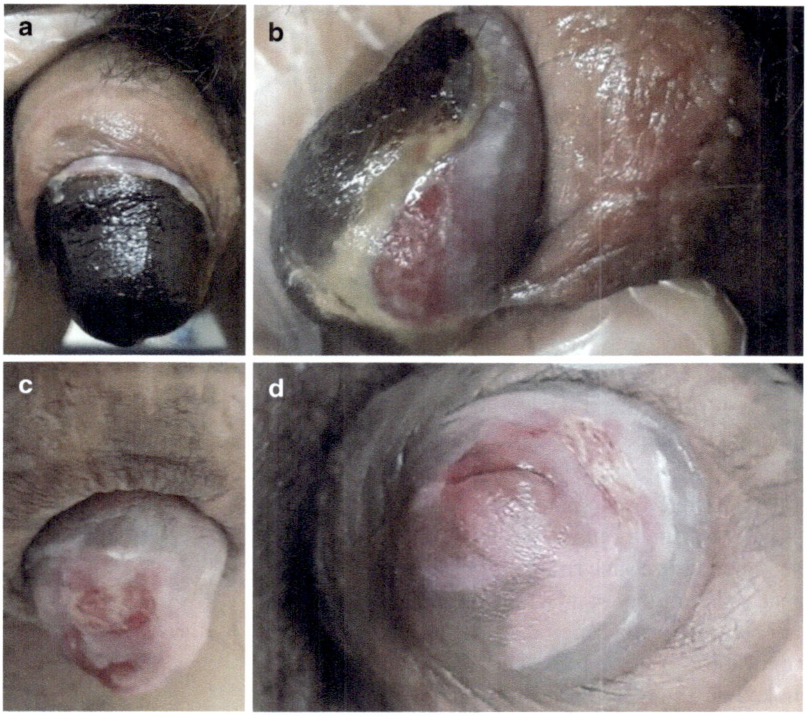

Fig. 18.9 The glans penis necrosis is observed after removal of the collagen scaffold used for indirect glans penis augmentation. (**a**) Patients presented with severe pain and dissatisfaction after indirect glans penis augmentation using Shaeer's glans augmentation technique. (**b**) Glans necrosis is observed after removal of implants. (**c**, **d**) Partial loss of glans penis with deformity can be observed at 2 months

18.19 Summary Table: Filler Types and Associated Complications

Filler type	Complication risks	Reversibility	Safety considerations
Hyaluronic acid (HA)	Minor swelling, undulation, rare granulomas	Yes (Hyaluronidase)	Safest option; reversible; technique-sensitive
Polyacrylamide hydrogel (PAAG)	Granulomas, infection, necrosis, deformity	No	Banned in many countries due to severe late complications
Bellagen	Pressure necrosis, hard nodules, resistant to enzymes	No	Cellular dermal fragments; resistant to hyaluronidase
Cross-linked Dextran (CD Gel)	Mucosal necrosis, inflammation, vascular compromise	No	Requires cautious use; volume and depth critical
Autologous fat	Resorption, asymmetry, fat embolism (rare fatal cases)	Partially (resorption)	High unpredictability; risk of deformities and embolism
Dermalive®/ Bio-Alcamid™	Chronic inflammation, granulomas, necrosis	No	Withdrawn from market due to severe adverse events
Rofilan (PAAG + HA derivative)	Necrotic ulcerations, granulomatous reactions	No	Severe complications reported; avoid use

18.20 Conclusion

Glans penis augmentation (GPA) using injectable fillers has evolved considerably since its initial introduction, offering both aesthetic and functional benefits to selected patients. While hyaluronic acid (HA) remains the most widely used and safest option due to its biocompatibility and reversibility, the use of alternative materials—particularly irreversible fillers such as polyacrylamide hydrogel (PAAG), Bellagen, and cross-linked dextran (CD) gel—has been associated with significant adverse events. These complications range from inflammatory responses and granuloma formation to vascular compromise and necrosis, some of which may result in permanent functional or aesthetic deficits.

To minimize such risks, careful selection of filler materials, mastery of injection techniques, and strict adherence to safety protocols are essential. Recent innovations in filler formulations, including cross-linked dextran gels, have shown initial promise but require further robust, long-term studies to confirm their safety and efficacy profiles.

Emerging clinical challenges underscore the need for ongoing evaluation of filler properties, their interactions with penile tissue, and the development of standardized protocols for GPA. Physicians performing these procedures must exercise meticulous judgment in patient selection, technical execution, and postoperative care to ensure optimal outcomes and patient satisfaction.

While GPA represents a significant advancement in penile augmentation, its long-term success depends on evidence-based practices, continued research, and a comprehensive understanding of the associated benefits and potential complications.

References

1. Du Geon Moon JWY, Bae JH, Han CS, Kim YK, Kim JJ. Sexual function and psychological characteristics of penile paraffinoma. Asian J Androl. 2003;5:191–4.
2. Lindau ST, Schumm LP, Laumann EO, Levinson W, O'Muircheartaigh CA, Waite LJ. A study of sexuality and health among older adults in the United States. N Engl J Med. 2007;357(8):762–74.
3. Kim J, Kwak T, Jeon B, Cheon J, Moon D. Human glans penis augmentation using injectable hyaluronic acid gel. Int J Impot Res. 2003;15(6):439–43.
4. Moon D, Kwak T, Cho H, Bae J, Park H, Kim J. Augmentation of glans penis using injectable hyaluronic acid gel. Int J Impot Res. 2003;15(6):456–60.
5. Kwak T, Jin M, Kim J, Moon D. Long-term effects of glans penis augmentation using injectable hyaluronic acid gel for premature ejaculation. Int J Impot Res. 2008;20(4):425–8.
6. Kwak TI, Oh M, Kim JJ, Moon DG. The effects of penile girth enhancement using injectable hyaluronic acid gel, a filler. J Sex Med. 2011;8:3407–13.
7. Yang DY, Ko K, Lee SH, Moon DG, Kim JW, Lee WK. Efficacy and safety of newly developed cross-linked dextran gel injection for glans penis augmentation with a novel technique. Asian J Androl. 2018;20(1):80–4.
8. Abdallah H, Abdelnasser T, Hosny H, Selim O, Al-Ahwany A, Shamloul R. Treatment of premature ejaculation by glans penis augmentation using hyaluronic acid gel: a pilot study. Andrologia. 2012;44:650–3.
9. Kim J, Kwak T, Jeon B, Cheon J, Moon D. Effects of glans penis augmentation using hyaluronic acid gel for premature ejaculation. Int J Impot Res. 2004;16(6):547–51.
10. Duffy DM. Complications of fillers: overview. Dermatologic Surg. 2005;31:1626–32.
11. Alijotas-Reig J, Fernández-Figueras MT, Puig L. Inflammatory, immune-mediated adverse reactions related to soft tissue dermal fillers. Semin Arthritis Rheum. 2013;43(2):241–58.
12. Moon DG, Kwak TI, Kim JJ. Glans penis augmentation using hyaluronic acid gel as an injectable filler. World J Mens Health. 2015;33(2):50–6.
13. Moon DG. General principles of GA. Penile Augmentation. Springer; 2016. p. 169–73.
14. Park TH, Seo SW, Kim JK, Chang CH. Clinical experience with hyaluronic acid-filler complications. J Plast Reconstr Aesthet Surg. 2011;64(7):892–6.
15. Daines SM, Williams EF. Complications associated with injectable soft-tissue fillers. JAMA Facial Plast Surg. 2013;15(1):66–71.
16. Vanaman M, Fabi SG, Carruthers J. Complications in the cosmetic dermatology patient: a review and our experience (part 1). Dermatologic Surg. 2016;42(1):1–11.
17. DeLorenzi C. Complications of injectable fillers, part I. Aesthet Surg J. 2013;33(4):561–75.
18. DeLorenzi C. Complications of injectable fillers, part 2: vascular complications. Aesthet Surg J. 2014;34(4):584–600.
19. Rohrich RJ, Ghavami A, Crosby MA. The role of hyaluronic acid fillers (Restylane) in facial cosmetic surgery: review and technical considerations. Plast Reconstr Surg. 2007;120(6 Suppl):41S–54S.
20. Klein AW. Soft tissue augmentation 2006: filler fantasy. Dermatol Ther. 2006;19(3):129–33.

21. Ahn ST, Kwak TI, Park KS, Kim JJ, Moon DG. Complications of glans penis augmentation. Int J Impot Res. 2019;31(4):245–55.
22. Gladstone HB, Cohen JL. Adverse effects when injecting facial fillers. Semin Cutan Med Surg. 2007;26(1):34–9.
23. Funt D, Pavicic T. Dermal fillers in aesthetics: an overview of adverse events and treatment approaches. Plast Aesthet Nurs. 2015;35(1):13–32.
24. Requena L, Requena C, Christensen L, Zimmermann US, Kutzner H, Cerroni L. Adverse reactions to injectable soft tissue fillers. J Am Acad Dermatol. 2011;64(1):1–34.
25. Artzi O, Loizides C, Verner I, Landau M. Resistant and recurrent late reaction to hyaluronic acid–based gel. Dermatologic Surg. 2016;42(1):31–7.
26. Perovic SV, Radojicic ZI, Djordjevic ML, Vukadinovic VV. Enlargement and sculpturing of a small and deformed glans. J Urol. 2003;170(4 Part 2):1686–90.
27. Okubo M, Hyakusoku H, Kanno K, Fumiiri M. Complications after injection mammaplasty. Aesthet Plast Surg. 1992;16:181–7.
28. Christensen LH, Breiting VB, Aasted A, Jørgensen A, Kebuladze I. Long-term effects of polyacrylamide hydrogel on human breast tissue. Plast Reconstr Surg. 2003;111(6):1883–90.
29. Cheng NX, Wang YL, Wang JH, Zhang XM, Zhong H. Complications of breast augmentation with injected hydrophilic polyacrylamide gel. Aesthet Plast Surg. 2002;26:375–82.
30. Chen B, Song H. Management of breast deformity after removal of injectable polyacrylamide hydrogel: retrospective study of 200 cases for 7 years. Aesthet Plast Surg. 2016;40:482–91.
31. de Bree R, Middelweerd MR, van der Waal I. Severe granulomatous inflammatory response induced by injection of polyacrylamide gel into the facial tissue. Arch Facial Plast Surg. 2004;6(3):204–6.
32. Liu Y, Cen Y, Xu XW, Duan WQ. Analysis of complications induced by polyacrylamide hydrogel injection for augmentation mammaplasty. Chin J Plast Surg. 2005;21(6):464–6.
33. Kang S, Zhang Z, Chou H, Zhai H. Complication of polyacrylamide hydrogel injection for facial plasty. Zhonghua Zheng Xing Wai Ke Za Zhi. 2003;19(5):325–7.
34. Brody HJ. Use of hyaluronidase in the treatment of granulomatous hyaluronic acid reactions or unwanted hyaluronic acid misplacement. Dermatologic Surg. 2005;31(8):893–7.
35. Hirsch RJ, Cohen JL, Carruthers JD. Successful management of an unusual presentation of impending necrosis following a hyaluronic acid injection embolus and a proposed algorithm for management with hyaluronidase. Dermatologic Surg. 2007;33(3):357–60.
36. Hirsch RJ, Brody HJ, Carruthers JD. Hyaluronidase in the office: a necessity for every dermasurgeon that injects hyaluronic acid. J Cosmet Laser Ther. 2007;9(3):182–5.
37. Bergeret-Galley C, Latouche X, Illouz YG. The value of a new filler material in corrective and cosmetic surgery: DermaLive and DermaDeep. Aesthet Plast Surg. 2001;25:249–55.
38. Park MK, Kim HK, Park KY, Li K, Seo SJ, Hong CK. Complications following BellaGen™ injection. Ann Dermatol. 2011;23(Suppl 3):S306–S9.
39. Sidwell R, Dhillon A, Butler P, Rustin M. Localized granulomatous reaction to a semi-permanent hyaluronic acid and acrylic hydrogel cosmetic filler. Clin Exp Dermatol. 2004;29(6):630–2.
40. Nicolau PJ. Long-lasting and permanent fillers: biomaterial influence over host tissue response. Plast Reconstr Surg. 2007;119(7):2271–85.
41. Rohrich RJ, Monheit G, Nguyen AT, Brown SA, Fagien S. Soft-tissue filler complications: the important role of biofilms. Plast Reconstr Surg. 2010;125(4):1250–6.
42. Christensen LH. Host tissue interaction, fate, and risks of degradable and nondegradable gel fillers. Dermatologic Surg. 2009;35:1612–9.
43. Bentkover SH. The biology of facial fillers. Facial Plast Surg. 2009;25(2):73–85.
44. Meire BP, Nílceo SM, Karime MH, Ediléia B, Sérgio T. A histologic study of adverse effects of different cosmetic skin fillers. Skinmed. 2005;4(6):345–9.
45. Życzkowski M, Prokopowicz G, Zajęcki W, Paradysz A. Complications following endoscopic treatment of vesicoureteric reflux with Deflux®–two case studies. Cent European J Urol. 2012;65(4):230–2.
46. Panfilov DE. Augmentative phalloplasty. Aesthet Plast Surg. 2006;30:183–97.
47. Kang DH, Chung JH, Kim YJ, Lee HN, Cho SH, Chang TH. Efficacy and safety of penile girth enhancement by autologous fat injection for patients with thin penises. Aesthet Plast Surg. 2012;36:813–8.
48. Niechajev I, Sevcuk O. Long-term results of fat transplantation: clinical and histologic studies. Plast Reconstr Surg. 1994;94(3):496–506.
49. Taş S, Top H. Reconstruction of hypoplastic glans and subglanular stricture with fat transfer and release. J Plast Reconstr Aesthet Surg. 2014;67(12):1744–6.
50. Perovic S, Scepanovic D, Vukadinovic V, Djakovic N, Djordjevic M. Penile disassembly technique: a new approach in the surgical reconstruction of hypospadias. Prog Urol. 1999;9(2):371–9.
51. Shaeer O. Shaeer's glans augmentation technique: a pilot study. J Sex Med. 2012;9(12):3264–9.

Indirect Glans Penis Augmentation (GPA)

19

Contents

19.1 Introduction

Augmentation phalloplasty has traditionally focused on two primary techniques: penile girth enhancement (PGE) and penile lengthening procedures. Until the early 2000s, however, no standardized method existed for glans penis augmentation (GPA) aimed at improving sexual function or aesthetic concerns. In the early 2000s, the author pioneered GPA using hyaluronic acid (HA) gel injections to address conditions such as subjectively small glans penis, disproportionate glans size following PGE, glans deformities, and postsurgical corrections after procedures like hypospadias repair.

Glans penis augmentation (GPA) has since emerged as a topic of growing interest and debate within andrological surgery. Its limited adoption can largely be attributed to the absence of high-quality supporting evidence and the technical challenges inherent to glans augmentation [1, 2]. Despite these limitations, patient demand for GPA continues to rise, positioning it as a "hot topic" among both patients and clinicians. Notably, GPA is widely accepted and uncontroversial in specific reconstructive contexts, such as in hypospadias repair, congenital micropenis, and secondary micropenis due to iatrogenic injury, infection, or trauma [3, 4].

Modern PGE techniques, while effective in increasing penile shaft girth, may inadvertently create aesthetic disharmony—resulting in a thickened penile shaft juxtaposed against a relatively smaller glans. This iatrogenic dispropor-

D. G. Moon, *Penile Augmentation with Injectable Hyaluronic Acid*,
https://doi.org/10.1007/978-981-95-5385-3_19

tion can provoke patient dissatisfaction, particularly in cases where poor glans tumescence during erection is observed [5]. Similarly, patients undergoing penile prosthesis implantation often present with inadequate glans size or rigidity, further highlighting the need for adjunctive GPA [6, 7].

Direct GPA, characterized by intradermal HA injections, primarily achieves surface elevation without providing total functional or volumetric enhancement of the glans [8]. This method faces inherent limitations, including technically demanding injection techniques, the need for precise material placement, and the time-limited nature of results due to gradual volume loss or graft resorption.

In contrast, indirect GPA modifies substructural anatomy by placing dermofat grafts or bioengineered scaffolds between the distal corpora cavernosa and glans base. This concept is rooted in Perović's penile disassembly technique [9] and refined by Shaeer's glans augmentation technique [1].

Introduction of dermofat grafts (2000s): Dermofat grafts were initially used for penile girth restoration but were soon adapted for glans projection by placing the graft between the glans mucosa and the corpora cavernosa. This method provided moderate volumetric enhancement but was hindered by donor site morbidity and limited durability [10].

Shaeer's refinement of indirect glans augmentation (2010s): Osama Shaeer refined this method using autologous dermofat grafts inserted into the periurethral space. His technique included ventral incisions along the coronal sulcus and glans flap dissection. A pilot study of ten patients showed a 16.6% initial increase in glans circumference, slightly decreasing to 14.2% at 12 months. Sensory preservation and functional integrity were noted, but invasiveness and long-term durability remained concerns [1, 8].

Advancements in scaffold technology (2010s to present): To overcome dermofat graft limitations, Korean surgeons developed a scaffold-based method using Lyoplant® (a collagen matrix). This technique involved dorsal access and placement of the scaffold between the glans and distal corpora cavernosa. While results were initially promising, scaffold resorption, painful induration, and glans necrosis have been reported [11].

Integration with penile lengthening techniques: Indirect GPA has also been combined with penile lengthening procedures to enhance distal glans projection and penile aesthetics. Though theoretically synergistic, the technique's invasiveness and lack of reproducible data have limited widespread adoption [1].

19.2 Historical Background

The evolution of indirect glans penis augmentation (GPA) reflects a series of innovative surgical techniques developed to address specific anatomical and aesthetic challenges in penile reconstruction. This section traces the milestones that shaped the concept of Indirect GPA.

19.2.1 Penile Disassembly Technique by Perovic (1990s)

Dr. Sava Perovic introduced the penile disassembly technique to allow structural modification of the distal penis. This approach enabled the creation of a potential space between the glans penis and the corpora cavernosa, allowing insertion of grafts or materials that indirectly elevated the glans. Although innovative, limitations included technical complexity and lack of long-term data [3, 9, 12] (Figs. 19.1 and 19.2).

19.2.2 Introduction of Dermofat Grafts (2000s)

Dermofat grafts were initially used for penile girth restoration but were soon adapted for glans projection by placing the graft between the glans mucosa and the corpora cavernosa. This method provided moderate volumetric enhancement but was hindered by donor site morbidity and limited durability [10].

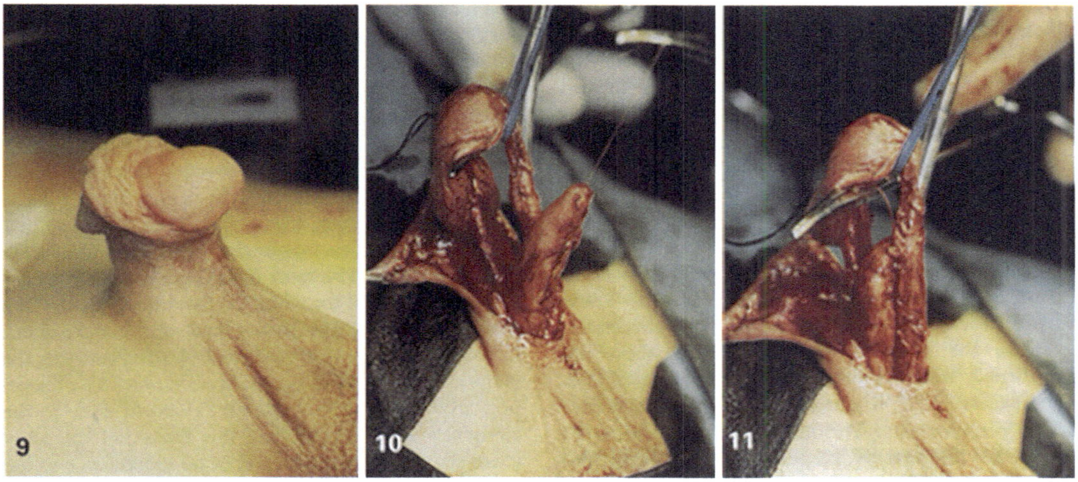

Fig. 19.1 Penile disassembly technique in hypospadias repair. (Adopted by Perovic, 1998)

Fig. 19.2 Penile lengthening adopted by Perovic, BJU International. 2000

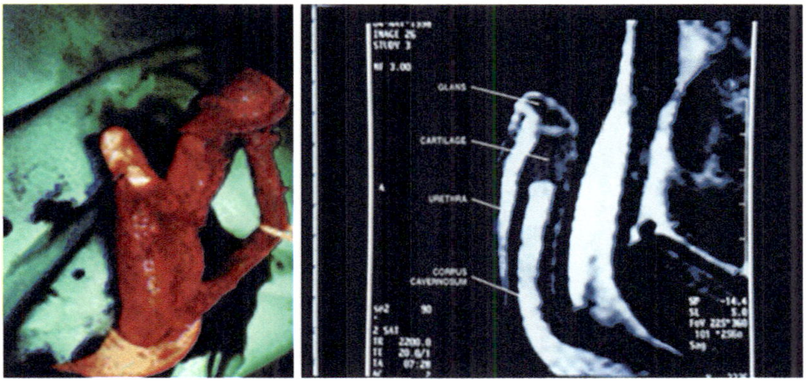

19.2.3 Shaeer's Refinement of Indirect Glans Augmentation (2010s)

Dr. Osama Shaeer further refined this method using autologous dermofat grafts inserted into the periurethral space. His technique included ventral incisions along the coronal sulcus and glans flap dissection. A pilot study of ten patients showed a 16.6% initial increase in glans circumference, slightly decreasing to 14.2% at 12 months. Sensory preservation and functional integrity were noted, but invasiveness and long-term durability remained concerns [1, 8] (Fig. 19.3).

19.2.4 Advancements in Scaffold Technology (2010s to Present)

To overcome dermofat graft limitations, Korean surgeons developed a scaffold-based method using Lyoplant® (a collagen matrix). This technique involved dorsal access and placement of the scaffold between the glans and distal corpora cavernosa. While results were initially promising, scaffold resorption, painful induration, and glans necrosis have been reported [11] (Fig. 19.4).

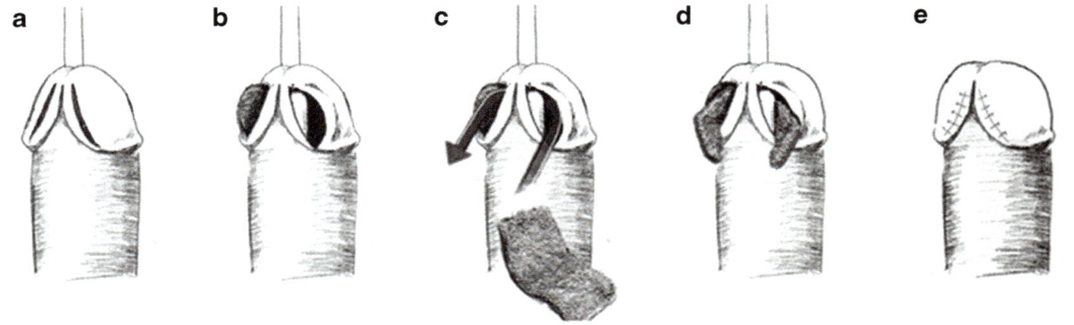

Fig. 19.3 Shaeer's surgical steps. (**a**) Incision, (**b**) dissecting glans flaps, (**c**) the periurethral plane, (**d**) graft insetting, and (**e**) incision closure

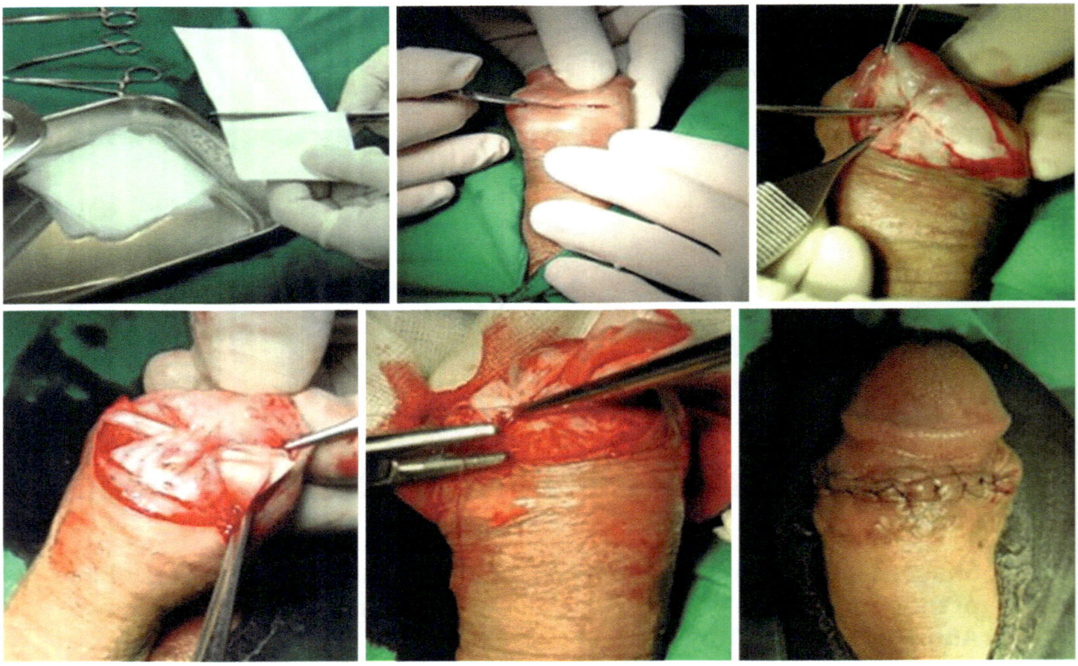

Fig. 19.4 Preparation and procedures for indirect glans penis augmentation by Lyoplant insertion

19.2.5 Integration of Lengthening Techniques

Indirect GPA has also been combined with penile lengthening procedures to enhance distal glans projection and penile aesthetics. Though theoretically synergistic, the technique's invasiveness and lack of reproducible data have limited widespread adoption [13, 14].

19.3 Objectives and Techniques

The main objective of Indirect GPA is to achieve distal glans projection by modifying the underlying anatomy without direct mucosal injection. This is particularly useful in patients with glans hypersensitivity or previous surgeries that preclude direct augmentation [5, 8].

Shaeer's technique involves dermofat harvested from the groin and inserted into the periurethral plane. Postoperative follow-ups showed high patient satisfaction and preserved function but highlighted donor site complications and procedural invasiveness [1, 8].

The Lyoplant-based approach uses bioengineered collagen scaffolds inserted via a dorsal incision. The scaffold indirectly elevates the glans by sitting between the glans base and the corpora cavernosa. Despite initial positive outcomes, resorption, vascular compromise, and necrosis have been documented [11].

Perovic's disassembly method offers a more extensive restructuring of penile anatomy and can complement glans augmentation. However, its invasiveness confines its application to complex reconstructive cases [3, 9].

19.4 Indications, Advantages, Limitations, and Risks of Indirect GPA

Indirect glans penis augmentation (GPA) finds its primary application in patients requiring distal glans elongation rather than superficial surface expansion. It is particularly suited for cases with structural imbalances where indirect augmentation offers a more harmonious and proportional result. Additionally, it provides a valuable alternative in situations where direct glans augmentation is contraindicated due to hypersensitivity, previous surgical interventions, or scarring that compromises the integrity of the glans [5, 8].

The advantages of indirect GPA lie in its ability to deliver natural and proportionate enhancement without direct manipulation of the glans mucosa. By modifying substructural anatomy, this approach reduces the risks commonly associated with intradermal filler injections, such as changes in sensitivity or surface irregularities. When executed with precision and supported by appropriate material selection, indirect GPA has the potential to provide stable and long-lasting aesthetic results. These qualities make it particularly attractive to patients seeking subtle improvements that preserve functional aspects of the glans.

Nevertheless, several limitations and challenges constrain the widespread adoption of indirect GPA. The requirement for surgical intervention introduces inherent risks and prolongs recovery compared to less invasive alternatives. The technical demands of precise graft or scaffold placement elevate the potential for asymmetry and unsatisfactory outcomes if meticulous attention is not paid to anatomical detail. Comprehensive preoperative counseling is essential to align patient expectations with the realities of the procedure, including the possibility of revision surgery. Furthermore, the current body of evidence supporting indirect GPA remains limited, with a paucity of robust long-term efficacy data [1]. Serious complications such as urethral injury, ischemic tissue loss, and graft contraction or necrosis further emphasize the need for cautious application and surgical expertise.

Complications specific to indirect GPA are notable and often more severe than those encountered in direct techniques. One of the most critical risks is glans mucosal necrosis resulting from vascular compromise during dermofat graft placement or scaffold substitution. Loss of blood supply can lead to ischemia, necessitating urgent surgical intervention to prevent permanent deformity or total glans loss [3]. Clinical reports have described cases where scaffold implantation resulted in painful hard masses within the glans, subsequently inducing vascular compromise and tissue necrosis [2, 11].

Other reported complications include chronic inflammation and fibrosis caused by foreign material reactions, leading to pain and distortion of penile anatomy. Graft or scaffold extrusion has also been documented, often requiring surgical removal and complex reconstructive procedures. Additionally, changes in glans sensation, ranging from partial to complete loss, may occur if neural pathways are inadvertently disrupted [1, 8]. Deep infections, though rare, can progress to abscess formation or systemic sepsis if not promptly managed. Even less severe complications, such as prolonged postoperative edema, have been noted; Shaeer's series reported delayed healing in approximately 15% of cases, requiring extended

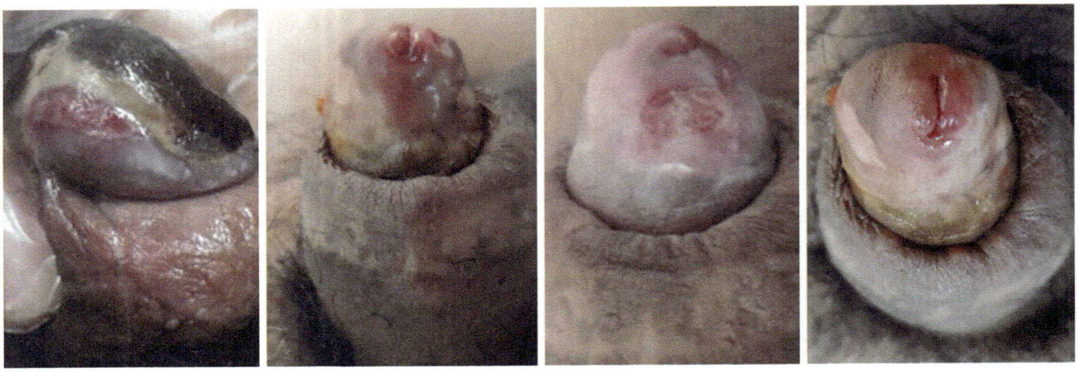

Fig. 19.5 Glans mucosal necrosis after Indirect GPA. This patient presented severe pain and unsatisfaction after indirect GPA by Shaeer's glans augmentation technique. Removal of implants showed the fate of scaffold implantation. Painful hard mass inside glans penis induced vascular compromise and eventual glans penis necrosis and deformity

periods of postoperative care [1, 8]. These risks underscore the necessity for surgical precision, judicious patient selection, and thorough preoperative counseling. While indirect GPA expands the surgical options for penile enhancement, its invasive nature and complication profile limit its applicability to highly selected cases managed by experienced surgeons (Fig. 19.5).

19.5 Conclusion

Indirect glans penis augmentation (GPA) represents a significant advancement in penile enhancement techniques, providing an alternative for patients where direct augmentation may not be ideal. By modifying the substructural anatomy beneath the glans, it achieves distal elevation and improved aesthetic harmony without directly altering the glans mucosa. Techniques inspired by innovative surgical approaches, such as Perović's penile disassembly method and refined by Shaeer's dermofat grafting, have contributed to the evolution of this concept.

The primary advantages of indirect GPA include its ability to deliver natural, proportionate enhancement and its reduced likelihood of affecting glans sensitivity compared to direct filler injections. However, these benefits must be weighed against the limitations inherent to its surgical nature. Indirect GPA primarily achieves structural elevation rather than comprehensive functional augmentation, and its demanding technical requirements necessitate a high level of surgical expertise. Additionally, challenges such as material resorption, vascular compromise, and the risk of glans mucosal necrosis highlight the importance of cautious patient selection and meticulous technique.

Ultimately, the success of indirect GPA depends on careful surgical planning, precise execution, and thorough preoperative counseling. By setting realistic expectations and educating patients about potential outcomes and complications, surgeons can optimize satisfaction and achieve lasting aesthetic results. Although indirect GPA expands the range of options in penile enhancement, its invasive nature and lack of robust long-term data currently confine its use to highly selected cases in specialized centers.

References

1. Shaeer O. Shaeer's glans augmentation technique: a pilot study. J Sex Med. 2012;9(12):3264–9.
2. Moon DG, Kwak TI, Kim JJ. Glans penis augmentation using hyaluronic acid gel as an injectable filler. World J Mens Health. 2015;33(2):50.
3. Perovic V, Djordjevic D. The penile disassembly technique in hypospadias repair. Br J Urol. 1998;81(3):479–87.
4. Perovic S, Djordjevic M. Penile lengthening. BJU Int. 2000;86(9):1028–33.
5. Ebbehøj J, Metz P. Lacking tumescence of glans during penile erection. J Urol. 1985;134(6):1220.

6. Montague DK. Penile prosthesis implantation: size matters. Eur Urol. 2007;51(4):887–8.
7. Chew K, Stuckey B. Use of transurethral alprostadil (MUSE)(prostaglandin E1) for glans tumescence in a patient with penile prosthesis. Int J Impot Res. 2000;12(3):195–6.
8. Shaeer O. Supersizing the penis following penile prosthesis implantation. J Sex Med. 2010;7(7):2608–16.
9. Perovic SV, Vukadinovic V, Djordjevic ML, Djakovic NG. Penile disassembly technique for epispadias repair: variants of technique. J Urol. 1999;162(3 Part 2):1181–4.
10. Park NC. Penile girth enhancement with dermofat graft. Penile Augmentation. 2016:57–63.
11. Ahn ST, Il Kwak T, Park KS, Kim JJ, Moon DG. Complications of glans penis augmentation. Int J Impot Res. 2019;31(4):245–55.
12. Perovic SV, Djordjevic ML, Djakovic NG. A new approach to the treatment of penile curvature. J Urol. 1998;160(3 Part 2) 1123–7.
13. Moon DG, Kwak TI, Kim JJ. Glans penis augmentation using injectable hyaluronic acid gel. Int J Impot Res. 2003;15(6):439–43.
14. Perovic SV, Djinovic R, Bumbasirevic M, Djordjevic M, Vukovic P. Total phalloplasty using a musculocutaneous latissimus dorsi flap. BJU Int. 2007;100(4):899–905.

Glans Penis Augmentation (GPA) with Distal Penile Girth Enhancement (PGE)

20

Contents

20.1 Introduction

The simultaneous application of glans penis augmentation (GPA) and distal penile girth enhancement (PGE) has emerged as an innovative strategy in penile augmentation, offering a comprehensive solution that addresses both aesthetic and functional concerns. This dual approach is gaining traction among clinicians and patients alike, as it provides proportional enhancement of the penis while accommodating individual anatomical variations and patient-specific goals.

Initially developed to correct small glans size and penile deformities, GPA using hyaluronic acid (HA) gel has since expanded in scope. The author extended its application to the management of premature ejaculation (PE), establishing a theoretical basis for its use in modulating glans sensitivity [1]. Supporting this concept, several studies have demonstrated the therapeutic efficacy of GPA using HA filler in improving PE-related symptoms [2–5]. More recently, findings from a clinical trial revealed that penile girth enhancement alone may also contribute to symptom improvement in PE [6]. Although the precise mechanisms underlying this effect remain unclear, it is hypothesized that the desensitizing properties of HA filler injections in the subcutaneous tissues may contribute, paralleling the mechanism proposed for GPA [7]. Building on this knowledge, the author recently conducted a pilot study evaluating the combined approach of GPA with distal PGE for PE management, with promising preliminary outcomes.

Supplementary Information The online version contains supplementary material available at https://doi.org/10.1007/978-981-95-5385-3_20.

D. G. Moon, *Penile Augmentation with Injectable Hyaluronic Acid*,
https://doi.org/10.1007/978-981-95-5385-3_20

20.2 Rationale for Combining GPA and Distal PGE Can Be Discussed in Three Aspects

The combination of glans penis augmentation (GPA) and distal penile girth enhancement (PGE) offers a synergistic approach that addresses both functional and aesthetic demands in penile augmentation. This integrated technique can be understood from three interrelated perspectives: aesthetic balance, functional benefits, and patient-oriented considerations.

From an aesthetic standpoint, the simultaneous application of GPA and distal PGE creates a seamless transition between the penile shaft and glans. This avoids the abrupt contour changes or "mushroom-like" appearance that can result from shaft-only PGE, particularly when filler migration leads to distal tapering or irregularities. By targeting the distal shaft, distal PGE restores symmetry and proportionality, ensuring a harmonious penile silhouette, especially in patients with naturally less prominent distal girth.

Functionally, the dual approach enhances not only the appearance but also the tactile qualities of the penile body. This contributes to improved sexual satisfaction for both the patient and their partner. The procedure may also provide therapeutic benefits by reducing hypersensitivity in key areas, such as the frenulum, potentially improving symptoms of premature ejaculation (PE) and supporting erectile function. These functional enhancements add a meaningful dimension to what was previously considered a primarily cosmetic intervention.

From a patient-centered perspective, combining GPA and distal PGE addresses multiple concerns in a single session, reducing the need for separate procedures and their associated recovery periods. This comprehensive approach aligns well with patient preferences for efficiency and minimizes the psychological and physical burdens of undergoing staged treatments. For patients seeking both aesthetic refinement and functional improvement, this strategy offers a tailored and time-effective solution.

20.3 Procedure Considerations

Patients with premature ejaculation (PE) who are seeking penile girth enhancement (PGE) represent ideal candidates for the combined procedure of glans penis augmentation (GPA) with distal PGE. Preoperative preparation mirrors that of standard GPA and PGE protocols, ensuring patient readiness for a dual intervention.

The procedure begins with GPA using hyaluronic acid (HA) gel, performed first to achieve uniform submucosal glans augmentation. Once GPA is completed, additional distal PGE is carried out using the back-and-forth linear threading technique to distribute the filler circumferentially along the distal shaft. Based on the author's experience, approximately 10 mL of HA filler is typically sufficient to achieve symmetrical coverage of the distal penile circumference.

A key difference from standard PGE is the inclusion of the ventral urethral and frenulum regions during filler injection. This approach targets frenular sensitivity, which plays a significant role in PE, offering a potential therapeutic benefit alongside aesthetic improvement. Post-injection, gentle manual molding is critical to ensure even filler distribution, prevent lump formation, and maintain a natural contour. Postoperative care follows the same guidelines as for GPA and PGE performed independently, focusing on edema management and maintaining filler symmetry during healing.

20.4 Pilot Study Results: GPA with Distal PGE

Introduction and Objectives GPA using HA gel has gained acceptance as a treatment option for PE unresponsive to conventional therapies. Separately, PGE has also demonstrated efficacy in increasing intravaginal ejaculatory latency time (IELT). This pilot study aimed to evaluate the combined application of GPA with distal PGE in improving PE symptoms, hypothesizing that the dual approach would provide superior outcomes compared to either procedure alone.

Methods Twelve patients diagnosed with PE (defined as IELT <3 min) were enrolled in the study. GPA was first performed using a submucosal injection of 4–6 mL of HA gel evenly distributed across the glans surface. IELT changes were assessed at 12 weeks post-GPA. Following this assessment, distal PGE was performed by circularly injecting 10 mL of HA gel around the distal penile shaft, including the ventral urethral and frenulum areas, to target frenular sensitivity. IELT was reassessed at 6 months (Fig. 20.1, Video 20.1).

Secondary outcomes included patient satisfaction with penile shape and sexual function, as well as documentation of adverse events. Hyaluronidase was made available for managing any residual HA or deformities.

Results All participants completed the study without dropout. Distal penile girth increased significantly, with a mean gain of 25.95 ± 13.71 mm. Mean IELT improved from a preoperative value of 101.54 ± 69.72 s to 251.4 ± 72.3 s after GPA alone. Following distal PGE, IELT further increased to 325.38 ± 120.76 s at 6 months.

Patient satisfaction was high: 90% of participants reported notable improvements in penile shape and sexual function. Among the seven patients with severe PE, all achieved IELT values exceeding 3 min by the 6-month follow-up. Hyaluronidase was successfully employed in a small number of cases to correct residual HA or minor initial deformities. No serious adverse events were recorded.

Conclusions This pilot study demonstrated that GPA effectively increased IELT in patients with PE and that the addition of distal PGE further enhanced outcomes. Importantly, distal PGE avoided the unsatisfactory displacement or distortion sometimes observed with total PGE. Hyaluronidase proved to be a valuable adjunct for managing residual or misplaced HA filler, contributing to the overall safety and adaptability of the procedure. These findings suggest that the combined approach of GPA with distal PGE offers a promising strategy for patients seeking both functional and aesthetic penile enhancement.

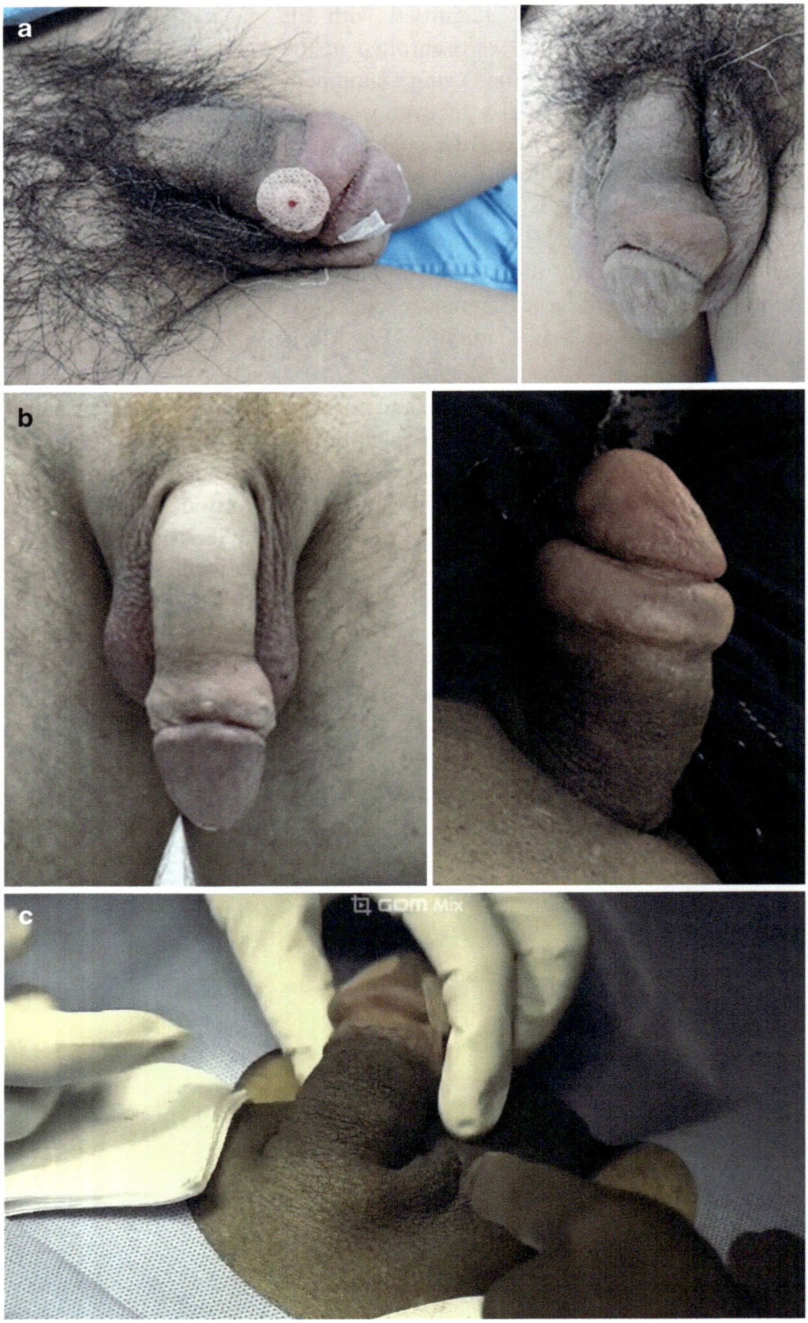

Fig. 20.1 GPA with distal PGE

20.5 Discussion

An understanding of penile neuroanatomy provides critical insight into the mechanisms by which glans penis augmentation (GPA) combined with distal penile girth enhancement (PGE) influences premature ejaculation (PE) and overall penile function. It is well established that one branch of the dorsal nerve runs along the dorsal midline and terminates in the glans, while other branches radiate laterally and ventrally over the penile shaft [8, 9]. Filler injected between Buck's fascia and the dartos fascia acts as a physical barrier to tactile stimuli, dampening sensory input to the dorsal nerve receptors and effectively raising the threshold for sensation [6]. This mechanism was observed in initial feasibility studies of PGE using HA fillers, where patients reported decreased tactile sensitivity of the shaft without adverse effects on sexual satisfaction [6].

The combination of GPA with distal PGE provides a comprehensive solution to several limitations inherent in GPA alone. While GPA effectively modulates glans sensitivity, it does not uniformly benefit all PE patients and may require retouching due to gradual volume resorption. The addition of distal PGE amplifies therapeutic outcomes by desensitizing the distal penile shaft, particularly the ventral region, and enhances the continuity of penile contour, avoiding the abrupt junction often seen between a thickened shaft and a smaller glans.

Distal PGE offers several advantages over total shaft PGE. Unlike total PGE, which carries a risk of filler migration and unnatural surface irregularities, distal PGE preserves a natural penile appearance by focusing augmentation on the distal shaft [10]. Moreover, it is functionally superior to mechanical alternatives such as silicone ring insertions, as HA fillers provide a softer, more physiologic effect and are readily reversible with hyaluronidase if needed.

From a surgical perspective, traditional principles of PGE emphasize avoiding filler placement near the urethral side to prevent complications. However, distal PGE using HA filler safely addresses the ventral shaft and frenulum regions without compromising function. This technique parallels the therapeutic rationale of frenuloplasty for PE, targeting one of the most sensitive zones of the penis to modulate ejaculatory control.

The frenulum, located on the ventral surface of the penis, is richly supplied by frenular vessels and innervated both by the dorsal nerve of the penis and a branch of the perineal nerve [8]. It is among the most densely innervated penile structures, playing a crucial role in sexual stimulation [9]. Frenectomy has been studied as a possible surgical therapy for PE because of the association of PE with a short frenulum, or frenulum breve [9].

Historically, the frenulum has been implicated as a contributing factor in PE. Since Gross's first description of "rapid ejaculation" in 1887 [11], there has been speculation within the urological community about a short frenulum (frenulum breve) as a risk factor for PE [12]. Waldinger outlined this historical evolution, noting that during the period between 1917 and 1950, some physicians attributed PE to anatomical abnormalities such as a short frenulum, advocating frenuloplasty or frenulectomy as treatment [13]. This condition can be congenital resulting from defects during sexual development or acquired secondary to excessive scarring occurring after rupture of a normal frenulum [8]. It hinders complete retraction of the prepuce during erection causing a ventral curvature of the glans. Nonetheless, there are plausible mechanisms by which frenulum breve may contribute to PE [14]. First, it can cause discomfort and a sense of traction during intercourse, leading to anticipatory ejaculation. Second, studies by Halata and Munger confirmed the frenulum's dense sensory innervation, identifying it—alongside the glans corona—as the most sensitive zone of the penis [9].

Importantly, frenulectomy has been shown to improve PE symptoms without significantly impacting glans sensitivity. As demonstrated by Yang and Bradley [8], the frenulum is innervated by a branch of the perineal nerve, while the glans receives input from dorsal nerve afferents to the pudendal nerves. This distinction allows frenulectomy to modulate ventral sensitivity without affecting dorsal glans sensation [15] (Figs. 20.2 and 20.3).

Recently, Perri et al. reported efficacy of one-shot hyaluronic acid injection into the frenulum of prepuce in lifelong premature ejaculation [16]. Similarly, the combination of GPA and distal PGE targets both sensory pathways: GPA modulates dorsal glans sensitivity, while distal PGE addresses ventral sensitivity, including the frenulum.

Compared to frenulectomy, distal PGE offers comparable safety and efficacy in managing

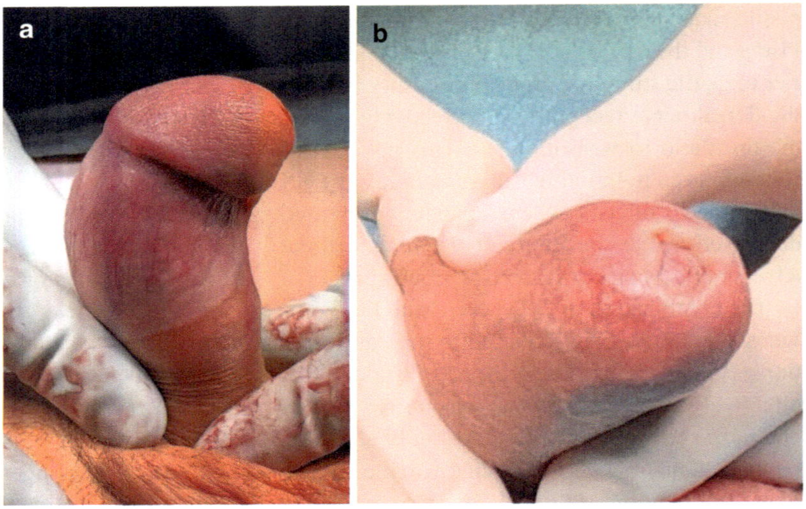

Fig. 20.2 Preoperative view of the penis. (**a**) Frenuloplasty performed due to ventral deviation of the glans combined with bothersome symptoms during sexual intercourse. (**b**) Circumcision combined with frenuloplasty due to balanitis xerotica obliterans

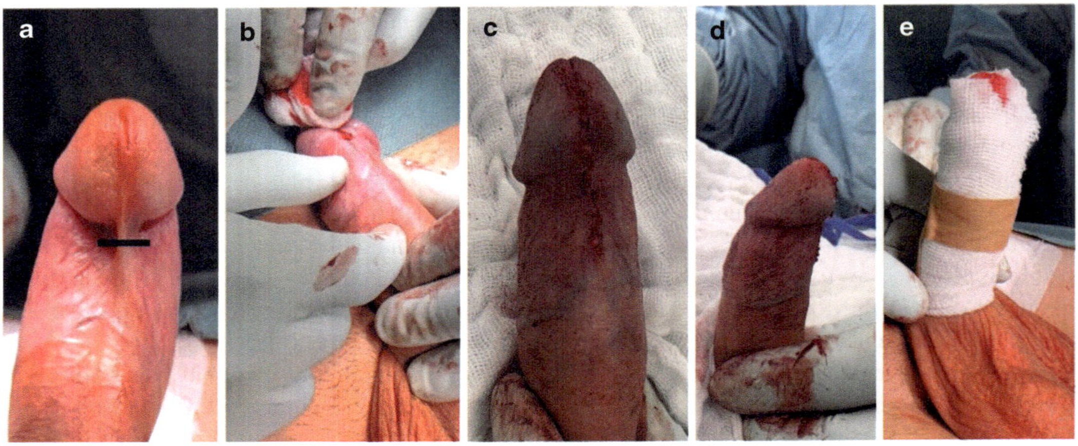

Fig. 20.3 Frenuloplasty for frenulum breve. (**a**) Superficial horizontal incision at the point of maximum tension. (**b**) Incision of frenulum with scalpel without coagulation. (**c**) Reconstruction of frenulum with interrupted 4–0 absorbable sutures. (**d**) Correction of the glans curvature. (**e**) Light compression dressing of the penis

PE. It is minimally invasive, is performed under local anesthesia with minimal discomfort, and requires no surgical incisions. Unlike frenulectomy, which removes tissue, distal PGE preserves anatomical integrity while modulating sensory input. This makes it an attractive alternative for patients seeking reversible and adjustable treatments (Fig. 20.4 and Table 20.1).

In summary, the combination of GPA and distal PGE represents a refined, patient-centered strategy for addressing PE. By targeting both dorsal and ventral penile sensory pathways, this approach provides comprehensive modulation of penile sensitivity, superior aesthetic outcomes, and high patient satisfaction.

Anatomical rationale for glans penis augmentation (GPA) and distal penile girth enhancement (PGE) using hyaluronic acid (HA) filler.

A. Dorsal view: Pink-shaded region indicates HA filler distributed within the submucosal plane of the glans penis for GPA, aimed at shielding dorsal nerve terminal branches. The blue-shaded region represents circular HA filler placement for distal PGE at the distal penile shaft.

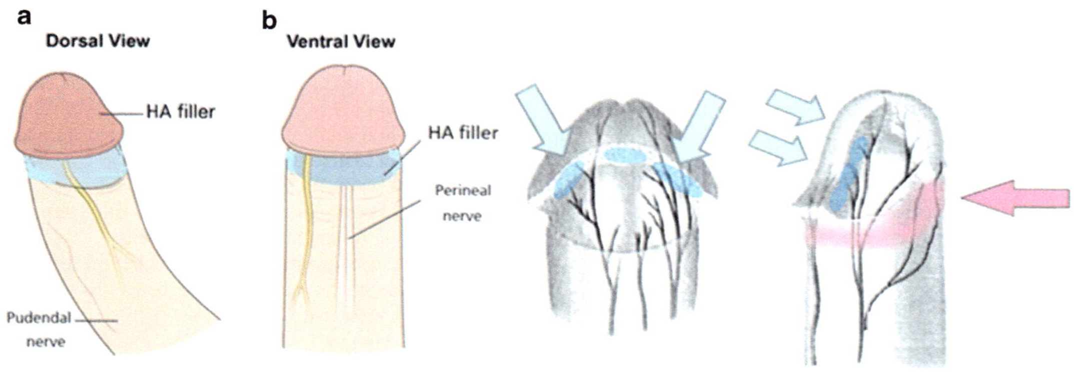

Fig. 20.4 Illustration of GPA with distal PGE. Proposed mechanism of glans penis augmentation (GPA) and distal penile girth enhancement (PGE) in modulating penile sensitivity

Table 20.1 Comparative features of GPA alone, distal PGE alone, and GPA combined with distal PGE

Feature	GPA alone	Distal PGE alone	GPA + Distal PGE
Increase in IELT	Moderate	Moderate	High
Improvement in satisfaction (penile appearance)	High	Moderate	Very high
Improvement in satisfaction (sexual function)	Moderate	Moderate	Very high
Risk of filler migration	Low	High	Minimal
Aesthetic outcome	Moderate	Variable (unnatural with time)	Natural
Need for retouching	High	Moderate	Low
Complexity of procedure	Simple	Moderate	Moderate

B. Ventral view: The same pink zone highlights HA filler within the glans. The blue-shaded filler zone beneath Buck's fascia encircles the distal shaft including the frenulum area, modulating sensory input from the perineal nerve.

Collectively, this dual-plane filler strategy is designed to desensitize both dorsal and ventral afferents and reduce hypersensitivity in patients with premature ejaculation.

20.6 Conclusion

The integration of glans penis augmentation (GPA) with distal penile girth enhancement (PGE) represents a sophisticated advancement in penile augmentation strategies. Clinical studies on PGE using hyaluronic acid (HA) fillers have already demonstrated its safety and efficacy, with notable improvements in penile girth and reductions in ejaculation-related symptoms. These findings highlight PGE as a promising therapeutic adjunct for managing premature ejaculation (PE).

The pilot study of GPA combined with distal PGE further supports the potential of this dual approach. By addressing both dorsal and ventral penile sensitivity zones, the combined procedure provides comprehensive modulation of penile sensation, resulting in significant improvements in intravaginal ejaculatory latency time (IELT) and high levels of patient satisfaction. Importantly, this method minimizes risks such as filler migration and maintains natural aesthetic outcomes.

While the results are encouraging, certain limitations must be acknowledged, including the reliance on subjective assessment tools such as the Premature Ejaculation Diagnostic Tool (PEDT) and the Premature Ejaculation Profile (PEP) questionnaires. Larger-scale studies with more objective endpoints are needed to validate these findings and determine the long-term safety and efficacy of GPA with distal PGE, particularly in patients with severe PE.

Ultimately, this dual procedure aligns with the evolving expectations of patients seeking not only aesthetic enhancement but also functional improvement. GPA combined with distal PGE offers a patient-centered, innovative solution that bridges the gap between cosmetic and therapeutic interventions in andrological practice.

References

1. Kim J, Kwak T, Jeon B, Cheon J, Moon D. Effects of glans penis augmentation using hyaluronic acid gel for premature ejaculation. Int J Impot Res. 2004;16(6):547–51.
2. Kwak T, Jin M, Kim J, Moon D. Long-term effects of glans penis augmentation using injectable hyaluronic acid gel for premature ejaculation. Int J Impot Res. 2008;20(4):425–8.
3. Alahwany A, Ragab MW, Zaghloul A, Abdallah H, Mostafa T. Hyaluronic acid injection in glans penis for treatment of premature ejaculation: a randomized controlled cross-over study. Int J Impot Res. 2019;31(5):348–55.
4. Chen K, Li Q, Xu T, Zhang X. Hyaluronic acid injection to coronal sulcus of the penis for the treatment of premature ejaculation: a retrospective observational study. BMC Urol. 2023;23(1):55.
5. Culha MG, Baran C, Erkoc M. Clinical efficacy and safety of hyaluronic acid gel injection in the glans penis for treatment of premature ejaculation: systematic review and meta-analysis. J Sex Med. 2024;21(10):878–88.
6. Ahn ST, Shim JS, Bae WJ, Kim SW, Kim JJ, Moon DG. Efficacy and safety of penile girth enhancement using hyaluronic acid filler and the clinical impact on ejaculation: a multi-center, patient/evaluator-blinded, randomized active-controlled trial. World J Mens Health. 2021;40(2):299.
7. Park NC. Penile girth enhancement with Dermofat graft. Penile Augmentation. 2016:57–63.
8. Yang. Neuroanatomy of the penile portion of the human dorsal nerve of the penis. Br J Urol. 1998;82(1):109–13.
9. Halata Z, Munger BL. The neuroanatomical basis for the protopathic sensibility of the human glans penis. Brain Res. 1986;371(2):205–30.
10. Kwak TI, Oh M, Kim JJ, Moon DG. The effects of penile girth enhancement using injectable hyaluronic acid gel, a filler. J Sex Med. 2011;8(12):3407–13.
11. Gross S. Practical treatise on impotens and sterity. Endinburgh: YJ Pentland; 1887.
12. Piediferro G, Colpi EM, Castiglioni F, Nerva F. Premature ejaculation. 1. Definition and etiology. Arch Ital Urol Androl. 2004;76:181–7.
13. Waldinger MD. History of premature ejaculation. In: Premature ejaculation: from etiology to diagnosis and treatment. Springer; 2012. p. 5–24.
14. Song B, Cai ZM. Possible function of the frenulum of prepuce in penile erection. Andrologia. 2012;44(1):23–5.
15. Pyrgidis N, Sokolakis I, Dimitriadis F, Hatzichristodoulou G. Frenuloplasty: from alpha to omega. Int J Impot Res. 2022;34(4):347–52.
16. Perri A, Lofaro D, Iuliano S, Bossio S, Rago V, Damiano R, et al. Effects of one-shot hyaluronic acid injection in lifelong premature ejaculation: a pilot study. Endocrine. 2022;3(3):538–44.

Clinical Case Series of Glans Penis Augmentation (GPA)

21

Contents

21.1 Introduction and Background

Indirect glans penis augmentation (GPA) was initially conceptualized as an alternative to direct filler-based augmentation in patients who were considered unsuitable for direct mucosal injection due to glans hypersensitivity or anatomical constraints. Among the pioneering efforts, Shaeer [1] introduced a technique termed "Shaeer's glans augmentation," which involved the insertion of a dermofat graft harvested from the groin into the periurethral space through a glans flap created via two incisions along the ventral coronal sulcus. In a pilot study involving ten patients, this approach demonstrated favorable outcomes, including stable glans volume at 1-year follow-up, preservation of tactile sensitivity, and absence of adverse effects on erectile function or ejaculation.

Despite its initial promise, the technique presented limitations such as surgical invasiveness, donor site morbidity, and a lack of long-term outcome data. Building upon this concept, a group of Korean andrologists developed a similar method of indirect GPA, initially employing dermofat grafts, but subsequently transitioning to collagen scaffold materials such as AlloDerm or Lyoplant to reduce procedural invasiveness. Although early cases showed aesthetic improvements, the indirect approach eventually revealed critical issues, namely, resorption of scaffold material, volume instability, and in some cases, glans tissue compromise, leading to mucosal thinning or necrosis.

Supplementary Information The online version contains supplementary material available at https://doi.org/10.1007/978-981-95-5385-3_21.

D. G. Moon, *Penile Augmentation with Injectable Hyaluronic Acid*,
https://doi.org/10.1007/978-981-95-5385-3_21

This chapter presents three representative cases that illustrate the evolution, refinement, and successful application of GPA, particularly when combined with distal penile girth enhancement (PGE), in diverse clinical scenarios.

21.2 Case 1. Correction of Glans Deformity Following Complication of Indirect GPA

Patient Summary

- 56-year-old male
- Presented in June 2017 with glans necrosis 2 weeks after undergoing indirect GPA at a local clinic (Fig. 21.1a, b, c).
- Observation approach was initially recommended; spontaneous healing occurred but left partial glans loss and deformity at 3 months, in Sep 2017 (Fig. 21.1d, e, f, g).

Treatment and Progress From February 2018 to October 2020, the patient underwent five sessions of HA filler injection to restore glans shape and volume. Early injections were challenging due to poor submucosal space integrity. However, repeated treatments progressively reestablished the submucosal plane, allowing elevation of the mucosal layer (Fig. 21.1h, I, j, k).

Despite the need for frequent reinjections every 3–6 months due to early volume loss, the

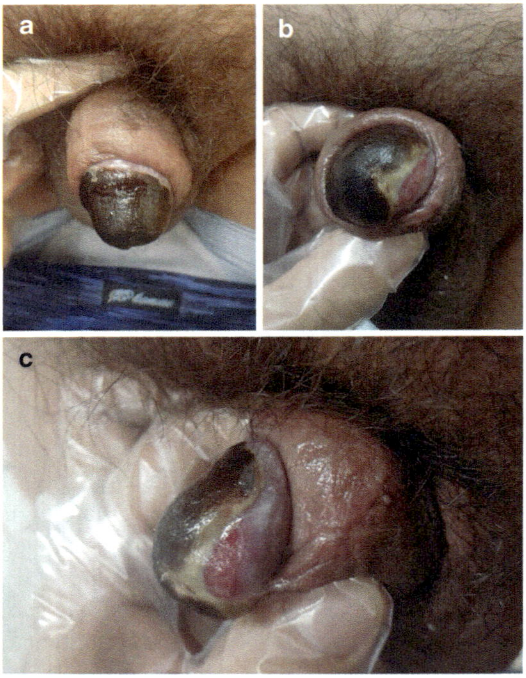

Fig. 21.1 Glans mucosal necrosis at 2 weeks after indirect GPA (**a**–**c**)
(**a**) Glans discoloration at dorsal view
(**b**) Glans mucosal necrosis with discoloration diff erentiated with underlying normal glans ventral view and (**c**) lateral view
Step 2: Glans deformity after spontaneous healing: (**d**–**g**)
(**d, e**) Partial loss of glans at Rt. Dorsum with deformity at 2 months
(**f, g**) Well-regenerated glans mucosa at frenular and left-side glans
Step 3: Five times of submucosal injection of HA corrected glans deformity gradually for 2 years (**h**–**k**)
(**l, m**) Final healing of glans mucosa with surface deformity

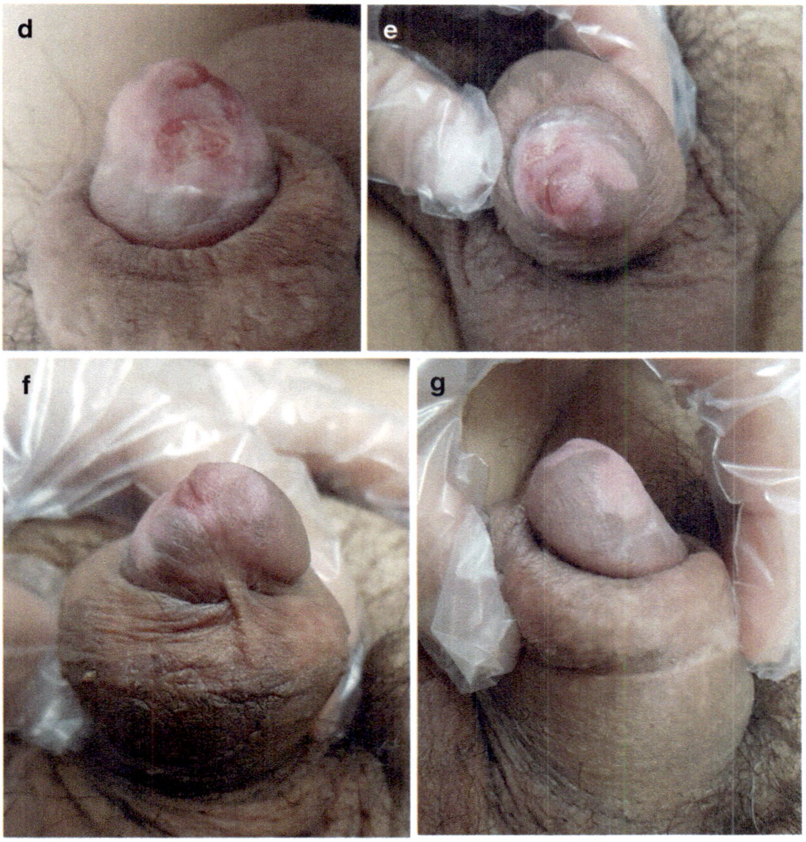

Fig. 21.1 (continued)

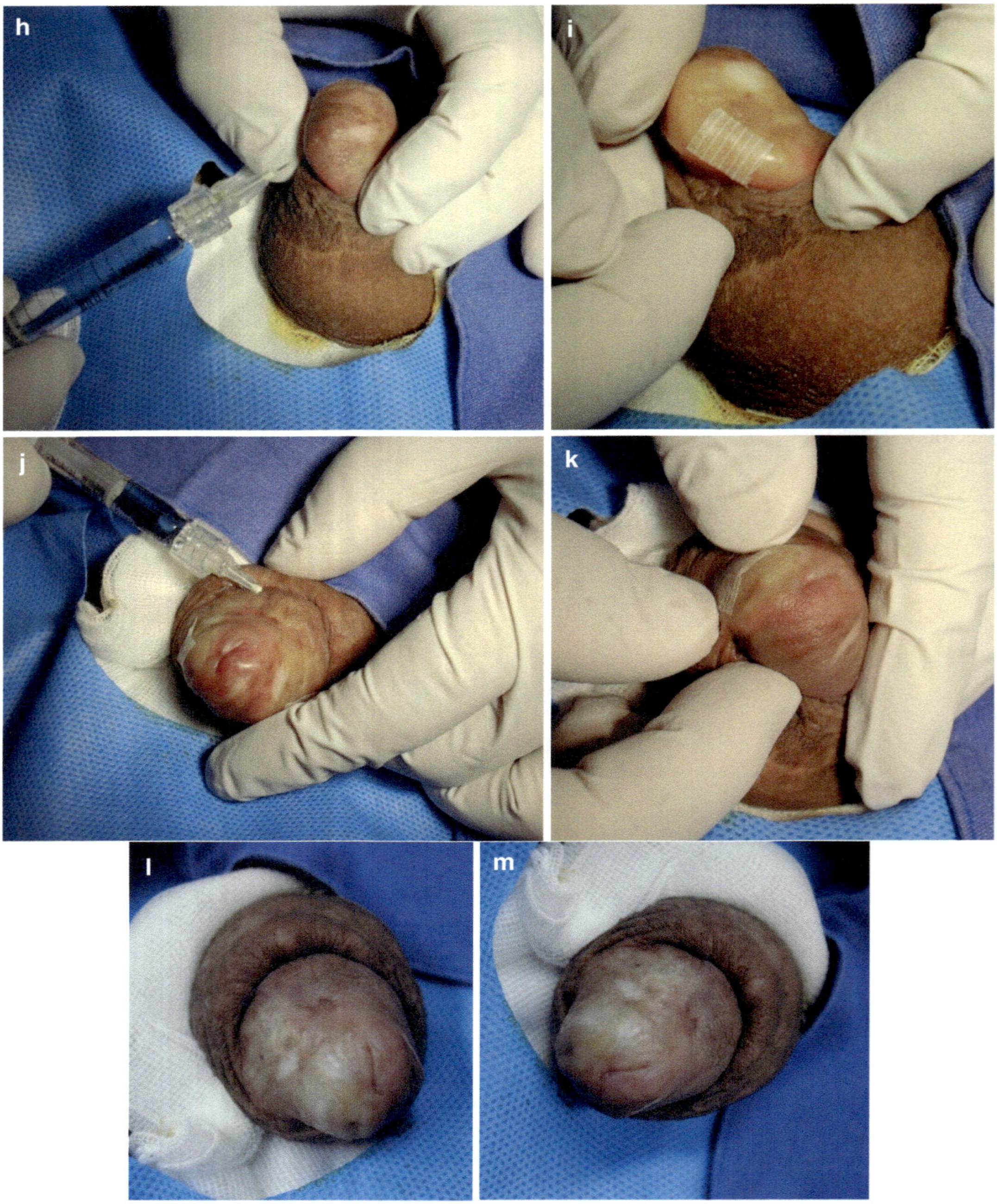

Fig. 21.1 (continued)

procedure achieved notable reconstructive success. Most of the necrotic and deformed glans tissue was restored, and the patient expressed high satisfaction despite incomplete regeneration of the mucosa (Fig. 21.1l, m).

Key Insight This case illustrates both the potential complications of indirect GPA and the efficacy of direct HA injection in reversing deformity. It emphasizes the importance of minimally invasive approaches and long-term follow-up.

21.3 Case 2. GPA with Frenulum HA Injection in a Patient with Intractable Premature Ejaculation

Background: Distal penile girth enhancement (PGE) offers functional and aesthetic benefits over full-shaft PGE by minimizing filler migration and preserving natural appearance. It also provides a physiological advantage over rigid alternatives like silicone rings. HA filler injection into the frenular area shares a therapeutic rationale with frenulectomy for PE, modulating one of the most sensitive zones on the penis. Unlike frenulectomy, HA-based distal PGE is reversible, is nonsurgical, and preserves anatomical integrity.

Patient Summary

- 44-year-old male, US citizen
- Chief complaint: lifelong PE with IELT of 2.5 min
- Previously underwent frenulectomy without improvement
- Consulted author after online search

Treatment Steps

- Step 1: GPA using 6 mL HA filler (Fig. 21.2a, b, c)
- Step 2: One week later, retouch procedure including targeted HA injection at the frenulum (Fig. 21.2d, e, f, g)

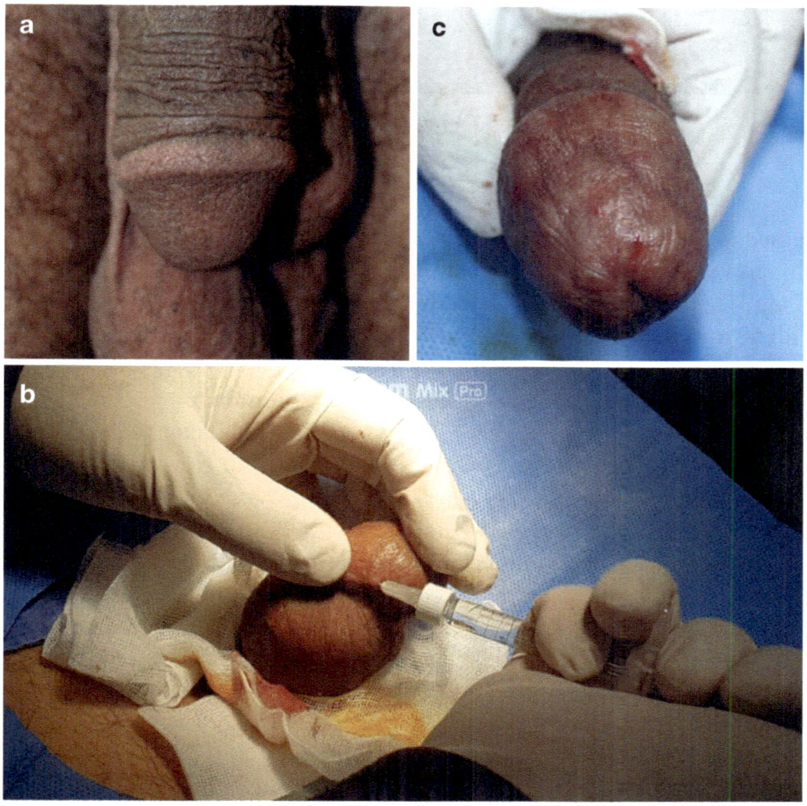

Fig. 21.2 Glans Penis augmentation with HA
Step 1: GPA using 6ml HA filler (**a**–**c**)
(**a**) Before augmentation Step 1. GPA with 6 mL HA injection
(**b**) Videoclip of GPA with HA
(**c**) Immediate after injection of 6 mL HA into whole glans evenly
Step 2. Retouch 1 week later with additonal HA injection (**d**–**g**)
(**d**) 1 week after GPA with HA, show some dimple area at mid glans
(**e**) Retouch filled vacant place and elevated dimple area
(**f**) HA injection at ventral glans below urethral orifice
(**g**) HA injection into the frenulum area
Step 3. His response after return to his country (**h**)
(**h**) Three months after GPA with HA, well-augmented glans without surface undulation or dimple

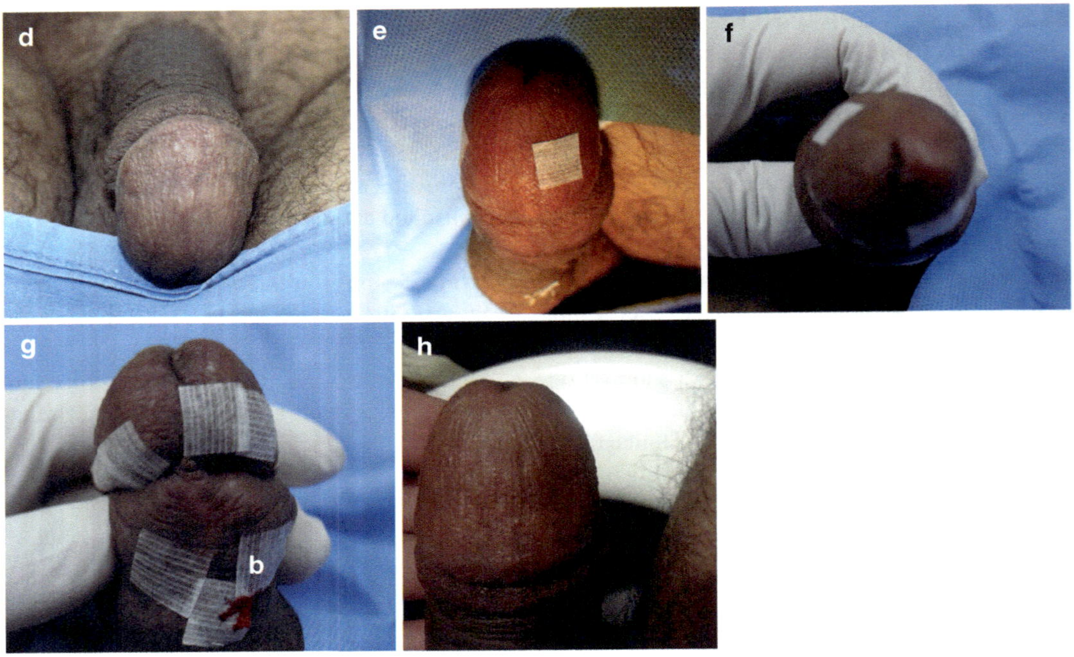

Fig. 21.2 (continued)

Outcome

- IELT increased to 8–9 min at 1 month
- Sustained improvement: 5–7 min at 3 months
- With 30 mg dapoxetine: IELT exceeded 10 min; with 60 mg: >20 min
- Patient expressed high satisfaction and sent photos and feedback after returning to the US (Fig. 21.2h).

Key Insight This case demonstrates the synergistic effect of GPA and frenulum-targeted distal PGE in modulating both dorsal and ventral penile sensitivity. It reinforces the role of filler-based interventions in refractory PE.

21.4 Case 3. GPA with Distal PGE in an International Patient

Background Neuroanatomical understanding reveals that dorsal nerve branches innervate both the glans and penile shaft. Filler injected between Buck's and dartos fascia desensitizes the shaft by raising tactile thresholds. GPA alone modulates glans sensitivity but may have limitations in certain PE patients. Combining GPA with distal PGE ensures comprehensive desensitization, eliminates abrupt glans-shaft transitions, and optimizes both function and aesthetics.

Patient Summary

- 39-year-old Italian male
- Presented in November 2022 for GPA due to PE

Treatment Steps

- *Nov 3, 2022:* Initial GPA
- *Nov 10, 2022:* GPA retouch + distal PGE
- *Jan 26, 2023:* GPA retouch + PGE
- *Feb 2, 2023:* PGE retouch

Outcome

- By March 7, 2023: IELT improved to 7–10 min
- Patient reported increased confidence, satisfaction with appearance, and positive psychological effects
- Expressed gratitude through messages and shared postoperative photos (Fig. 21.3a, b)

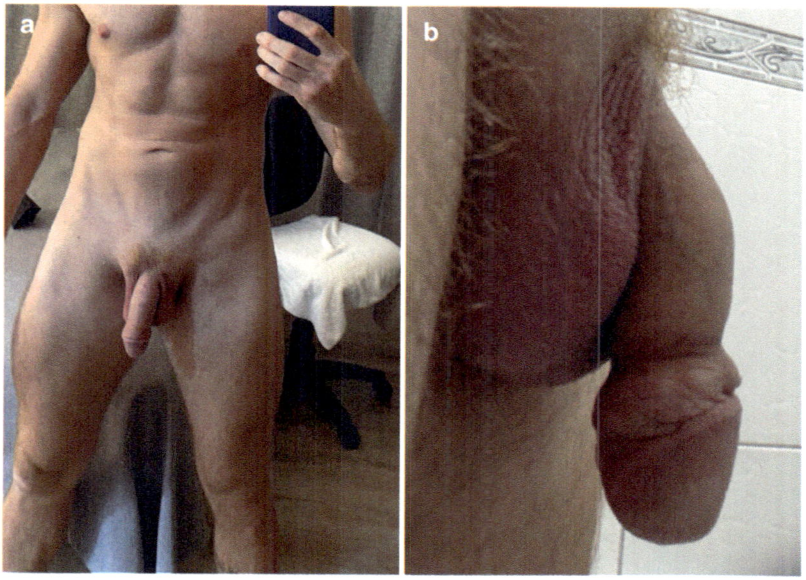

Fig. 21.3 (a) The patient sent his bodyshot focused enhanced penis with confidence and gratitude. (b) Rt. lateral view of penis shows enhanced penile body with prominent enhancement of distal circle just below the glans

Key Insight This case highlights the effectiveness of GPA combined with distal PGE for PE and aesthetic improvement. It also demonstrates excellent results in an international patient, confirming the reproducibility and appeal of this approach.

21.5 Case Summary Table

Case	Age	Chief complaint	Intervention	Key steps	IELT outcome	Patient feedback
1	56	Glans necrosis after indirect GPA	GPA with repeated HA injections	Five sessions (2018–2020)	Volume restoration, shape improvement	High satisfaction despite partial mucosal loss
2	44	Lifelong PE, failed frenulectomy	GPA + frenulum HA injection	Initial GPA + retouch with frenulum injection	2.5 → 3–9 min (1 mo), >10 min (with dapoxetine)	Very satisfied, sent photos and follow-up
3	39	PE and interest in aesthetic result	GPA + Distal PGE	Initial GPA + PGE retouch (Nov 2022–Feb 2023)	7–10 min by March 2023	Improved confidence and sexual function

21.6 Conclusion

These three cases collectively demonstrate the versatility and efficacy of HA-based GPA and distal PGE in real-world clinical practice. Whether correcting deformities, managing intractable PE, or enhancing both sensitivity and appearance in international patients, this evolving technique offers a safe, customizable, and patient-centered solution.

Future directions include protocol standardization, long-term efficacy monitoring, and broader clinical adoption in specialized urological practice.

References

1. Kim JJ, Moon DC, Park S-J, et al. Glans penis augmentation with hyaluronic acid for premature ejaculation. Int J Impot Res. 2016;28(4):163–8.

GPSR Compliance

The European Union's (EU) General Product Safety Regulation (GPSR) is a set of rules that requires consumer products to be safe and our obligations to ensure this.

If you have any concerns about our products, you can contact us on ProductSafety@springernature.com

In case Publisher is established outside the EU, the EU authorized representative is:

Springer Nature Customer Service Center GmbH
Europaplatz 3
69115 Heidelberg, Germany

Batch number: 10732809

Printed by Printforce, the Netherlands